Praise for Juan Carlos "JC" S

"*JC's Total Body Transformation* is a must-have book for anyone looking to enhance performance and transform their body! All the programs you could ever want, in one location, built by an industry leader in fitness!"

Cliff Edberg
Senior National Program Manager (Personal Training) for Life Time

"Juan Carlos Santana is one of the true thought leaders in strength and conditioning. *JC's Total Body Transformation* is a must for anyone seeking to improve their fitness."

Jose Antonio, PhD
Sports Scientist at Nova Southeastern University and
CEO of International Society of Sports Nutrition (ISSN)

"If you are looking for a one-stop shop for functional training and fitness, look no further than *JC's Total Body Transformation*!"

Douglas Kalman, PhD, RD, FACN, FISSN
Adjunct Professor at Nova Southeastern University

"The practicality and usefulness of *JC's Total Body Transformation* for directing others in their pursuit of optimum conditioning are second to none."

Darryn S. Willoughby, PhD, CSCS, CISSN, EPC, CNS, FACSM, FISSN, FACN, FASEP
Professor of Exercise/Nutritional Biochemistry and Molecular Physiology at Baylor University

"Whether you are an expert or a beginner, young or old, serious or casual about fitness, *JC's Total Body Transformation* is the one book you should have on your shelf. Read it, absorb it, do it, and BE TRANSFORMED."

David Woynarowski, MD
Expert in Longevity and Regenerative Medicine and Coauthor of *Immortality Edge* and
"Stem Cells Targeting Inflammation as Potential Anti-Aging Strategies and Therapies"

"If you're seeking a complete body transformation or a dramatic improvement in athletic performance, you must follow JC's training methodologies. He is a master at program design, creating safe and effective workouts that deliver serious results."

Carla Sanchez, CSCS
Owner of Performance Ready Fitness Studio, Two-Time Ironman, and IFBB Pro

"JC Santana has been at the apex of functional training in the fitness industry for over 25 years! The training methods in *JC's Total Body Transformation* provide you, the fitness professional, with a dynamic, essential text, including exercises and pertinent information to train active individuals. Teaching at the university level for many years, I would recommend this book to all of my students and university athletes, plus as a text for any strength training systems course."

B. Sue Graves, EdD, FACSM, ACSM CEP
Department of Exercise Science and Health Promotion, Florida Atlantic University

"JC brought me back from the brink of disaster with his training. I had a back injury resulting in eight screws in my lumbar spine! Using many of the protocols in this book, I'm now one of the top 15 fighters in the UFC middleweight division! Get this book in order to train like a champion."

Cezar "the Mutant" Ferreira
MMA Fighter–UFC Middleweight Contender,
Three-Time Brazilian Jiu-Jitsu World Champion,
Winner of Globo's The Ultimate Fighter: Brazil

"The training methods in this book have helped me compete at the highest level in the UFC. JC has a way of making the complex very simple to understand and that allows me to get the most out of my training. Get this book and experience what I experience every week—the IHP way!"

Gilbert "Durinho" Burns
MMA Fighter–UFC Lightweight Contender,
Three-Time Brazilian Jiu-Jitsu World Champion

"I have trained under JC's care for four years, and that experience has launched me into the top rakings of the middleweight division. The training found inside *JC's Total Body Transformation* has allowed me to go from a good amateur to a top prospect in pro boxing! This book is the real deal! No fluff here."

Luis "Cuba" Arias
Top-Ranked Professional Boxer, USBA Middleweight Champion

"To climb the seven summits, you have to be in tip-top shape, psychically, emotionally, and physically. The spiriemotional coaching and training protocols JC shares in *JC's Total Body Transformation* played a pivotal role in each of my summits! Follow the path this book sets and summit your next climb!"

Ruben Payan, Jr.
Seven Summiter

"I'm a busy mother of two and for the last eight years I have trusted JC's training methods to keep me looking better at 41 than I did in high school! I have used many of the protocols in *JC's Total Body Transformation* to get me ready for my photo shoots and stay lean and firm. I can only tell you one thing—they work!"

Gina Bussani

JC's Total Body Transformation

The <u>Very</u> <u>Best</u> Workouts for Strength, Fitness, and Function

Juan Carlos "JC" Santana

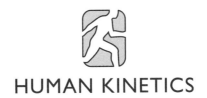

HUMAN KINETICS

Library of Congress Cataloging-in-Publication Data

Names: Santana, Juan Carlos, 1959- author.
Title: JC's total body transformation : the very best workouts for strength, fitness, and function / Juan Carlos "JC" Santana.
Other titles: Total body transformation
Description: Champaign, IL : Human Kinetics, 2019.
Identifiers: LCCN 2018039301 (print) | LCCN 2018054827 (ebook) | ISBN 9781492572763 (epub) | ISBN 9781492563181 (PDF) | ISBN 9781492563174 (print)
Subjects: LCSH: Physical fitness. | Exercise.
Classification: LCC GV481 (ebook) | LCC GV481 .S264 2019 (print) | DDC 613.7--dc23
LC record available at https://lccn.loc.gov/2018039301

ISBN: 978-1-4925-6317-4 (print)

This publication is written and published to provide accurate and authoritative information relevant to the subject matter presented. It is published and sold with the understanding that the author and publisher are not engaged in rendering legal, medical, or other professional services by reason of their authorship or publication of this work. If medical or other expert assistance is required, the services of a competent professional person should be sought.

Senior Acquisitions Editor: Michelle Maloney; **Senior Developmental Editor:** Cynthia McEntire; **Managing Editor:** Miranda K. Baur; **Copyeditor:** Michelle Horn; **Proofreader:** Ivonne B. Ward; **Senior Graphic Designer:** Joe Buck; **Cover Designer:** Keri Evans; **Cover Design Associate:** Susan Rothermel Allen; **Photograph (cover):** Top, Juan Carlos "JC" Santana; left, Pollyana FMS/ Moment/ Getty Images; middle, Ozimician/ iStock/ Getty Images; right, g-stockstudio/ iStock/ Getty Images; **Photographs (interior):** © Juan Carlos "JC" Santana; **Photo Production Manager:** Jason Allen; **Senior Art Manager:** Kelly Hendren; **Illustrations:** © Human Kinetics; **Printer:** Sheridan Books

We thank the Institute of Human Performance in Boca Raton, Florida, for assistance in providing the location for the photo shoot for this book.

Human Kinetics books are available at special discounts for bulk purchase. Special editions or book excerpts can also be created to specification. For details, contact the Special Sales Manager at Human Kinetics.

Printed in the United States of America

10 9 8 7 6 5 4 3 2 1

The paper in this book is certified under a sustainable forestry program.

Human Kinetics

P.O. Box 5076
Champaign, IL 61825-5076
Website: www.HumanKinetics.com

In the United States, email info@hkusa.com or call 800-747-4457.
In Canada, email info@hkcanada.com.
In the United Kingdom/Europe, email hk@hkeurope.com.

For information about Human Kinetics' coverage in other areas of the world, please visit our website: **www.HumanKinetics.com**

E7272

I dedicate this book to my parents, Arnaldo and Celerina Santana, for being the guiding light of our entire family.

Contents

Acknowledgments

Over time I have observed the importance of practice and experience, as opposed to formal education. Although I certainly value formal education, I now fully understand that education without experience is just information. Therefore, I acknowledge and treasure all that my former teachers, coaches, colleagues, and friends have shared with me. I am especially grateful to the Institute of Human Performance (IHP) for being a cauldron of creative energy for almost 18 years.

Considering the many social and cultural changes I witnessed in my life, I feel blessed to have been born during an era when old values and principles still drove social culture. My parents, Celerina and Arnaldo Santana, just celebrated their 65th wedding anniversary. That's just one small indication of the character these two angels have modeled for me and our family. To them I dedicate all of my works, for they are the reason I developed my work ethic, perseverance, and never-ending dedication to my family and career. They instilled in me my greatest virtues. Without a doubt, my parents are the finest people I know, which reminds me how lucky I am every day. I will never write a book in which I don't acknowledge them with this much passion.

My sisters Belkis and Moni (Godchild) have been with me through every up and down. They have been sources of comfort, strength, laughter, and accountability. They nurtured me and never let me get away with not being accountable. Accountability has always been at the forefront of our family, and these two have always held my feet to the fire with love. I thank them for their love and support, and credit them for helping me become and stay strong.

My parents taught me that family was number one, and my firstborn, Rio, helped me truly understand what that meant. Rio came into my life when I needed him the most and made a man of me, not with pain, but with laughter and amazement. I will always love him for the gift he is. Now I have the pleasure of working with him every day, watching him turn into a man while running the family business. This is another gift IHP gave me—a safe haven and a bright future for my son. My three other children—Caila, Dante, and Mia—are equal gifts. All are brilliant and special in their own way. Caila is my beautiful hippie, a loving, artistic, independent gift in my life. She is now working at IHP, and I hope she falls in love with it like Rio has. Dante is my engineer, blessed with a brilliant mind and a sense of humor. He keeps all of us in stitches with his memorized movie quotes. I'm amazed by how much information his brain holds and how bright he is. He is true gift to the family. Mia is the queen of elegance and likely a future attorney. She can argue her case well (reminds me of someone else I know). Mia gets along with everyone, is very loving and funny, and is gifted in all sorts of conversation. These four angels are my driving force, and I thank them for being that. Happily, I take great pride in that they see me as somewhat of a dinosaur. They claim everything with me turns into a lesson or lecture of some kind. I remind them that my job is to educate them on the essentials of human character, which means calling out the craziness I often see in today's society. I hope one day they will truly know and feel my undying love for them. Everything I do is to secure their future and teach them what is possible with hard work. Finally I cannot mention my children without giving due credit to the great women who helped raise them. Annie Aponte (Rio's mom) and Debbie Santana (Caila, Dante, and Mia's mom) have been instrumental in caring for our children, and I owe them a lifetime of gratitude for the love and support only mothers can bring to the upbringing of children. Thank you both.

For many years, my huge family in Miami served as a support community. The strength of this community was especially clear during major holidays. For three decades, our reunions were epic. Now, many of the old wise ones have passed on and the little ones started their own families. Our get-togethers are less frequent. Thank you to all of my aunts, uncles, nieces, nephews, and cousins for being part of my upbringing and the foundation of my family values. You, too, are part of this work and its success.

I have had the great pleasure and honor of sharing the stage with some of the brightest minds in the fitness industry. I have followed in the steps of giants. My coaches and teachers also played a huge role in shaping me into the man I am. From my wrestling coach (Andy Siegel) to my professional role models (e.g., Steve Cannavale, Dr. Anthony Abbott, Jose Antonio, Dr. Doug Kalman, Stu McGill, and Gary Gray), from my college professors (e.g., Dr. Graves, Dr. Whitehurst) to NSCA beacons such as Lee Brown, I thank you all for your knowledge, wisdom, and support. There has never been a call they did not answer, and for that I will forever be grateful. I thank Perform Better and Chris Poirier for giving me my start. Thank you, Chris, I will never forget my beginnings with you and PB.

A man is nothing without great friends and partners. Thank you, G, for coming into my life at the right time, and for the patience, laughter, fun, conversations, and support especially during my heavy schedule. From my Callahan Plaza friends to my new additions, I thank all of you for being part of my life. You always took care of me, made me laugh, allowed me to laugh and love without fear. You all were the light and beacons I needed to stay on the right path during life's biggest challenges and helped me get to the other side without a scratch. The list is long and distinguished, but here is the short list: Mark B., Pierro and Gina B., Rocky D., Guy F., Scott G., Jeff H., Mark M., Roly O., Carlos P., Barry P., Lizzi R., Billy R., Scott S., Kado T., Dave W., and members of the band Heaven!

My deepest gratitude goes to my IHP family, who served as models and assisted in the creation of this book. Guys, we got this done. You rock! Thank you to Rio, Adam, Andy, Katie, Jordan, Gandhi, Braden, Michelle, Rodrigo, Jess, Luis, and our photographer Emily Rollin. I want to thank IHP international for carrying our message far beyond the borders of the United States: Ruben Payan, Fernando Jaeger, Juan Pablo Perez, Juan Andres Garcia, Eduardo and Kimberly Poveda, Justo and Marisa Aon, Connie Beaulieu, Luis Noya, and Joel Proskowitz. They have been instrumental in launching the IHP global family. Together we have made IHP a worldwide brand. Thank you.

Introduction

Most trainers, athletes, or fitness consumers learn by doing. They don't necessarily want to be taught how to create workouts or programs. Therefore, this book contains battle-tested workouts that readers can immediately use and then tweak according to their preferences. The art and science of workout design and periodization were covered extensively in my previous book, *Functional Training* (2016, Human Kinetics). As the name implies, that book thoroughly defines functional training, explains the important concepts that surround it, and describes the periodization model and hybrid programming used to avoid overtraining and achieve peak performance. It also provides more than 110 functional exercises, more than 20 traditional strength exercises, yearly programs for 11 sports categories, and ready-to-go express protocols. This text expands on the programs provided in *Functional Training* and emphasizes the safe and effective workouts that have been proven inside the Institute of Human Performance (IHP), on the field, and on the road. I strongly recommend getting *Functional Training* as a reference and foundation for this book.

People choose to train for many reasons, including developing a better-looking body, getting rid of pain, enhancing performance in an activity or sport, rehabilitating an injury, reducing stress, improving health, or simply improving overall quality of life. The two most common client goals I see in my training facility are better looks and better athletic performance, with the former being the most common reason. This has certainly been our collective experience at IHP and my experience as I teach around the world. For this reason, this book is focused on body transformation workouts for both sexes. I also provide a good dose of performance workouts that include everything from conditioning to jump training and agility to speed training. There are more than 100 workouts in this book. Readers will find a workout they can start with now. There is no need to learn how to create workouts, and these workouts have already worked for someone else.

This book includes the mind-set and spiritual evolution that are part of the execution of these workouts and improved performance or body sculpting. As we say at IHP, "The IHP trainer resets the barometer of the human will." This mind-set and awareness model, called the Spiriemotion Paradigm, not only improves the training process and allows one to get more out of training but also can crossover into all aspects of life, thus enhancing the quality of life. This is true core training or, as we used to call it, training from the inside out.

Bringing a new and much-needed approach to training was a huge impetus behind writing this book. Part of this new approach is understanding the value of tirelessly repeating the basics. This attitude to training is in stark contrast to the entertainment value of "do something different every day" and muscle confusion philosophies that dominate the fitness market these days. If you are going to learn anything from this section, learn this: Training is not meant to be entertaining! It is meant to be repetitive and physically, mentally, and spiritually demanding. It leads to optimizing an intended outcome. Training is designed to be effective and obtain results!

Anyone can come up with a workout, but if the workout is so complicated that nobody understands it or few can perform it easily, it becomes another useless workout in a magazine or video on social media. Likewise, you can go with the muscle confusion nonsense and do something different every day to better stimulate muscle or to avoid getting bored with training. However, this approach will never get you the results you want; muscle responds to the manipulation of training variables (volume, intensity, frequency), not confusion, and any skill is learned by millions of repetitions. If you don't believe this, look at any elite athlete or world-class performer. One thing you will consistently find is that they are all excellent at tirelessly repeating the basics; they don't get bored or suffer from muscle confusion. As Geoff Colvin explains in his book, *Talent Is Overrated: What Really Separates World-Class Performers from Everybody Else* (2008, Portfolio), the road to excellence is paved with a lot of deliberate practice (e.g., 10,000 hours or 10 years' worth). Training is no different.

The workouts in this book involve relatively high volumes of basic exercises. I stayed with the basics because they allow you to get the learning out of the way so you can start to load the exercise and get more work done. Then the training can do what it's supposed to do: get you strong, get you toned, get you big, get you in shape, or perfect a skill. If you are constantly learning or perfecting an exercise, you never get to complete the right volume with the right load or speed, and therefore you will never get the results you are looking for. Only by perfecting an exercise can you start to work in the effective training zone. As I say, "In order to start the real training, you have to get the learning out of the way." All the workouts in this book are based on performing high numbers of sets or repetitions. In other words, we will be doing work.

As a trainer, I always explain the importance of repetition and basics to my client. Although athletes are used to grueling repetitions, I still harp on the importance of deliberately practicing the basics. I did not coach people back from comas, get athletes ready for competition, or train the U.S. Army Special Forces with lies and false promises. I am very straightforward with all my clients and athletes.

- I'm a performance coach and personal trainer and am very proud of the title. I'm not here to amuse or entertain. I'm here to coach clients through the necessary steps that will get them to the goals they outlined when they hired me.

- We are here to do the right amount of work to get the job done, with an emphasis on the words *right* and *work*.

- These workouts are based on science but driven by results. This means we are guided by sound scientific principles and are perfecting the basics that have proven successful over time. No pie-in-the-sky exercises or routines.

- There is more to training and performance than the physical. Training is as much a spiritual evolution as it is a physical transformation.

If you are a personal trainer or a strength and condition coach, I suggest you consider this professional no-nonsense approach to training your clients and athletes. If this is your position, then you will attract these types of clients. If you are a client or athlete, I highly recommend you look for a trainer or coach who has this philosophy to get you to your destination quickly and safely. The workouts in this book will help you implement the repetitive basic concepts because they are very effective and easy to understand and perform. Fitness aficionados, athletes, trainers, and coaches will find they can immediately use the workouts laid out in this book and safely embark on an effective training journey.

This book is organized into parts and chapters that include transformation workouts, performance workouts, and conditioning workouts. I created a book that could boast more than 100 workouts for everything you need. It is designed to be so comprehensive that I could say, "If it's not in this book, you don't need it." With that intent, I pored through my folders, studied the last 17 years of programming at IHP, and collaborated with some of the best in the world to deliver what I think is the best programming and workout book on the market.

However, the real jewel of this book is not the workouts; it's how we look at training. This new perspective on how to view and coach training is what really has taken IHP's training to another level. I have been working on this new paradigm and its effect on coaching for the last seven years. After reading this book and performing the routines in it with a different mind-set and perspective, your life and training will never be the same. Let's go over this new training and coaching paradigm.

IHP Spiriemotion Paradigm (Spirit + Emotion + Motion)

When you got this book, you were expecting to read about exercise, training, physical transformation, and being physically ready for anything, and all that will still happen. But you will get much more. You will become aware of something that's organic and intuitive, yet you probably never heard it put into words before. You will learn about the IHP Spiriemotion Paradigm, the model we use to coach clients and athletes to higher levels of performance and, more importantly, a higher level of being. This new awareness will improve not only your workouts but also every other aspect of your life.

After 45 years as an athlete and coach, I realized the transformations I witnessed in training went beyond the physical. Yes, some who wanted a better body or to win a championship got the body of his or her dreams or won the trophy. But the truth is, most people did not end up with a six-pack or with a championship belt. Although the external changes most people witnessed with training may not have been dramatic, their internal changes were nothing short of miraculous. Our fighters stayed the same weight (outside of the obvious weight cut) and looked the same for years, but their performances went through the roof and many fought their way into top-10 world rankings. My NFL players looked the same for their entire careers but had better on-field performance and lives with each year they trained at IHP. Our personal training clients, many of whom were once sedentary and some even depressed, were now happy and running 5K or 10K races and even triathlons. In most cases, the performances were beyond the visual appearance of the transformation. The "skill versus will" phenomena can be seen everywhere in life, but sport provides a magnifying glass that allows everyone to clearly see it. Everyone has witnessed a well-prepared athlete just collapse mentally and physically under the stress of the moment.

After seeing great athletes choke and often seemingly lesser athletes persevere, I started to wonder what drives the body to win or lose, or endure or surrender. I contemplated the important mechanisms of the action of the spirit, the will, the faith, and even the famous placebo effect accounted for in scientific studies yet so misunderstood. More importantly, I started to look at the connection between the spiritual, emotional, and physical, and thereby the connection between physical training and spiritual evolution or the fortification of the human will. Now, let's look at the similarities of training and many of the practices used today for the fortification of the human will—or spiritual evolution as I like to call it. Understanding this will change the way you train, the way you look at training, and what you get out of your training. Understanding these changes and how they are applicable to all aspects of life in turn changes your life.

Body, Mind, and Soul Connection

This section may be the most important in terms of changing your life. After reading it, you'll see training as a form of meditation that fortifies the human will. You will be able to use these tools in all areas of your life. Pay attention.

The mind, body, and soul are the three components of a person's being often expressed in music, literature, and art, and intuitively we accept these components of our being as self-evident. We know that if we are ready to perform and get a call with bad news, we could shut down and not be able to perform. Well, what shuts down? The emotions (i.e., the mind) shut down the central nervous system, preventing effective communication to the muscles (i.e., the body), leading to a lack in performance. What shuts down the emotions and the mind? The spirit, the will, the soul. What is the will, spirit, soul, or whatever controls the emotions?

A saying in some spiritual teachings is, "The past casts a shadow on the present to ensure the future will not change." This means that if we constantly operate with old and outdated and limiting beliefs (i.e., an outdated, or limited, workout), we will never evolve, and the future will be the same as the past; history repeats itself if you don't learn. What we are (our very being) is the result of our life's experiences (i.e., the past). Some of these experiences were great learning points in our lives and helped us evolve. However, some experiences were not so great and left impressions and perceptions (e.g., insecurity, fear, and anger) that may keep us stuck. These perceptions and old programming are like clouds that stay above us throughout our lives and keep us from seeing the truth, dealing with issues, and accepting things and working on our flaws. This spiritual stagnation keeps us from evolving. So how do we get rid of the clouds that keep us in the dark? How do we get rid of this old baggage and update our approach to training? And more importantly, what does training or this book have to do with this spiritual evolution and resetting the human will? Let's start answering these questions.

The measure of a person is not seen when things are great and going as planned. True character is on display when someone is at his or her worst, when things are not going right, and when stress is high. Stress is one of the primal triggers that makes us react according to what we have been taught (i.e., our old approach to training)—the good, the bad, and the ugly. Therefore, overcoming stress can be used as a tool for growth.

For these reasons, many religious disciplines have used stress (e.g., physical pain or discomfort) to transcend the physical and evolve spiritually. One needs only to look at some of the painful religious ceremonies around the world to see how withstanding pain and discomfort has been used throughout history to facilitate some form of spiritual transcendence. Simply observing yoga classes reveals an incremental difficulty in the yoga positions as the practitioners progress from novice to expert classes. What do the more advanced positions achieve? The more advanced yoga positions obviously increase psychological stress by increasing physical stress. This tolerance of physical and psychological discomfort forges a deeper connection with the present moment and the self. One can only endure what seems impossible by redefining what is possible, resetting the barometer of the human will. Therefore, one can conclude that many traditions use discomfort to facilitate spiritual transcendence or spiritual evolution.

Exercise and training normally are seen as activities that improve fitness, performance, health, and general well-being. We talk about the positive impact that exercise has on our fitness and our states of mind due to its effect on the neuromuscular and hormonal systems. This is one of the many reasons exercise has a "feel good" or antidepressive effect. But just like in religious ceremonies and other spiritual practices, exercise is a self-imposed discomfort, pain, or stress that can serve as a vehicle to spiritual transcendence if we simply understand the process and use the feeling of effort as a vehicle to fortify our will.

Think about it: When you exercise hard, you start breathing heavily to provide the extra oxygen the working muscles need. You may have to slow down or stop so you can catch up on your oxygen supply. In essence, that feeling of not having enough oxygen due to exercise is a form of voluntary suffocation that's no different than water-boarding; you know you are not going to die, but it certainly feels like you will, and you succumb (react) to the sensation. Lack of oxygen (suffocation) triggers a primitive reaction that always tests the human will. Therefore, when exercise intensity reaches a specific point, some individuals will grunt, grimace, cry, complain, or quit. We can use our reaction to the stress of exercise to analyze how we interpret and project stress in general. Learning to constantly deal with the emotions associated with the stress of exercise can teach strategies to better deal with any emotion and transcend beyond our current belief system.

At IHP, we use the sensations of suffocation and physical stress to deliberately discipline the mind and access the spirit (i.e., the will). This process creates an awareness of how we have allowed our limiting beliefs to stagnate our view and approach to life's challenges. Changing how we see exercise, effort, and the stress of training allows us to begin to change all things related to stress and redefine what we are willing to accept and endure. This process of using exercise (motion) to reset the barometer of the human will (emotions and spirit) is the IHP Spiriemotion Paradigm. Like in all religious disciplines, through specific coaching and practice (i.e., repetitive and deliberate training), clients learn to see what was once considered painful, limiting, or unpleasant is just an experience with no value or judgment attached to it. In many spiritual teachings, this is referred to as staying in the present moment. Eckhart Tolle, author of *The Power of Now: A Guide to Spiritual Enlightenment* (2004, Namaste Publishing), calls the stillness of the present moment "the Now." This Spiriemotion Paradigm has set IHP coaching apart and has allowed our training take on a whole new meaning.

Summary of IHP's Spiriemotion Paradigm

Using training to learn to deal with all components associated with the stress of exercise, one can learn to do the following:

- Accept emotions without reacting to them, putting a value on them, or judging them. The feelings of discomfort from exercise have only the meaning you give them. They are not good or bad; they simply are.
- Relax. Stay in the present moment, avoiding unnecessary projections into the future. Staying relaxed and focused during each repetition prevents sabotaging the next few reps.

Staying connected and relaxed in the moment is, in my opinion, the biggest training adaptation everyone makes. People change on a very deep level and stay cool with no judgment in the presence of a big challenge, a discomfort, a new sensation, or an unknown. This is IHP's Spiriemotion Paradigm, and it's the essence of true core training because it changes people at their cores. In practical terms, the paradox is that it changes people from the inside out by driving a stimulus from the outside in.

Principles and Process of the IHP Spiriemotion Paradigm

The sum of the experiences of people's lives sets the level of discomfort at which they will start hurting and eventually quit. How people define risk versus reward, pain versus pleasure, pride versus shame, strength versus weakness, and success versus failure are all part of what determines how people respond to training intensity, how hard they are willing to push, and to what point they will go before they mentally fail and quit. These perceived emotions and eventual actions have more to do with learned behaviors than physiological mechanisms.

When the training gets hard, most people start to show reactions to stress. The most common sign is a grimace or other facial expression that shows stress, pain, or anguish. They suddenly quit and don't even want to discuss it. The sign of stress (e.g., the grimace on the face) is consistent with and comes from past experiences: This is uncomfortable, this is painful, the end is soon coming, and I should be stopping now to avoid even more pain. The decision to react and eventually stop the discomfort of exertion just because of a feeling based on old beliefs is an example of how old limiting beliefs and false judgment can project into the future and sabotage the present moment. The fear of feeling even worse makes people stop. FEAR can be seen as False Evidence Appearing Real. Fear is the cloud from the past that casts a shadow on the present to ensure the future will not change; you learned to quit when you felt like this; therefore, you will always quit when you feel this. This faulty paradigm ensures one never evolves. At the grimace or first expression of panic or stress, we say, "Relax your face, stay in the moment, stay with me." No judgment, no past false beliefs, no sabotage. What you are feeling is just a feeling—this is what accelerated metabolism feels like. Observe it neutrally. Review the various sensations, feelings, or voices in your head and see them as a series of floats and people in a parade. Observe them as they pass without jumping into the parade. The essence of presence and peace is not to clear your mind of thoughts, but to know you are not your thoughts and to allow your thoughts to pass as floats pass during a parade.

The intensity and the feeling associated with the level at which people decide to stop or quit are never their maximum intensity but rather a percentage of that maximum intensity they are willing to endure. By repeating the training that elicits this feeling, people get used to it, and the feeling is reinterpreted, losing its initial meaning and impact. The repetitive nature of training helps us neutralize these feelings, not giving them the weight they once had. We learn that feelings by themselves never killed anyone and really never hurt anyone; they are just feelings. It's what we made of the feeling that affected our lives. The feeling of exercise and intense effort is simply normal accelerated metabolism; that's it. So, the experience is redefined; this is just the feeling associated with this form or level of training, just like the sun is associated with daylight and morning, and its absence is not a reason for panic because it simply indicates night.

This process of repeatedly experiencing the discomfort associated with high-intensity training allows one to feel the experience without projecting into the future and sabotaging the present moment. This means you don't quit just because training gets hard because your perception of hard and how you learn to just observe it constantly changes. Over time, what you are *willing* to endure constantly changes, thus redefining your will. By using training and its process as a teachable moment in redefining the human will (and thereby the spirit), we can teach and learn the parallel impact this evolution has on all aspect of our lives. If that is not a spiritual evolution, then I don't know what would be.

Applying the Spiriemotion In and Out of Training

In summary, the IHP Spiriemotion Paradigm uses training to not only fortify the body and teach good movement pattern but also reset the barometer of the human will (spiritual evolution). This latter adaptation is the fastest and biggest adaptation training produces, especially if we know how to teach or learn the coaching associated with it. When training, a person will feel all the normal training sensations, especially at intense levels. At higher training intensities, everyone changes their demeanors, such as their facial expressions. When some outward facial expression shows up in response to the effort of training, you will hear an IHP coach say, "Relax your face, stay with me; you are almost done, and 9 and 10. You are done. Great job." After that set is over, the teachable moment is at hand. The IHP trainer coaches the client (John, in this example) through this process: "John, as you can see, 10 reps were no problem. But, at about rep number seven, you began to interpret the sensations you were feeling according to old beliefs and values. (i.e., the drama), and you fell right into it with the grunting and faces of anguish. Ten easy reps were made harder than needed, and all over nothing—just an old story. This happens in all aspects of life, we assume, we project, and we sabotage experiences that could be easy and even enjoyable and make them nightmares over nothing (i.e., old stories). This next set is the most important set of our session. I want you to complete the next set without reacting to anything in your head. No drama for 10 reps. The feeling you will experience at about rep seven is not hard or easy, it's not good or bad, and you don't like or hate it. The feeling is a natural part of getting to 10 reps, which is no mystery because you have already done it, and rather easily, may I add. Stay present and understand that what you feel is just accelerated metabolism. I will guide you through reps 7 to 10. Just keep your face relaxed and stay in the moment—you got this."

Without fail, John gets through 10 reps without any grunting or facial expressions. It may take a little reminding to relax the face from our coach through reps 7 to 10, but eventually you see all the IHP-trained clients with expressionless faces when they are going through their toughest reps.

Through mindful physical training, you will be able to separate yourself from your thoughts or feelings. In essence, your mindful training actually becomes mindless or neutral—you stay out of the drama that lives in your mind. This practice is particularly important when it comes to negative thoughts, the "he said, she said" drama in your mind. If you react to all the negative thoughts that can creep into your mind, such as fear, envy, insecurity, jealousy, or inadequacy, your life becomes a drama-filled reality show. Not good! Learning not to react to the stress of exercise by not judging or using old negative stories but seeing it as just a state of being and just a feeling will teach you to do the same with the other stresses in your life. As you train yourself to detach from your old story of how much training hurts, how tired you are, and how you want to quit, you will also detach from the other sabotages you practice in your daily life. You will not only catch yourself when you judge others but also when you judge yourself and when you sabotage situations based on your old workout. As you relax your face in training, so too you will relax your face in life. When you start "relaxing your face" under stress, that shadow of the past will clear and allow you to finally see the reality of this moment, the reality of the now, the only reality. Then you will begin to be free of the old programs holding you back and free yourself to further evolve as a person.

So relax your face when the training stress appears and you want to grimace. Stay in the moment, finish what you started, and practice our Spiriemotion every repetition, every set, and every workout. Finish the few repetitions left, the few seconds left, or the few yards left with no emotions or judgments attached. Practice this discipline in your everyday life. When you practice staying in the moment every repetition of training, you practice present-moment awareness many times per week, close to a thousand times, in some cases. It is hard for this conscious training not to affect your subconscious and seep into other aspects of your life. You actually become aware of this phenomenon and start catching yourself wanting to react to something and relaxing your face, breathing, just letting it go, and observing it without becoming it. This practice improves your quality of life more than any other adaptation physical training offers. This is how training helps you spiritually evolve, clearing the clouds of the past from the now so you can evolve and your future can change for the better.

Simple and Repetitive

In these days of marketing-driven sales, social media explosion, and shocking sales bylines, you hear all kinds of crazy catchphrases. *Muscle confusion*, the *insanity workout*, and workouts with the word *extreme* in the titles are just some of the catchy phrases being used. Then, of course, you have the booty, abs, and shredding Instagramers offering the latest in diet secrets, specialized workouts, and quick results. Finally, you have the YouTube channels, where everyone is the star of his or her own video universe and can claim anything and become anyone for a few minutes on camera. However, if you were to meet some of these people, it would hit you: There is no substance, no system, no method, no nothing. The one-hour rap is up.

If you are going to get one thing out of this book, it is this: Nothing will work better than the basics. Nothing has changed when it comes to developing excellence in anything. Show me every great performer who has lasted a couple decades at the world level, and I will show someone who invested his or her time in perfecting the basics. How does a golfer perfect a 320-yard drive? How does a basketball player develop a 90 percent average from the free throw line? How does a musician perfect his instrument? How do weightlifters continue to break records year after year? How do bodybuilders develop the incredible bodies we see today? They all master the basics. When performance and careers are on the line, the pros don't fall for the gimmicks; that is left for the amateurs. Why are the basics so important, and how do they relate to the content in this book? Let's explore that further.

From a performance standpoint, the basic patterns of movement must be engrained in the central nervous system (CNS) in order for the perfect movement to be available without thought or special effort. The perfect movement must become more of a reflex than a conscious decision, as if that's the only way the body knows how to do it. From a structural standpoint, the efficiency and stability associated with great movements are also crucial. The more aligned, stable, and efficient the movement becomes, the more perfect it is. This stability and efficiency allow more weight to be used and more volume (i.e., more work) to be performed. With more strength and more work, the body must change accordingly. Just look at athletes and how their bodies change over time, even if changing how the body looks is not a goal. There is also the Spiriemotion Paradigm we just discussed. In order to deal with emotions and develop the spiritual connection, you must be able to focus and relax your face. You can't do the inner work if you are too busy perfecting the exercise or dealing with the novelty of new training every session. Novelty is good for entertainment, not training. For this reason, I have purposefully kept the workouts in this book simple. I need you to concentrate on connecting your brain (i.e., the CNS) to the movement and the muscles without overthinking. In other words, let the CNS fire up and drive the body as you quiet the mind. Don't let your mind tell you how bored you are, how much it hurts, how hard it is, how tired you are, or how good it would feel to stop. That is your old story, and it no longer serves you. Working hard on the basics and the simple stuff allows you to get more out of your training without creating drama out of your training. This repetition and perfection of the basics transfers to life. Concentrate and be grateful for the basics and simple things in life such as love, health, family, friends, laughter, peace, a sunrise, a sunset, a great conversation, or a child's first step. These are the simple basics of life, and every appreciation is a good solid repetition. Stay simple, my friends. Stay simple.

Programming Functional Training

Training has come a long way in the last four decades. In the past, the only reason people trained hard was to prepare for sport or battle. Then the bodybuilding revolution hit, and people trained to look a certain way as well. Now people train for all sorts of reasons. Therefore, workouts are diverse and many factors are considered to maximize results.

It is very important to know exactly why you are doing something, but often people just do things without really understanding why. Part I looks at the various reasons people train and the role of those goals when selecting the right approach, mental attitude, and workout. This simple analysis can help a person avoid the endless "lift more for the sake of lifting more" war that ends up crippling thousands of gym goers.

Part I also provides a detailed account of the workouts throughout the book and their classifications. Variety, intensity, and safety are discussed because it is important to understand these factors when designing a workout.

Finally, part I introduces the difference between periodization and programming and the variables to consider when designing and progressing any workout over weeks. A biomechanical assessment is provided to assist you in determining if you have any major deficiencies. I conclude with a discussion on the concept of conscious training and performing a quality repetition. Part I sets the tone for the rest of the book, so enjoy.

CHAPTER 1

Train for Results

What are you training for, performance outside the gym or inside the gym? When people come to Institute of Human Performance (IHP) to train, I ask commonsense questions, but I seem to go in a different direction than most. I actually stay on task while I see many trainers ignore the actual answers to their questions. This is where the awareness of the real issues at hand begins. Let's deal with the basic reasons people buy a training book or go to a gym.

Reasons to Train

Why do people train? Well, when we ask people why they come into IHP or why they are taking up a new training program, it's usually for looks, health, rehabilitation from an injury or surgery, performance in a specific sport, or just a better quality of life. Although IHP is a very different commercial gym (i.e., young and high-level athletic clientele), the main reason people come into IHP is the same as most other gyms: to look better. The athletic population wants to look better when they win, the rehab population wants to look better after they rehab, and everyone who is working for a better quality of life wants to do so looking better! That is one of the reasons that the body transformation portion of this book is as dense as it is. However, even within the transformation section, we have workouts with carryover to function. Therefore, don't feel like you have to compromise between function and looks—you can have them both.

We should also briefly discuss the impact exercise has on the physical appearance of the body. The stimulus for muscle growth or strength is rather simple, and few things work better than the good old-fashioned bodybuilding workouts in this book. Therefore, the complexity of routines and special workouts must be questioned. Muscles do only one thing: They change length while under tension. The muscle simply responds to the distance, the tension, and the speed at which it contracts and lengthens. It's rather a simple process. When muscles are exposed to tension, the fibers and cells undergo a disruption. The muscle does not care what created the tension (i.e., a sandbag, a barbell, a band, or a machine). Microtears occur when a muscle works against tension (i.e., a resistance) with significant intensity. Immediately following the cellular disruption, there is an inflammatory response (i.e., the pump) that is felt during the training, but some partial and prolonged swelling lasts for some time after the initial stimulus. Depending on the level of muscle damage, the swelling can last for days, like the swelling left after a contusion to your thigh. This inflammation and other repair mechanisms are followed by the remodeling process, and this makes the muscles stronger and bigger. This is an oversimplified description of how a muscle is toned or gets bigger. Therefore, to think that a magical exercise, routine, or piece of equipment alone will change your body, or a muscle, is really fictional. That idea has to be reconciled if you are going to concentrate on the most important thing, which is proper training intensity and volume. You simply have to learn to manage your perception of training, stay focused, and keep loading and stimulating the muscle to grow. That's how bodybuilders and other athletes do the same exercise and training year in and year out and keep getting bigger, faster, and stronger. With these athletes, the exercise mode doesn't change much; the loads and intensity are increased until the point of diminishing return or optimal strength is reached. The exercises and workouts in this book will be all you need to get the body you want or perform at your best. You simply have to execute the training at a higher level than you have before. Using the Spiriemotion Paradigm explained in the introduction, you will take your training to levels you never even imagined, and your body will reflect this new level of execution.

Since we have given the transformation portion of this book such emphasis, it should be noted that virtually all transformation programs require a significant nutritional intervention. Most people want to drop weight (i.e., fat) to look better; a small number of people are hard gainers who have to battle genetics, age, or some other limitation to put on weight. Even muscle gain has a nutritional component to it. I would say the fat-loss component most people desire is 80 percent nutrition and 20 percent training. After all, most people will tell you they don't want to look like a bodybuilder; they want to look athletic and toned. The physical training needed to tone a muscle is minimal. Anyone can train—that's the easy part! However, the 24/7 dieting or eating lifestyle that goes with reducing the fat and allowing the beautiful human anatomy to show is a different story. Like training, nutrition has more to do with emotions and spiritual makeup than it does nutritional know-how. Why people eat is more important than what people eat because the why usually controls the what. We will address the nutritional component later in chapter 16.

People who are looking for better health and even those rehabilitating some form of trauma often think that some special training needs to be considered. We have used many of the transformation workouts in this book to rehabilitate bodies or bring them from the lowest levels of function imaginable to perfect health. The only variable dramatically altered is the weight used in an exercise. Range of motion is also an important variable to consider when dealing with very low levels of function. However, regardless of whether you are manipulating load or range of motion, many of the transformation workouts provided in this book make great health and rehabilitative workouts.

Athletes want that edge on the competition, so they are easy to sell on the next gimmick. Athletes will try anything to gain a competitive edge, but like everyone else, they eventually have to come back to repeating the basics to get ahead of the competition. Additionally, we have found that even though they come in asking for higher vertical jumps, more speed, or faster changes in direction, most athletes need relentless conditioning. For this reason, included in this book are many of the metabolic protocols and conditioning drills we have used over the last 18 years. When you go through some of the metabolic and conditioning workouts, you will understand why IHP athletes outlast the competition.

Point of Diminishing Returns

Every training has a risk-to-reward ratio to consider, as well as a point of diminishing returns. I see many individuals at the gym just looking to lift heavier weights. To these people, I ask why and how much strength is enough for what you need? I'm all about getting stronger for a reason, but when I see senseless weight being pushed around for no reason other than lifting heavy stuff, then I start to wonder how much of the workout the ego is running and how much of it the brain is running (i.e., logical and purposeful training). Before, I used to ask, What's the most I can train to get the results I want? Now I ask, What is the minimum effective training I can undertake to get the maximum results? I have changed my position on training because apart from basically destroying my body and not wanting anyone else to go through what I have, the high-intensity training needed at the highest level of performance has a sinister side few talk about.

The high-performance training necessary to excel in sports today is usually inversely proportional to long-term health and wellness. The harder you train, the more the chances you will run into problems in your 40s and beyond. Strongmen, strength and power athletes, bodybuilders, football players (especially linemen and linebackers), fighters, and many other athletes involved in hard, intense training don't typically live long and healthy lives when compared to the average population. Additionally, if we look at the orthopedic issues many of these athletes experience, often as early as their mid-30s, it's obvious that heavy training also has a heavy price. This is why I try to keep my training simple and manipulate my intensity and volume to perfection. I never recommend anyone train *through* pain and very rarely train to failure. Effort is one thing, but pain and total exhaustion is another, and for the most part, not necessary!

At 59, I have many battle scars to show for my decades of "badass" training or ego-centered stupidity. After two hip replacements, two arthritic knees, and intermittent shoulder issues, I can tell you that heavy training is overrated and mostly unjustified from a scientific and practical standpoint. Yes, it's cool to pound your chest with Olympians and world champions—I did it for more than 20 years. There is a sense of accomplishment and ego boost when you can do what most people can't. I would be a liar if I did not admit that there is a certain air of confidence that comes from walking into a room, with people knowing you are a badass. But I would also be a liar if I told you that had anything to do with anything except the ego. In retrospect, I know that 80 percent of my training could have been lighter yet more intense and specific, less damaging, and more effective. Perhaps if an older and wiser JC Santana had advised me when I was young, I would have not needed my surgeries and would be enjoying a healthy and pain-free body now. This is one of the reasons I love my job so much. I know that my philosophy, training, and teachings are preventing damage, prolonging careers, and improving quality of life into the later decades of life.

Since I competed in Olympic weightlifting and powerlifting and these are popular methods of training, let's take a look at their training methods and why they may not always be the best option for building muscles or improving performance. Now, I competed at the state and national levels in both sports, qualifying and competing in the American Open Series (Olympic weightlifting) in 1998 at almost 40 years old. I have been coached by two Olympic coaches (Rafael Guerrero and Leo Totten). I also hold a level 2 coaching certification with USA Weightlifting. I don't give this information to brag, but to show that I love the sports and enjoyed them with excellent coaching and technique. I'm well qualified to make the statements I'm about to make.

Let's start by saying the efficacy and safety of many lifts and training methods depend greatly on how a person is built and not necessarily the technique used. For example, if you are not designed to full squat, you may full squat while you are young or for a few years but eventually, in some form, your body will collect the biomechanical debt you have accumulated. In my case, I believe many of my issues were brought on by the extreme ranges of motion and heavy loads of the Olympic lifts. If the knees, hips, and shoulders are not made for the loads and ranges of motion needed for the correct execution of the Olympic lifts, these will put a beating on these joints, even with good form. If you add bad form to the equation, then you will pay the price that many have paid!

Powerlifting is much more forgiving on the flexibility side, but the loads needed to be competitive end up eating up the body. If you want to bench 300 to 500 pounds, squat 500 to 1,000 pounds, and deadlift 500 to 1,000 pounds, then be ready to pay for this heavy training at some point. The human body was not made for this abuse (loads and ranges of motion), and although some may apparently get away with it, most pay with their joints. Yes, some people may survive it for a few years and a rare few for life, but the majority won't. This is why you will not see any of this extreme and questionably effective training in this book. We will use simple and basic exercise, concentrating on great form and intense work output. This approach will allow us to train heavy enough for what we want and develop as much muscular mass as we need, all with minimal to no damage.

Right now, heavy and intense training is very popular. One example is CrossFit. I don't have anything against the sport, and as a sport, CrossFit is no more abusive than MMA. However, I witnessed a Wodapalooza (CrossFit competition) in January of 2017, at Bayfront Park in downtown Miami. I saw two days of competition and spent a ton of time in the therapy tent and witnessed the injuries, both acute and chronic injuries. I was horrified at the lack of proper form I saw during the competition in full back squatting, snatching to failure, and overhead squatting. To add insult to injury, all were done in a fatigued state. I kid you not—it was an orthopedic surgeon's dream. I see this training going on in many gyms around the world, and outside of competing in CrossFit, this training has nothing to do with anything except pretty much guaranteeing people will have unnecessary injuries. That is my experience with this style of training, from being not only present at competitions, but also in over 30 CrossFit gyms all over the world. In my humble opinion, there are better alternatives to achieve performance enhancement and body transformation. I have witnessed many of the people training in these gyms doing exercises they don't know how to perform and may not even be built for. I fear if they keep it up, they will end up just like me, with metal parts all over their bodies and often in some pain or discomfort. Trust me, that's no way to live, and there are better training options.

Training Variables

If repeating the same thing is effective, then what manipulations are needed to keep the muscles and body constantly changing? The basic variables we manipulate are intensity, volume, and frequency. Manipulation of these variables stimulates muscles and the motor learning system to adapt and get us the results we are really looking for. These variables and how they are changed through different periods will be covered in chapters 2 and 17. A more comprehensive explanation on the manipulation of these training variables and the principle of periodization can found in *Functional Training*, and I refer you there for a complete review on this topic.

You may ask if changing up the routine is not a good thing? The answer to that question is not as easy as you would think because it all depends on why you are changing the routine. If you are changing the routine because you hit a plateau or are bored, chances are changing the routine is not the issue; lack of planning and hitting the right intensity is. So, changing the routine without changing your focus, intention, perspective, and progressive manipulation of the basics variables will do little to nothing for you. It may entertain you for a few weeks, but in the long run, you will end up with the same issue: Your training will not get you the results you want. If you are a personal trainer and your clients are bored, it's because *you are bored,* and your clients are reflecting your energy back at you. If you are bored with your routine, then you have to ask the deeper question of why? If you are uniformed, then you have this book, and that will no longer be the case. If someone is bored because they lack knowledge, then that knowledge must be acquired and applied. Otherwise, no workout will get someone out of a rut, and the cycle continues. Ignorance is one of the main reasons the cloud from the past (same thoughtless thinking) is allowed to cast a shadow on the present (stay stuck), and if something does not change (awareness and evolution), the future does not change (you repeat the same mistake again).

So, what are some good reasons to change a routine? I understand it will take changing things up to add some fire into a career or a yearly training program. I get it! Something new can add more confidence and a new look. But these changes just for excitement must be rare and after establishing a foundation on the basics. Other than that, there are still some good reasons to change things up. If you are changing your routine because the old one is causing you pain or discomfort, then you have a very good reason to look for a new routine, one that uses training methods that don't hurt your body. If, after you have a base, you are changing your routine for a better routine with a purpose and more specific training, then that also is a great reason to try something new. If you are changing your routine as part of a periodized program that allows specially designated peaks and valleys in order to let the body recover and peak in an organized fashion, then it is the best reason to change a program.

To summarize, although something new can be positive, changing things up is best after establishing the basics. Changes should be centered on specifically progressing the training, to get out of pain, or to deliberately follow a periodized program. Other than that, you are changing things up because you need to be entertained, and that's no way or reason to train.

CHAPTER 2

Program Framework

The workouts in this book are separated into three basic categories: transformation, movement, and endurance. Since most of what is promoted in gyms, popular magazines, and books centers on physical transformation, I provide a hefty section on this topic. The transformation section consists of 60 workouts for six body parts, with workouts for men and women in each chapter. The transformation workouts vary in equipment needs. Some workouts require no equipment, using your body weight as the only resistance. Others require minimal equipment such as dumbbells, bands, medicine balls, and stability balls. I even include bodybuilding workouts that use the standard equipment available in most commercial gyms.

The movement section consists of 20 workouts divided into four different performance-oriented abilities, each with five workouts. These workouts also require simple equipment, and some don't require any equipment at all.

The final workout section is the endurance section. There are 20 conditioning workouts for four body parts, each with five workouts. As a bonus, I have solicited the help of some of the top people in the industry to provide some of their favorite workouts and expertise so you will be introduced to some of the workouts the giants in the industry use with their clients or athletes. Including the base workouts in each chapter, the additional workouts courtesy of my fitness colleagues, and the weekly workouts, this book contains about 120 workouts. If it's not in this book, you likely don't need it.

Program Classifications

IHP is well known throughout the world for its cutting-edge, intense yet simple training. We do not adhere to the outdated norms set by traditional dogma. For example, we don't believe in women training versus men training, youth training versus older people training, or athlete training versus nonathlete training. At IHP we train abilities, not gender, age, status, or any other social classification. If you have the ability, then we want you to reach your potential in that ability. Many IHP women train harder than many men I have seen in other gyms. We have seen some clients who would be considered nonathletes (e.g., attorneys, doctors, pilots) outtrain some of our world-class athletes. We have also watched men in their 50s and 60s wipe the floor with teenagers and young studs in their 20s. So, at IHP we don't play the gender, age, or classification game as a way to limit or stifle anyone. There are no victims at IHP; come to play or stay home. The workouts in this book have been used by a wide array of clients at various training levels. These workouts can be performed at crushing intensities or a more moderate pace to provide a decent level of fitness and even rehabilitation.

Even though we don't differentiate between men and women when training at IHP, we have divided the transformation workouts in this book by sex. Why did we do that? First, ease of use and classification. Not everyone can come to IHP and be coached professionally through these workouts or have the workouts perfectly adjusted for them. Many people, especially women, have misconceptions of what training is, what it will do, and what it won't do. After all, how many times have we heard a woman say, "I don't want to lift weights because I don't want to get big and look like a man" or something similar? Likewise, how many times have we heard coaches or men say, "In order to get big, you need to lift heavy loads for few repetitions (e.g., 3 repetitions)?" These myths, fears, and lack of education create the need for simple education and classification so people can understand and trust the information in the absence of knowledge. This is one of the reasons we separated the men's and women's transformation workouts.

Another obvious reason is the different goals between men and women. Whether it's a specific body part or a specific look, men and women differ quite a bit. For example, for the most part, women don't care how much they bench, but men do. Men want to get big and strong, while women want to be slender and toned. Women want the backs of their arms, butts, and thighs tight, while men want the big V, with the chest and the guns on display. Generally speaking, the women's workouts will be higher volumes with lower weights and the men's workouts will provide more work with heavier loads. However, a man can certainly use one of the exercises from a woman's workout and use the light loads and high repetitions as a flush set or as a finishing exercise. Likewise, a woman can take a workout from the men's section and use it to gain strength and accelerate the increase of bone density to combat osteoporosis. Therefore, there is a ton of carryover between the men's and women's workouts in this book, and we will expand on this in the workout chapters. All other workouts basically are the same for both men and women; conditioning and athletic skills have no gender bias. Each workout will provide basic progressions, regressions, and alternatives. You will get enough variety to make any adjustment you need.

Variety

Within the context explained earlier, we can easily mix and match workouts as well as exercises within a workout. This means we can put half of a back workout and half of a chest workout together and create an awesome upper-body workout. We can also take a chest workout and exchange one or two exercises from another chest workout to create a unique workout that better suits you. Finally, most compound exercises (i.e., exercises that move multiple joints at the same time) lend themselves to different repetition ranges, so feel free to take an exercise listed for a repetition range of 15 to 20 and turn it into a strength exercise by adding weight and dropping the repetitions to 4 to 6.

The equipment suggested in the workouts can also be substituted. Remember, a muscle only knows resistance; it does not care where the resistance comes from. Therefore, feel free to try different exercises with different equipment and in different positions. For example, if you like a routine that normally calls for dumbbells, but you are traveling and don't have dumbbells, don't be afraid to try the routine on the road with the JC Traveler or Predator Jr. bands. This means you can take a dumbbell bench fly and substitute it for a standing band fly. These kinds of changes allow you to not only stay consistent with your workout but also provide a different stimulus to the muscle being worked and make the exercise more functional by bringing in other synergistic muscle systems.

Intensity and Safety

No programming should be without a clear discussion about intensity and safety. We have already touched on topics related to intensity when we talked about resetting the barometer of the human will. However, this discussion is more focused on the mechanics and programming end of exercises and training. We want to make sure that anyone can alter the intensity of any exercise without using weight as an intensity parameter. Let's take a look at some simple techniques that can be used to alter the intensity of any functional exercise.

In functional training, we often use just body weight or light equipment that requires a system to vary resistance without adding an external load. The IHP functional training system describes four tweaks that can make any exercise a little harder (progression) or easier (regression). The four tweaks are base of support, lever arm, range of motion, and speed. Following is a brief summary of these tweaks. We refer you to *Functional Training* for a more complete review of this topic. In time, you will learn to use each tweak and combine multiple tweaks in order to keep your programming progressing consistently, effectively, and safely.

Base of Support

The base of support provides two things: surface area and fixed points of contact to react with the ground. Without these two important features, it's hard to establish the body and express any significant force production. This need for stability and ground reaction must be understood in today's age of unstable training environments that actually hinder strength development. Increasing the base provides more stability and shares the training load over the bigger surface or more points of contact. Both features make any exercise easier. Reducing the base simply increases the instability factor and puts more load on the structures contacting the ground, therefore making any exercise harder. When reducing the base to make things harder, you have to ensure that those remaining base structures can stabilize the system so it can be properly loaded. If one loses load (i.e., the weight used) to balance requirements, strength development suffers. An example of how to reduce the base to increase loading but not lose the load to balance can be seen in the single-leg anterior reach. If you want to increase the loading parameter of a single leg, but you can't balance on a single leg, stand in a staggered stance so most of the weight is on the front foot and the rear foot lightly taps the ground to stabilize the position. Even if the front foot takes on 80 to 90 percent of the load, you will be able to use greater loads and do more work; 80 to 90 percent of a huge number is better than 100 percent of a small number. So, reduce the base but make sure it is stable enough to load the system appropriately.

Range of Motion

Range of motion is another good tweak to manipulate the amount of intensity and work performed in an exercise. The longer a mass (e.g., medicine ball) travels, the more work is done; it's that simple. There is also a mechanical concern that involves the eccentric portion of the exercise, which is when the muscle lengthens while producing force or the negative portion of the contraction. The eccentric portion of a muscular contraction is when most muscle damage takes place, and thus it is a strong stimulus for growth. The longer the range of motion, the larger the eccentric component, and therefore the more stimulus for muscle growth and strength. Now, this does not mean that isometric contractions and partial-range-of-motion training are not effective; they are. These strategies can be employed when specific strength is needed at specific angles or ranges of motion. However, range of motion is strongly associated with the amount of work done and the eccentric component of training.

Lever Arm

The lever arm is another great tweak to organically manipulate the intensity of an exercise. The longer the lever arm (i.e., the distance between the pivot point or axis and the load), the harder the exercise becomes. That's why when you elevate a push-up, it becomes easier, and the further the dumbbell is from the shoulder, the harder the lateral raise is. The lever arm is also the difference between a bench and a dumbbell fly. This is a great tweak to use when you have limited loads or equipment to work with but still need to get some intensity out of the load.

Speed

The last tweak is the speed. Speed is a very diverse tweak because either fast or slow speeds can be used to make an exercise easier or harder. That is, doing something fast can make some things easier and other things harder. For example, speed creates momentum that is hard to generate, but once it's generated, an activity like throwing, jumping, or running becomes easy. Generally, if you are training to generate dynamic movements (e.g., explosive push-ups, jump squats, and speed repetitions), going fast can increase the training intensity, especially if it's done for high repetitions. This tweak is used to develop power and power endurance.

Now, if you want to make a moderately loaded exercise harder, you can use the time-under-tension principle and slow it down. This puts the muscle under tension for a longer time, thereby increasing the work the muscle performs. This tweak is excellent for developing strength and hypertrophy while keeping the loads to a modest level. Bodybuilders often use this approach to add muscle while sparing joints.

Equipment Needed for the Workouts

The workouts in this book are very diverse and so is the equipment needed. There are bodyweight workouts that require nothing but heart and attitude. There are band workouts that are perfect to take on the road. There are workouts that can be done with a single weight plate, and they are perfect for the garage or back yard. There are functional workouts that require small functional equipment, such as bands, medicine balls, stability balls, dumbbells, kettlebells, or an adjustable bench, and they're perfect for that home workout everyone wants. Finally, there are straight-up bodybuilding workouts for the meathead in many of us. These workouts are designed for a commercial gym that has standard bodybuilding equipment, such as machines, cables, barbells, and dumbbells. Each workout will list the equipment needed and some possible alternatives just in case you don't have access to one piece.

Basic Programming and Periodization

One of the reasons books like this one are very popular is because programming is such a difficult area to master, in part because much of the scientific literature about programming and periodization had to be translated from Russian and other languages and dealt with the training of elite athletes, not the development of general fitness. The workouts in this book cover a wide array of application, from toning to total-body metabolic power. Following is a brief review of periodization and program design. For a more comprehensive discussion on the theory and practice of periodization and program design, I refer you to *Functional Training*.

Periodization is the manipulation of training variables during different periods of time; thus its name. Training variables include intensity, volume, and frequency. Our version of periodization includes four periods that progressively train a body to peak at a specific time. The four periods are conditioning or hypertrophy, strength, power, and power endurance. Each of these periods can be 4 weeks long, making an entire training block 16 weeks. Depending on the time line available, each period can be made shorter and, in some cases, avoided altogether.

The transformation workouts in this book use a higher volume of work, and for that reason they can be used for conditioning or hypertrophy. Any hypertrophy or conditioning workout is easily converted to a strength workout by increasing the weight so that four to six repetitions become challenging. Although there are many ways to develop power, the athletic performance workouts in this book have a huge power component and can certainly be used for that cycle.

Finally, athletic endurance workouts are, in essence, metabolic power workouts and are perfect for the final stage of athletic preparation, the power endurance cycle. With the workouts in this book, you will be able to effectively train through any period inside of a periodized training scheme. *Functional Training* has a complete explanation of the periodization and programming component and over 70 programs covering all applications and phases or cycles of training. I strongly recommend you make that book part of your library; it's a perfect supplement to this one.

CHAPTER 3

Assess and Progress

One of the most complicated areas of personal training and even program design is knowing where to begin. Many people want some kind of evaluation to know where to start. In my humble opinion, that does not even exist. For example, most people who start a jogging program don't perform a $\dot{V}O_2$ test to figure out how long and how fast to run on their first training session. Likewise, most people who join a gym don't go through a bunch of one-rep maximum tests to start at specific percentages of that maximum lift. Even if they did, that maximum lift goes up every week when first beginning an exercise program; therefore all the percentages would be off in the second to third week. In most of these cases, people start a new training program on intuition and trial and error. For example, if you sit on a bench press machine for the first time and don't know how much you can handle for eight repetitions, you start with a weight you feel you can do and adjust up or down from there. Eventually you get to a weight you can manage for the eight repetitions desired. All beginners start at a level they feel they can manage and go from there. Yes, sometimes some people get a bit overzealous and start too intense, and in about 24 hours or so, delayed onset muscle soreness (DOMS) reminds them of their indiscretion for a few days. Believe me, they don't make the same mistake twice.

Basic Assessments

When we assess, we come more from a biomechanical and performance basis than from a programming basis. We want to know what is weak and where problems may be lingering. Safe training relies on the integrity of the major muscle systems of the body. Since our movement model is the four pillars of human movement, we use eight movements to assess and train the four pillars. That's why we say, "The assessment is the exercise, and the exercise is the assessment." Both the assessment and the training should improve at the same time as the target activity. This means the assessment must be part of the training, and as both the training and assessment improve, so should the target activity. The day your training gets better and the target activity does not, you are past your optimal strength and conditioning and training for other reasons, not function.

Table 3.1 shows the pillars, associated assessment movements, compensations to look for, and potential weaknesses associated with the compensation. The exercises used in the following assessments were thoroughly discussed in *Functional Training*, and I strongly recommend that text as a foundational resource to help you get the most out of this book. For those not familiar with that text, here is a summary of some of the basic movement assessments we use with our clients. We also provide some general ranges and performance levels to assign to specific repetitions completed.

Table 3.1 Biomechanical Assessments and Protocols

Number	Exercise	Pillar	What to look for	Problem
1	Single-leg CLA (contralateral arm) anterior reach	Locomotion	Front: Knees cave in or out Side: Heels up, knees forward, hips tucked in Back: Hips move right or left, hike up, or hike down	Weak back core muscles (glutes, paraspinals, hamstrings)
2	Single-leg squat	Locomotion	Front: Knees cave in or out Side: Heels up, knees forward, hips tucked in Back: Hips move right or left, hike up, or hike down	Weak back core muscles (glutes, paraspinals, hamstrings)
3	Bodyweight double-leg squat	Level change	Front: Knees cave in or out Side: Heels up, knees forward, hips tucked in Back: Hips move right or left, hike up, or hike down	Weak back core muscles (glutes, paraspinals, hamstrings)
4	Bodyweight alternating lunge	Level change	Front: Knees cave in or out Side: Trailing hip flexes Back: Hips move right or left, hike up, or hike down	Weak back core muscles (glutes, paraspinals, hamstrings)
5	Bodyweight push-up	Push/pull	Front: Unstable or winging scapula, poor shoulder and hip alignment Side: Sagging core and unstable or winging scapula	Weak front core muscles (hip flexors and abs), push mechanics, and scapula control
6	Recline pull (row)	Push/pull	Front: Rounded or shrugging shoulders due to unstable scapula Side: Hips drop and unstable or protracting scapula	Weak back core muscles (glutes, paraspinals, hamstrings), pull mechanics, and scapula control
7	Rotation with pivot	Rotation	Knee of the base leg rotates externally due to decreased internal hip rotation	Poor hip internal rotation
8	Rotation without pivot	Rotation	Hips shake due to decreased core stiffness	Lack of core stiffness

The way to use these assessments is simple. Master these exercises before going on to a more advanced version. For example, before doing a barbell squat, you must perform a bodyweight squat perfectly and do several sets of 20 or so repetitions without suffering any DOMS the day after. The same goes for all the other exercises in this assessment group. These are the major functional progressions all people should master before moving to more advanced functional training.

Table 3.2 shows the assessment exercise or major progression, the repetition range, and corresponding level. The number represents the number of repetitions that can be performed (for each limb in the case of unilateral exercises).

Getting Started

Once you master the general movement pattern of any exercise, the next thing is to start at the right intensity. This is especially true when you are starting a workout program after a long layoff or for the first time. Starting off too hard can leave you paralyzed with muscle soreness for a couple of days, and we have all been there—not fun. I remember practically stumbling down the stairs while in college one day after

Table 3.2 Levels and Repetition Ranges for Assessment Exercises

Level	Beginner	Intermediate	Advanced	Elite athlete
Exercise	Repetitions	Repetitions	Repetitions	Repetitions
Single-leg CLA anterior reach (per leg)	3-5	6-10	11-15	15 +
Single-leg squat (90 to 110 degrees of knee flexion)	1-3	4-5	6-10	10 +
Bodyweight double-leg squat (to parallel)	10 (in 10 sec)	11-15 (in 11-15 sec)	16-20 (in 16-20 sec)	20 + (1 per sec)
Bodyweight alternating lunge (per leg)	3-5 (in 9-15 sec)	6-10 (in 18-30 sec)	11-15 (in 33-45 sec)	15 + (in 45 sec)
Bodyweight push-up (from feet)	1-9 men 1-5 women	10-20 men 6-10 women	21-30 men 11-20 women	30 + men 20 + women
Recline pull (row) (back is 1 ft off ground at full arm extension)	1-9 men 1-5 women	10-20 men 6-10 women	21-30 men 11-20 women	30 + men 20 + women
Rotation with pivot	10-15	16-20	21-30	30 +
Rotation without pivot*	10-15 (no hip movement)	16-20 (no hip movement)	21-30 (no hip movement)	30 + (no hip movement)

* The rotation without pivot is an easy assessment exercises that uses no equipment. Once the athlete is good at the basic movement, we add weight with a band or pulley (BP) and it becomes the BP short rotation exercise.

a crazy leg day at the gym. Starting at the right intensity is not only safe but saves us from hobbling around unnecessarily.

I wish I could give you a magic formula, assessment, or protocol that would allow you to begin an exercise program at the perfect intensity, but I'm afraid that easy solution does not exist. This is where each person must take responsibility and exercise common sense or, at best, will be really sore, and, at worst, will be injured. So, buyer beware. These are my strong recommendations to everyone who will use this book.

- Make sure you are healthy and ready to work out. *If in doubt, get clearance from your doctor.* A medical clearance is especially important if you have any orthopedic or chronic conditions, such as lower-back pathology, high blood pressure, or diabetes.

- If at any time you feel uncomfortable pressure or pain, stop because the exercise or amount of load is probably not appropriate for you.

- If you are inexperienced or don't have a good training base (training constantly for one year), start these workouts at 50 percent of the sets described and use a light load (weight or resistance) that allows you to easily complete the repetitions. This will ensure you are not too sore the next day and that the training experience is a pleasurable one. There is always next week to increase the load a bit. Trust me: I'm a great coach not because of my knowledge of exercise science; it's the ability to creep up slowly every week so that my athletes become cyborgs without ever feeling like they got demolished in any one session. Be patient; slow progression wins the race.

- If you don't have years of proper training experience, it's always a great idea to hire a certified personal trainer to show you how to properly perform the exercises in any workout. A half hour is enough to show you four or five exercises and discuss the workout. Of course, if you can afford consultation for a longer period, then do it. At the minimum, invest in a half hour with a qualified trainer to make sure you are safe.

If you follow these recommendations and are patient at the start of a workout, you will make faster progress and stay safe while doing so. The biggest error I see in fitness is not enough patience and progressing too fast. Everyone has the "more is better" mentality; I have also been guilty of it, so don't feel bad. However, we must all be accountable and responsible for our actions. Follow the recommendations I have provided and use common sense. You will be just fine.

Signs of Overtraining

The topic of stress and when to back off is a complicated one, and much attention is being dedicated to it in the life-extension circles. A more comprehensive discussion of proper recovery and restoration is provided in chapter 16. However, I want to address some of the obvious signs of overtraining and recommend when to slow down or even back off. Having this information and following these recommendations will prevent layoffs and possible doctor visits due to doing too much too fast.

Overtraining is not just a potential obstacle to working out, it can affect everyday life as well. Overtraining is just simply overstressed; you are putting more stress on your body than it can take. This applies to the mechanical stresses the body experiences through exercise as well as all stresses from life. For example, whether you are the CEO of a company, a parent juggling kids and a busy home, or a full-time college student holding down a part-time job, you can suffer from overtraining symptoms without ever stepping foot in a gym. Now, add working out, an additional stress, to the mix, and you could create a recipe for disaster. Therefore, you need to learn to recognize the symptoms of overtraining or overstress. Let's keep this discussion on overtraining related to working out, and we can deal with the other issues surrounding recovery in chapter 16.

The sequence to overtraining is fairly straightforward and almost always follows the same order. The first step in overtraining is that the person feels constantly tired and lacks the energy to train. Often people try to remedy this feeling through discipline, by grinding through a workout, or by consuming an energy drink. An occasional tired feeling is OK, and there are many causes for feeling tired. However, chronic fatigue is something else and often an indication something is wrong. Another symptom of overtraining is chronic pain that won't go away (the "-itis"). This is especially true of joint pain. Muscle pain usually goes away, but pain closer to the joints is something else. Pain that does not go away is not normal and can indicate overtraining. After persistent pain comes insomnia. People who are chronically overtrained start having problems sleeping. Since you do most of your recovery when you sleep (due to a series of hormonal processes), lack of sleep marks the beginning of the end when it comes recovery. Finally, we have upper respiratory infections (URIs). When your body is not recovering, your immune system is compromised. When that happens, viruses and infections, especially URIs, are a natural outcome. Therefore, the take-home message is you are better off undertrained than overtrained. A rested person can pull out a miracle performance because his or her will is intact, but a beaten person does not have the will to summon his or her best.

Ideas for Progression

Progressing the intensity (loads) of weighted exercise is easy; simply add more weight. Manipulating the intensity of functional training is not as easy but certainly doable. We went through the tweaks of functional training exercises in chapter 2 (i.e., base of support, range of motion, lever arm, and speed). These tweaks also work with traditional exercises, especially those using dumbbells, barbells, and cables. Weight training is all about levers, range of motion, and speed of training. These variables can change the intensity of an exercise in a second.

One cool way to progress is by changing equipment and machines to do the same exercise. Although I'm a huge fan of repeating the basics, I understand the value of jumping between two machines that do the same thing. Small angles and even a different angle can make a huge difference in the quality of a muscular contraction. For example, going from a cable row to a machine row can change the way you feel an exercise in your entire back. Likewise, going from heavy pull-downs to pull-ups can change the training stimulus for the entire back musculature. The new feel of an exercise can certainly change a host of mechanisms that can lead to greater strength and muscle growth.

One of the best ways to add to the progressive nature of training is how one sees a repetition, especially when looking at the weight training designed around hypertrophy. My good friend and former Mr. USA, John DeFendis, has a great five-step contraction model he calls the stretch-flex-drag-contract-negative model (SFDCN).

John designed this system because he felt traditional eccentric and concentric contractions did not truly capture the essence of the perfect muscle hypertrophy stimulus. I feel the DeFendis rep adds an awareness to training that allows one to get more hypertrophy stimulus using less weight and, more importantly, with less wear and tear on the joints. Here are the five steps of a DeFendis rep.

1. **Stretch:** Begin the exercise in the stretched position with tension on the muscle, but you're not yet ready to perform the exercise. For example, for a triceps pressdown, hold the bar at the top by your chest and keep your elbows in to feel the stretch before you start the exercise.

2. **Flex:** Flex the triceps and tuck your elbows in tight to your sides, creating tension to get ready to slowly press the weight down.

3. **Drag:** Slowly drag the weight and use only the triceps to press the weight down. Do not throw the weight. Feel the triceps through the entire movement.

4. **Contraction:** Lock out at the bottom of the movement and squeeze the triceps so you feel an intense contraction almost to the point of a cramp.

5. **Negative:** Now slowly bring your arms back to the original position while feeling the triceps through the negative part of the movement.

I consider the DeFendis rep the perfect form when performing any hypertrophy exercise. Just being aware of these steps improves your training from OK to purposeful and effective training. Some strength training may also show benefits from the Defendis rep model. However heavier loads and training cycles often require an explosive approach to muscular contraction.

One last idea on progressing your training is to understand that plateaus are not necessarily bad. They may be an indication you have hit the point of diminishing returns in a certain attribute or body part. Instead of beating your body into submission and putting in a ton of work for very little return, keep your strength by putting your body in maintenance mode and concentrate on an attribute or body part that needs more work. We all love to work on our favorite body parts or attributes, but changing the emphasis and addressing the weak areas allows you to improve your physique and performance.

I hope these ideas on progressing your training will always keep you moving in the right direction. Remember that training is not self-punishment but rather a nurturing of your physical, mental, and spiritual beings. Always ask, Why am I doing this? It doesn't matter if you have to ask that question three times in a row to get three layers deep as to why you are training. Keep the DeFendis rep consciousness in mind when you are training for muscle growth; you will find that you will get more out of your training without using more weight. Finally, enjoy your favorite training, but don't keep pounding it into the ground. Start going after your weaker areas and create a more balanced you, physically, mentally, and spiritually.

\

PART II

Body Transformation

The workouts in this book take 60 to 90 minutes to complete at their highest levels. They are also very high in volume, and you must make sure to give your body enough time to adapt before moving on to the next stage. For example, if you get to the second week and can barely finish the workout or feel very sore the next day, perform the second week again as many times as necessary until you can complete the workout with good form and with some energy in the tank after the workout. There is no need to rush or train to exhaustion to get great results. In fact, staying healthy throughout the workout allows you to complete a higher volume of work, providing better results. Be patient and don't overdo it. Stay in any one week as many weeks as necessary to create a great training base, adapt, and get stronger. Then proceed to the next week.

The transformation workouts in part II are listed in complimentary pairs so you can work in a circuit. This strategy saves time and prefatigues muscles so you can stimulate them into growing without using heavier weight in follow-up sets. Circuits 1 and 2 are usually the essentials; circuit 3 usually is made up of finishers. The finishers are higher volume and are made to flush the area with lots of blood to provide a nice finishing pump. Remember, you don't have to finish the volumes noted within the workouts. For example, if you are on week 4 and are told to complete four or five sets, but you don't have the energy or time to complete that prescribed volume, it's fine to perform two or three sets. You are working to your safe capacity or in the time allotted and will still get great results. So, do what you can and add a little every week. The volumes noted in these workouts are just guidelines, not rules set in stone.

The paired circuit strategy is particularly effective for women, since most women we have worked with respond better to higher volume (i.e., sets and repetitions) as opposed to higher intensity (i.e., loads). The circuit format not only stimulates growth but also has a great impact on caloric expenditure, cardiovascular conditioning, and time efficiency. All these benefits are big positives in this very busy and sedentary world. However, depending on the time you have to train, you may prefer to perform the workouts in succession or sequences. When you perform exercises in succession, you finish all sets of one exercise before going to the next exercise. When you perform exercise in sequence, you do one set of each exercise then go on to the next, performing the determined number of exercises as a giant circuit.

Speaking of giant sets, these workouts can be performed in a class or group format. Therefore, if you are a personal trainer and have a "booty class" for women, two women's leg workouts can easily handle 8 to 10 women. If you are a coach handling a male basketball team, two of the leg workouts duplicated inside a gym can handle the entire boys team on leg and hip days.

We are always looking to make the body adapt to more work by getting bigger and stronger. But remember, your body does not want to acquire muscle mass. It has mechanisms against that (e.g., myostatin gene). Therefore, we always have to try to increase the work the muscles see. Sometimes we do this with more volume (more sets and repetitions) and keep the load the same. Sometimes we reduce the volume from one week to the next but increase the weight. Therefore, if you see a drop in repetitions from one week to the next, feel free to increase the weight (usually by 5-10%) so that the muscle is forced to adapt by lifting a heavier load for fewer repetitions. For example, if week 3 calls for three sets of 15 repetitions of a chest press, and week 4 drops the volume of the chest press to four sets of 10 repetitions, increase the load of the 10 repetitions of the chest press by 5 to 10 percent. If the exercise is not weight-dependent, such as a SB bridge, use a speed, base, or lever arm tweak to make the exercise harder while performing fewer repetitions. For example, if you are doing 15 repetitions of a two-leg SB bridge and you want to increase the load as you drop to 10 reps, you can perform the exercise slower, move the SB closer to the feet, or you can go to a single-leg progression to give the 10 reps the right level of intensity.

One final note on recovery and avoiding overtraining. The workouts included can be reduced in volume and intensity to accommodate most people, and they can be completed as they are written and really push extremely fit individuals. If you complete a four- to five-week program as it is written in this book, you have completed a great deal of work, and I recommend a week of cross-training before going to the next workout. After completing each workout, take it easy on that body part or on the entire body if you are combining several of these workouts in one week. Fill the recovery week with lighter work, BioFoam rolling, biking, walking, swimming, or any other activity that will allow your body and mind to recover from the high volume of work you just completed.

I have addressed this before, but I never get tired of stressing it—never train through pain. All movements must be free of pain, not free of effort. If it's hard and causes you to exert yourself, that's awesome. Relax your face and stay in the moment. Allow yourself to experience effort with no value or judgement. The awareness of what is normal high-intensity effort and what is detrimental pain is the biggest awareness you will gain from training. Accepting effort without judgement and not projecting panic into the future is the biggest adaptation of physical training and the essence of redefining the human will. Likewise, the awareness and understanding when you are hurting your body is also part of training wisdom. This wisdom is more important than the ability to drive hard through four weeks of grueling work.

Perform all exercises in a slow and controlled fashion. Remember, the transformation workouts are about putting stress on the muscle, and nothing puts stress on a muscle like time under tension. Unless otherwise specified, try to feel every angle of the range of motion; feel the DeFendis rep: stretch, flex, drag, contraction, negative. As a general recommendation, you can take 0.5 to 1.5 seconds for each positive and 0.5 to 1.5 seconds for each negative, depending on the amplitude of the exercise. For additional muscle stimulation, pause for 0.5 to 1 second at the bottom (loaded) and squeeze 0.5 to 1 second at the peak contraction of each move. This pause kills reflexes and momentum that can make the work more efficient biomechanically but less effective from a toning or hypertrophy standpoint. The squeeze at the top, or pause at bottom, makes all the difference in the world. If you are performing circuits, you may move from one exercise to another with a 15- to 30-second pause between each exercise. Rest 60 to 120 seconds between circuits or individual exercises that are performed in succession.

If you are looking for more athleticism or function from a toning exercise, speed up the movement and don't pause at the bottom. This dynamic quality takes the emphasis off a single muscle and has the tendency to bring in other muscle systems. Dynamic movement also uses more reflexes and physical qualities, such as momentum, to make the body more efficient. Don't think that because a movement is dynamic and more functional it will not provide tone. It will. It just won't stimulate muscle growth as much as it does when it is performed slow and controlled. Combat athletes have chiseled bodies made to move; none of them perform traditional hypertrophy training out of fear of adding extra muscle that would put them in a higher weight class.

CHAPTER 4

Legs and Hips

The legs and hips workouts in this chapter run the gamut from travel workouts that will keep your fitness levels high while you're on the road to banging-and-clanging gym workouts sure to put some muscle behind your hustle. Some of the industry giants known for their leg development workouts have chimed in to make this one of the best chapters in this book. You are in for a real treat.

These workouts are in a specific order. We start each of the men's and women's sections with some band-only workouts that have slowly become my favorite supplemental home and travel glute workouts. Then we have the glutes-only workouts that use weight but spare the knees. I love both of these glute-dominated workouts because my arthritic and injured knees limit the amount of heavy squatting I can do and just about prohibit me from doing lunges and step-ups. We then move on to the functional workouts that are great for people who want a level of tone and fitness without necessarily adding huge size to the lower body. We add more advanced workouts that can be done in commercial or home gyms to the mix and end with professional-grade workouts. I provide volume ranges for beginners and advanced users so everyone can safely enjoy the workouts by choosing an appropriate volume to match his or her abilities. I strongly urge you to stay conservative in your approach. If in doubt, do less. Go lighter, not heavier. More training lies ahead.

The legs and hips are the motor of the body, where all the power comes from. This is especially true if you understand that the legs and hips are the base of the core and are the limbs that react with the ground to propel the body in any direction. Often the training load is on the shoulders or in the hands. The core is the bridge connecting the hips to the shoulders, so the core is trained as well. The legs and hips are a key feature for the aesthetic appeal of the body. Sports usually require lower-body speed and power, so lower-body training is at the forefront of any athletic strength and conditioning program.

Although we have divided this chapter into his and her workouts, a muscle does not know gender; it only understands intensity, volume, and frequency. Therefore, feel free to mix and match workouts and exercises. A man who wants to try a larger volume of work when training the legs and hips should adopt one of the workouts from the *her* section. A woman looking for extra bone density or muscle should feel free to try one of the *his* workouts.

As mentioned, some of the top guns in the fitness industry have contributed some of the workouts they use with their athletes and on themselves to compete at the highest levels of sport (e.g., bodybuilding and figure, American football). I want to give a special shout-out to the glute guy, Bret Contreras (http://bretcontreras.com), for the enormous amount of work he has put into the area of hip training. Much of the glute work I do and present in this book was inspired by Bret's work and our communications. Thank you, Bret.

All the workouts in this chapter assume you can do four sets of 20 repetitions of bodyweight squats, completing each set in 20 seconds and resting about a minute between each set without any pain during or a day after the workout (i.e., DOMS). If you are not there, please make sure you can complete the following workout. You may start anywhere along this progression you feel is appropriate. Please be conservative at the beginning and take your time to develop a base if you have not exercised in more than a month or two.

Week 1: 2 sets of 10 squats, rest 2-3 minutes between sets, 3 times per week

Week 2: 3 sets of 15 squats, rest 2 minutes between sets, 3 times per week

Week 3: 3 sets of 20 squats, rest 1-2 minutes between sets, 3 times per week

Week 4: 4 sets of 20 squats, rest 1 minute between sets, 3 times per week

Most people will do fine with the first two weeks of most of these workouts. If you are combining legs with another body part for a single day, the volumes of the first two weeks work perfectly. Most people working legs multiple times a week also will do fine with the volume of the first two weeks. The last two weeks are for elite athletes and highly-trained individuals who have experienced these volumes of work before. Before attempting these high volumes for the first time, seek the guidance of a nationally-certified fitness professional.

A Special Note From JC and Bret Contreras

Some exercises in this chapter may be seen as "feminine" or "girly" exercises. However, we urge you to rethink training and leave egos and preconceived notions off the training floor. We both have used these workouts and all the exercises in this chapter to help us stay strong and fit. Bret got a 620-pound deadlift done using these exercises. JC is 58 and not interested in heavy lifting anymore due to all the damage his body has taken over the years, but these exercises allowed him to squat and deadlift for repetitions with more than 300 pounds and perform hip thrusts for sets of 10 with 400 pounds. This is after two hip replacements and arthritic and scoped knees. You will also find Dwayne "The Rock" Johnson and James Harrison (NFL's strongest man) showing off their hip thrusts and many of the exercises in this chapter on their Instagram and YouTube channels to help their performances and keep their bodies looking in top shape. The Rock says hip thrusts help his body feel better so he can keep training. James Harrison believes these exercises help his explosion off the line. These are arguably the two manliest men on the planet. This advice applies to the hip circle band exercises as well. We have taken all of the abduction and adduction and related hip exercises and presented them as hard isometric, slow eccentric, high tension, low reps, and explosive protocols. Squats and deadlifts are going through the roof! If you want bigger lifts, use the hip circle band exercises to grow stronger while saving your back. Don't be scared to do these exercises, guys. They are not just for women. They are made for all glutes.

HIS LEGS AND HIPS 1: GLUTES, BAND ONLY

This 4-week program is a glute workout using only a band. This program uses a circle band (such as the IHP circle band) for all exercises, making it a perfect home or travel workout. This is a great way to add glute training to your existing leg and hip program or to train your hips while you are rehabilitating a knee or back injury and can't do traditional leg training. Depending on your natural capacity and training history, weeks 1 and 2 can be repeated twice to reduce the 4-week volume and provide more time to adapt. The higher-volume ranges of weeks 3 and 4 are for the advanced trainee.

Equipment

IHP circle band (or substitute with a super band)

Notes

Weeks 1 and 2: Perform 2 times per week.

Weeks 3 and 4: Perform 1 or 2 times per week.

Table 4.1   His Legs and Hips 1: Glutes, Band Only

Exercise	Photo	Description	Weeks	Sets × reps
1a. Band squat abduction (3 sec pause at abduction)		Place band around your legs, below or above the knees, whichever is more comfortable. Assume a squat stance, your feet slightly wider than shoulder-width apart. Abduct and roll on the outside of your feet. Adduct your legs and flatten your feet. Repeat for prescribed reps.	Week 1	1 × 10
			Week 2	2 × 15
			Week 3	2 × 20
			Week 4	3 × 20
1b. Band standing hip extension and abduction		Place band around your legs, below or above the knees, whichever is more comfortable. Stand in front of a sturdy structure and hold it for support, your feet hip-width apart, a slight forward lean, and flexed knees. Extend your left leg back and out about 30 degrees, slightly externally rotating your foot during the hip extension. Repeat for prescribed reps, then repeat with other leg.	Week 1	1 × 15 per leg
			Week 2	2 × 20 per leg
			Week 3	2 × 25 per leg
			Week 4	3 × 30 per leg
2a. Band hip-hinge abduction (3 sec pause at abduction)		Place band around your legs, below or above the knees, whichever is more comfortable. Assume a high deadlift position, with your knees slightly bent, shoulders over feet, feet about shoulder-width apart, and knees slightly inside your feet (adducted). Keeping your back straight, abduct your legs, rolling slightly to the outside of your feet. Hold for 3 sec. Adduct your legs and flatten your feet to return to the starting position and repeat. Perform prescribed reps.	Week 1	1 × 10
			Week 2	2 × 15
			Week 3	2 × 20
			Week 4	3 × 20

(continued)

Table 4.1 His Legs and Hips 1: Glutes, Band Only *(continued)*

Exercise	Photo	Description	Weeks	Sets × reps
2b. Band quadru- ped hip extension		Place band around your legs and get on your hands and knees, with one end of the band under your right knee and the other above your left knee. Extend your left leg back and out about 30 degrees, slightly externally rotating your foot during the hip extension. Bring your left leg back down to the starting position and repeat for prescribed reps. Perform with your right leg.	Week 1	1 × 15 per leg
			Week 2	2 × 20 per leg
			Week 3	2 × 25 per leg
			Week 4	3 × 30 per leg

HIS LEGS AND HIPS 2: GLUTES, WEIGHTS ONLY

This 4-week program is a glute-only training program. This is a perfect workout for people interested in adding strength and volume to their glutes or for people who need a lower-body training program that doesn't vertically load the spine or tax the knees. We have successfully used this workout with people in knee rehab and with those suffering from arthritis in the knees. Since this workout uses inexpensive equipment, like a set of JC Predator Jr. and IHP circle bands, it is a great option for a quick workout at home. Depending on your natural capacity and training history, weeks 1 and 2 can be repeated twice to reduce the volume and provide more time to adapt. The higher ranges of weeks 3 and 4 are for the advanced trainee.

Equipment

Circle band or superband, stretch band (such as a JC Predator Jr.) or cable machine, hip thruster bench, weight bench, 45-degree extension bench or stability ball, barbell, weight plate, or dumbbell.

Notes

Weeks 1 and 2: Perform 2 times per week.

Weeks 3 and 4: Perform 1 or 2 times per week.

Table 4.2 His Legs and Hips 2: Glutes, Weights Only

Exercise	Photo	Description	Weeks	Sets × reps
1a. Barbell hip thrust		Sit on the ground and rest your upper back against a bench. Roll a bar over your hips. (You may use a pad between the bar and your hips.) Bend your knees and keep your feet flat on the ground between hip- and shoulder-width apart. Securing the bar with your hands, extend your hips and bridge up until they are fully extended. Lower until your glutes almost touch the ground. Repeat.	Week 1	2 × 10
			Week 2	3 × 12
			Week 3	4 × 10
			Week 4	5 × 8
1b. Band squat abduction		Place band around your legs, below or above the knees, whichever is more comfortable. Assume a squat position, your feet slightly wider than shoulder-width apart. Abduct and roll on the outside of your feet, then adduct your legs and flatten your feet. Perform prescribed reps.	Week 1	2 × 10
			Week 2	3 × 15
			Week 3	4 × 20
			Week 4	5 × 15

Exercise	Photo	Description	Weeks	Sets × reps
2a. BP deadlift		Stand in a parallel stance with handles to a low cable in each hand. Keeping your core and knees slightly bent, flex at the hips and reach with both hands toward the cable (anchor point) until you feel a comfortable stretch in your hamstrings. Come back to the starting upright position and repeat desired reps.	Week 1	2 × 10
			Week 2	3 × 12
			Week 3	4 × 15
			Week 4	5 × 10
2b. Band hip thrust (2 sec pause at top)		Sit on the ground and rest your upper back against a bench. Secure a band on each side of you so the band stretches over your hips. (You may use a pad between the band and your hips.) Bend your knees and keep your feet flat on the ground between hip- and shoulder-width apart. Extend your hips and bridge up until they are fully extended. Pause for 2 sec. Lower until your glutes almost touch the ground. Repeat.	Week 1	2 × 8
			Week 2	3 × 10
			Week 3	4 × 10
			Week 4	5 × 8
3a. 45-degree weighted back extension (toes out)		Place your feet on the footplate of a 45-degree angled bench. Point your toes out and secure the thigh pads on your thighs below the hip bone. Hold dumbbells or weight plate at your chest. Keeping your back straight, flex at the hips until you feel a comfortable stretch at the glutes and hamstrings. Extend your hips to the starting position. Repeat.	Week 1	2 × 10
			Week 2	3 × 12
			Week 3	4 × 15
			Week 4	5 × 15
3b. Seated band abduction (10 sec count)		Place band around your legs, below or above the knees, whichever is more comfortable. Sit on a bench or chair, your feet slightly wider than shoulder-width apart. Abduct your legs and roll on the outside of your feet. Adduct your legs for a 10 sec count until your legs close and your feet are flat on the ground. Repeat for prescribed reps.	Week 1	2 × 10 sec
			Week 2	3 × 10 sec
			Week 3	4 × 10 sec
			Week 4	5 × 10 sec

HIS LEGS AND HIPS 3: FUNCTIONAL

This 4-week program is a pure functional training program that focuses on developing muscle tone and athleticism. This is a perfect workout for the young athlete or for someone with less training experience who wants to be introduced to functional training and is looking to get into shape. It's a perfect home routine because the equipment involved is minimal and inexpensive.

Depending on your natural capacity and training history, weeks 1 and 2 can be repeated twice to reduce the 4-week volume and provide more time to adapt. The higher-volume ranges of weeks 3 and 4 are for the advanced trainee.

Equipment

Medicine ball, dumbbells, cable machine or resistance band (such as a JC Sports Band or Predator), stability ball

Notes

Weeks 1 and 2: Perform 2 times per week.

Weeks 3 and 4: Perform 1 or 2 times per week.

Table 4.3   His Legs and Hips 3: Functional

Exercise	Photo	Description	Weeks	Sets × reps
1a. MB diagonal chop		Stand with your feet slightly wider than shoulder-width apart and your knees slightly bent. Hold a medicine ball above your right shoulder. Shift your weight to your left leg and chop diagonally while pivoting your right foot until the medicine ball is to the left of your body between your left knee and hip. Return to the starting position. Perform to the other side of the body.	Week 1	2 × 10 per side
			Week 2	3 × 12 per side
			Week 3	4 × 10 per side
			Week 4	5 × 10 per side
1b. MB/DB alternating front reaching lunge		Stand with your feet hip-width apart and your knees bent. Hold a medicine ball or a dumbbell in both hands. Keeping your core tight, take a big step forward with your left leg, bending your left leg slightly. Keeping your back straight and stable, flex your hips your hips and reach toward your left foot until you feel a comfortable stretch in your hamstrings. Return to the starting position and repeat to the right side.	Week 1	2 × 7 per leg
			Week 2	3 × 10 per leg
			Week 3	4 × 12 per leg
			Week 4	5 × 10 per leg
2a. BP staggered stance CLA deadlift		Stand in a staggered stance, your left foot forward. Hold the handle to a low cable in your right hand. Keeping your core straight and tight, flex your hips and reach your right hand toward the cable (anchor point) until you feel a comfortable stretch in your right hamstrings. Return to the starting position and repeat for the desired reps. Switch stance and arm, and repeat.	Week 1	2 × 10 per leg
			Week 2	3 × 12 per leg
			Week 3	4 × 10 per leg
			Week 4	5 × 8 per leg

Exercise	Photo	Description	Weeks	Sets × reps
2b. SB single-leg bridge		Lie flat in a supine position. Place your left leg on top of a stability ball, keeping your right leg slightly flexed and in the air. Raise your hips and squeeze your glutes at the top, then lower the hips until just short of the ground. Repeat for the desired reps. Switch legs and repeat.	Week 1	2 × 7 per leg
			Week 2	3 × 10 per leg
			Week 3	4 × 12 per leg
			Week 4	5 × 15 per leg
3a. 45-degree calf pump		Lean against a wall with both hands on the wall, both heels up, and your body leaning at about 45-70 degrees. Raise your left knee. Keep your knee and left toes up. Perform quick right ankle pumps using a short range of motion. Repeat ankle pumps on the left.	Week 1	2 × 15 per leg
			Week 2	3 × 20 per leg
			Week 3	4 × 30 per leg
			Week 4	5 × 40 per leg

HIS LEGS AND HIPS 4: WEIGHTS AND FUNCTIONAL

This 4-week program is a functional training program with a metabolic blast at the end. This workout can be tailored for the intermediate or advanced trainee, depending on what weeks are completed. It's a perfect home routine since it involves minimal inexpensive yet effective exercise equipment. Depending on your natural capacity and training history, weeks 1 and 2 can be repeated twice to reduce the 4-week volume and provide more time to adapt. The higher-volume ranges of weeks 3 and 4 are for the advanced trainee.

Equipment

Step (8-14 in. [20-36 cm]), medicine ball, dumbbells, cable machine or band (such as a JC Sports Band or Predator), circle band, stability ball

Notes

Weeks 1 and 2: Perform 2 times per week.

Weeks 3 and 4: Perform 1 or 2 times per week.

Table 4.4 His Legs and Hips 4: Weights and Functional

Exercise	Photo	Description	Weeks	Sets × reps
1a. Loaded step-up		Stand in front of a step (8-14 in. [20-36 cm]) with your feet hip-width apart. Hold a medicine ball in both hands or dumbbells in each hand. Keeping your core tight, step onto the step with your left leg. Extend your left knee, step on the step, and finish with your left leg extended. Step back down and repeat for desired reps. Repeat with the right leg.	Week 1	2 × 10 per leg
			Week 2	3 × 12 per leg
			Week 3	4 × 15 per leg
			Week 4	5 × 10 per leg

(continued)

Table 4.4 His Legs and Hips 4: Weights and Functional *(continued)*

Exercise	Photo	Description	Weeks	Sets × reps
1b. BP deadlift		Stand in a parallel stance, the handles of a low cable or band in each hand. Keeping your core tight and your knees slightly bent, flex your hips and reach with both hands toward the cable until you feel a comfortable stretch in your hamstrings. Return to the starting position and repeat.	Week 1	2 × 5 per leg
			Week 2	3 × 7 per leg
			Week 3	4 × 10 per leg
			Week 4	5 × 15 per leg
2a. Lateral alternating reaching lunge		Stand with your feet hip-width apart. Hold a medicine ball or dumbbell in both hands. Keeping your core tight, take a big lateral step with your left leg, bending the left knee slightly. Flex the hips and reach toward your left foot until you feel a comfortable stretch in your left hamstrings. Return to the starting position and repeat to the right side.	Week 1	2 × 10 per leg
			Week 2	3 × 15 per leg
			Week 3	4 × 20 per leg
			Week 4	5 × 20 per leg
2b. Band squat abduction		Place the band around your legs, below or above the knees, whichever is more comfortable. Assume a squat position with your feet slightly wider than shoulder-width apart. Abduct your legs and roll on the outside of your feet. Adduct your legs and flatten your feet. Perform prescribed reps.	Week 1	2 × 10 per leg
			Week 2	3 × 15 per leg
			Week 3	4 × 20 per leg
			Week 4	5 × 20 per leg
3a. Single-leg SB leg curl		Lie in a supine position. Place your right foot on top of a stability ball, keeping your right knee flexed at 90 degrees. Lift your left leg in the air while keeping your left knee flexed at 90 degrees. Raise your hips, squeezing your glutes at the top. Keeping your hips elevated, flex and extend your right knee for the prescribed reps. Repeat with the left leg.	Week 1	2 × 10 per leg
			Week 2	3 × 15 per leg
			Week 3	4 × 20 per leg
			Week 4	5 × 15 per leg
3b. 45-degree calf pump		Lean against the wall with both hands on the wall, both heels up, and your body leaning at about 45-70 degrees. Raise your right knee, keeping the knee and toes up. Perform quick left ankle pumps using a short range of motion. Repeat ankle pumps on right leg.	Week 1	2 × 10 per leg
			Week 2	3 × 15 per leg
			Week 3	4 × 20 per leg
			Week 4	5 × 30 per leg

Exercise	Photo	Description	Weeks	Sets × reps
4. Leg crank		Perform 24 squats, 24 lunges (12 per leg), 24 split jumps (12 per leg), and 12 squat jumps (84 total reps).	Week 1	1 set
			Week 2	1 or 2 sets
			Week 3	2 or 3 sets
			Week 4	3 or 4 sets

HIS LEGS AND HIPS 5: BRET'S WEIGHTS WORKOUT

This 6-week leg and hip workout is a heavy-duty workout right from the glute guy himself, Bret Contreras. The idea is to stay with the same set and rep scheme indicated (or as close as possible) but go up in weight each week. Don't go too fast; that is the biggest mistake people make with this kind of workout. For the first week, start with a weight that allows you to easily complete the exercises as indicated. Add 2.5%-5% each week. That is a lot of increase over 6 weeks! The goal is to get stronger but not get stuck at weeks 3 to 5. If that happens, you progressed too fast. This is a killer workout, especially the last 2 weeks, so try to get 2 or 3 days of rest between day 1 and 2 workouts. This rest period will allow your legs and hips to recover so you can get the most out of this workout.

Equipment

Weight bench, 45-degree bench, barbell, power rack, circle band, dumbbells

Notes

Add some of the calf work from workout 4 if desired. Perform the program for 6 weeks.

Table 4.5 His Legs and Hips 5: Bret's Weights Workout

Exercise	Photo	Description	Sets × reps
DAY 1			
Barbell hip thrust		Sit on the ground and rest your upper back against a weight bench. Roll a barbell over your hips. (You may use a pad between the bar and your hips, if desired.) Bend your knees and keep your feet flat on ground between hip- and shoulder-width apart. Securing the bar with your hands, extend your hips and bridge up until they are fully extended. Lower until your glutes almost touch the ground. Repeat.	3 × 10
Barbell back squat		Using a power rack, safely place a barbell on your back, right on the trapezius muscles. Stand with your feet at about shoulder-width apart. Keep the core tight and the back straight throughout the entire movement. Flex your hips and knees until you reach a sitting position about chair level. Return to the starting position. Repeat.	3 × 6

(continued)

Table 4.5 His Legs and Hips 5: Bret's Weights Workout *(continued)*

Exercise	Photo	Description	Sets × reps
DAY 1 (CONTINUED)			
Barbell Romanian deadlift		Stand in front of a barbell in a shoulder-width stance, toes pointing forward. Keeping your core tight and your knees slightly bent, flex your hips and knees and grab the bar with your hands hip- to shoulder-width apart. You may use an alternating or a pronated grip. Drive through your heels, extending your legs and hips simultaneously until you are standing fully erect. Reverse the sequence and lower the bar to the floor. Repeat.	3 × 8
Band lateral walk		Place band around your legs, below or above the knees, whichever is more comfortable. Stand in a semisquat position with your feet hip-width apart. Try to keep your back straight. Lean forward slightly. Take a lateral step to the right until your feet are wider than shoulder-width apart. Step your left foot toward the right foot until your feet are hip-width apart. Perform the prescribed reps to the right, then switch and repeat to the left.	3 × 20 per side
DAY 2			
Barbell glute bridge with band		Sit on the ground with a circle band around your legs right above the knees. Roll a barbell over your hips. (You may use a pad between the bar and your hips, if desired.) Lie down and bend your knees, keeping your feet flat on the ground between hip- and shoulder-width apart. Secure the bar at the hips with your hands and keep your legs open, your knees lining up with your feet. While holding the bar in position, extend your hips and bridge up until they are fully extended. Lower until the glutes are about to touch the floor and bridge again. Repeat.	3 × 15
DB walking lunge		Stand with your feet parallel to each other and hip-width apart. Hold a dumbbell in each hand, hands by your sides. Keeping your core tight, take a big step forward with your right leg and drop your body into a split squat. Rise and take a forward step with your left leg to return to the starting position. Repeat the sequence, lunging with your left leg.	3 × 20 total (10 per leg)
DB back extension (toes out)		Place your feet on the footplate of a 45-degree bench, your toes pointing out and the thigh pads set on your thighs below the hip bone. Hold a dumbbell or weight plate at your chest. Keeping your back straight, flex at the hips until you feel a comfortable stretch in the in the glutes and hamstrings. Extend your hips to the starting position. Repeat.	3 × 10

Exercise	Photo	Description	Sets × reps
		DAY 2 (CONTINUED)	
Extended range side-lying hip abduction		Lie on a stable and secured weight bench on your left side, resting on your left elbow. Hold the bench with your right hand for support. Bend your left knee at the end of the bench and let your right leg hang fully extended over the end of the bench, your toes pointing to the ground. Abduct your right hip, raising your right foot. Squeeze the right glute at the top of the movement and lower to the starting position. Repeat desired reps then switch sides and repeat on the other side.	3 × 20 per leg
		DAY 3	
Barbell hip thrust (3 sec pause at top)		Sit on the ground and rest your upper back on a weight bench. Roll a barbell over your hips. (You may use a pad between the bar and your hips, if desired.) Bend your knees and keep your feet flat on the ground between hip- and shoulder-width apart. Securing the barbell with your hands, extend your hips and bridge up until they are fully extended. Pause for 3 sec at the top of the movement. Lower until your glutes almost touch the ground. Repeat.	3 × 5
Barbell sumo deadlift		Stand in front of a barbell in a wide parallel stance, your feet pointing out. Keeping your core tight and your knees slightly bent, flex your hips and knees and grab the bar with your hands hip- to shoulder-width apart. You may use an alternating or a pronated grip. Drive through your heels, extending the legs and hips simultaneously until you are standing fully erect. Reverse the sequence and lower the bar to the ground. Repeat.	3 × 6
Barbell front squat		Using a power rack, safely place a barbell on your front shoulder muscles. Stand with your feet about shoulder-width apart. Keep the core tight and torso as vertical as possible throughout the entire movement. Flex at the knees and hips until you reach a sitting position about chair level. Return to the starting position. Repeat.	6 × 4
Band seated hip abduction		Place band around your legs, below or above the knees, whichever is more comfortable. Sit on a bench or chair with your feet about shoulder-width apart. Abduct your legs and roll on the outside of your feet. Adduct your legs and flatten your feet. Repeat for prescribed reps.	3 × 20

HIS LEGS AND HIPS 6: GET MASSIVE

This 4-week program is a heavy-duty hypertrophy program that will tax your resolve and recovery. It has the best of parallel- and unilateral-stance training, addressing strength imbalances between the right and left legs. As with the previous Bret Contreras workout, for the first week, start at a weight that allows you to easily complete the workout. Then add 2.5%-5% each week. You will feel this increase over 4 weeks! The goal is to get stronger but not get stuck at any week, especially weeks 3 and 4. If that happens, you've progressed too fast.

Equipment

Power rack, barbell, dumbbells, plyometric box or weight bench, cable machine, 45-degree back extension bench, stability ball

Notes

Weeks 1 and 2: Perform 2 times per week.

Weeks 3 and 4: Perform 1 or 2 times per week.

Table 4.6 His Legs and Hips 6: Get Massive

Exercise	Photo	Description	Sets × reps
Barbell squat		Using a power rack, safely place a bar on your back, right on the trapezius muscles. Stand with your feet about shoulder-width apart. Keep the core tight and back straight throughout the entire movement. Flex your hips and knees until you reach a sitting position about chair level. Return to the starting position.	3 × 8-12
Barbell deadlift		Stand in front of a barbell, your feet shoulder-width apart and your toes pointing forward. You may use any style grip. Keeping your core tight and your knees slightly bent, flex your hips and knees and grab the bar with your hands hip- to shoulder-width apart. Drive through your heels, extending your legs and hips simultaneously until you are standing fully erect. Reverse the sequence and lower the barbell to the floor. Repeat the lifting motion.	3 × 8-12
DB/KB lateral reaching lunge		Stand upright with your feet hip-width apart. Hold a dumbbell in each hand. Keeping your core tight, take a big lateral step with your left leg, landing in a slight lunge. Flex your hips and reach toward your left foot until you feel a comfortable stretch in your left hamstrings. Return to the starting position and repeat on the right side.	3 × 8-10 per leg

Exercise	Photo	Description	Sets × reps
DB Bulgarian squat (may also use Smith machine; split squat with rear foot elevated)		Hold dumbbells by your sides. Stand on your right leg and place your left foot on top of a box or bench behind you. Keeping your core tight, perform a split squat, your right foot on the ground in front you and your left foot on a box or bench behind you. Return to the starting position and repeat the split squat for the prescribed reps. Repeat on the left leg.	3 × 8-12 per side
BP low-to-high chop		Stand with your feet shoulder-width apart. Hold a cable handle in both hands in front of you. The cable should be in the lowest position available and to your right. Keeping your arms straight and the core tight, rotate to the right while sinking into the right hip and lowering the cable handle toward the cable pulley. Return to the starting position and complete all reps. Switch to the other side and repeat.	3 × 12 per side
45-degree weighted back extension (toes out)		Place your feet on the footplate of a 45-degree angled bench, your toes pointing out and the thigh pads set on your thighs below the hip bone. Hold a dumbbell or weight plate at your chest. Keeping your back straight, flex at the hips until you feel a comfortable stretch in the glute and hamstrings. Extend your body to the original position. Repeat.	3 × 15-20
SB triple threat burn		SB bridge (lie supine with your feet on a stability ball; raise and lower hips for reps indicated). SB leg curl (without lowering your hips, flex and extend your knees to perform leg curls). SB hip lift (without lowering your hips, walk the ball down until the stability ball is under the balls of your feet; perform short hip lifts). Return to starting position and repeat for the prescribed number of reps.	2-3 × 15 + 15 + 15

HER LEGS AND HIPS 1: GLUTES, BAND ONLY

This 4-week program is a monster high-volume glutes-only program and makes a great home or travel program. This is one of my favorites when I only have about 15 minutes to work out; nothing pumps your glutes more than this one. This workout uses 2 circuits of 3 exercises each. Go from one exercise to the other until the circuit is completed. Everything is done in a smooth but dynamic fashion. Depending on your natural capacity and training history, weeks 1 and 2 can be repeated twice each to reduce the volume and provide more time to adapt. The higher ranges in weeks 3 and 4 are for advanced trainees.

Equipment

Circle band, weight bench or elevated surface

Notes

Weeks 1 and 2: Perform 2 times per week.

Weeks 3 and 4: Perform 2 or 3 times per week if this is the only glute training you are doing. If you are using this workout to supplement your leg training, perform 1 or 2 times per week.

Table 4.7   Her Legs and Hips 1: Glutes, Band Only

Exercise	Photo	Description	Weeks	Sets × reps
1a. Band squat abduction		Place band around your legs, below or above the knees, whichever is more comfortable. Assume a squat position with your feet about shoulder-width apart and your knees slightly inside your feet (adducted). Abduct (open) your legs, rolling slightly to the outside of your feet. Adduct your legs and flatten your feet to return to the starting position. Repeat for prescribed reps.	Week 1	2 × 10
			Week 2	2 × 20
			Week 3	3 × 20
			Week 4	3 × 30
1b. Band hip-hinge abduction		Place band around your legs, below or above the knees, whichever is more comfortable. Assume a high deadlift position with your knees slightly bent, your shoulders over your feet, your feet about shoulder-width apart, and your knees slightly inside your feet (adducted). Keeping your back straight, abduct (open) your legs, rolling slightly to the outside of your feet. Adduct your legs and flatten your feet to return to the starting position. Repeat for prescribed reps.	Week 1	2 × 10
			Week 2	2 × 20
			Week 3	3 × 20
			Week 4	3 × 30

Exercise	Photo	Description	Weeks	Sets × reps
1c. Band seated three-way abduction		Place band around your legs, below or above the knees, whichever is more comfortable. Sit at the end of a bench with your feet on the ground about shoulder-width apart. Keeping your back straight, abduct (open) your legs, rolling slightly to the outside of your feet. Close your legs and flatten your feet to return to the starting position. Repeat for the prescribed reps in each position continuously: position 1, lean back and place hands on bench for support; position 2, sit upright; position 3, lean forward, keeping back straight.	Week 1	2 × 15 per position
			Week 2	2 × 20 per position
			Week 3	3 × 25 per position
			Week 4	3 × 30 per position
2a. Band glute bridge		Place band around your legs, below or above the knees, whichever is more comfortable. Lie on the ground, your knees bent and your feet flat on the ground. Put your feet between hip- and shoulder-width apart. While keeping your legs open and knees lined up with your feet, extend your hips and bridge up until your hips are fully extended. Holding the extended position, perform abduction and adduction of the legs for prescribed number of repetitions.	Week 1	2 × 15
			Week 2	2 × 20
			Week 3	3 × 25
			Week 4	3 × 30
2b. Band bridge abduction		Place band around your legs, below or above the knees, whichever is more comfortable. Sit on the ground with your knees bent, keeping your feet flat on the ground and between hip- and shoulder-width apart. While keeping your legs open and your knees lined up with your feet, extend your hips and bridge up until your hips are fully extended. Lower until the glutes are about to touch the floor and bridge again. Repeat.	Week 1	2 × 15
			Week 2	2 × 20
			Week 3	3 × 25
			Week 4	3 × 30
2c. Frog pump		Lie on your back with knees flexed, legs open, the bottoms of your feet together, and your heels as close to your glutes as possible. Tuck your chin in as if you were going to start an abdominal crunch. Raise your hips to perform a short bridge, then lower short of touching the ground. Repeat. I suggest performing this exercise facing a wall away from gym traffic.	Week 1	2 × 15
			Week 2	2 × 20
			Week 3	3 × 25
			Week 4	3 × 30

HER LEGS AND HIPS 2: BRET'S AT-HOME WORKOUT

This is a simple at-home workout designed by my buddy, Bret Contreras, the glute guy. Don't think that just because it's a home workout it's easy and won't work. This is a serious glute workout for anyone! This workout can be done anywhere, even while on a vacation, so no excuses!

Equipment

Low box, step, or medicine ball; weight bench (optional); stability ball

Notes

Add calf work from his leg and hips workout 4 if desired. Perform program for 6 weeks.

Table 4.8 Her Legs and Hips 2: Bret's At-Home Workout

Exercise	Photo	Description	Sets × reps
DAY 1			
Single-leg glute bridge		Lie flat in a supine position. Keeping your left knee flexed at 90 degrees and right leg in the air, raise your hips, squeezing your glutes at the top. Lower your hips short of reaching the ground. Repeat. Perform to the other side.	3 × 12 per leg
Bulgarian split squat		Stand on your left leg and place your right foot on top of a box, bench, or chair behind you. Keeping your core tight, perform a split squat with your left foot on the ground in front you and your right foot on a box or bench behind you. Return to the starting position and repeat the split-squat motion for the prescribed reps. Repeat on the right side.	3 × 12 per leg
Quadruped hip extension (1 sec squeeze at the top)		Get on your hands and knees. Extend your left leg back and out about 30 degrees, slightly externally rotating your foot during your hip extension. Lower your left leg to the starting position and repeat for the prescribed reps. Perform with the right leg.	3 × 12 per leg
Side-lying hip raise		Lie on your right side, resting on your right elbow, and put your left hand on the floor for support. Your body is straight and both knees flexed 90 degrees throughout the entire movement, supporting your lower body on your right knee. Simultaneously raise your hips and open your legs as much as you can. Lower to the starting position and repeat for the prescribed reps. Perform on the left side.	3 × 12 per leg

Exercise	Photo	Description	Sets × reps
DAY 2			
Frog pump		Lie facing up with your knees flexed, your legs open, the bottoms of your feet together, and your heels as close to your glutes as possible. Tuck your chin in as if you were going to start an abdominal crunch. Raise your hips to perform a short bridge. Lower short of touching the ground. Repeat. I suggest performing this exercise facing a wall away from gym traffic.	3 × 30
Reverse lunge		Stand tall with your feet hip-width apart. Keeping your weight on your left foot, take a big step back with your right foot. Lower your body by bending your knees until your left thigh is parallel to the floor. Step forward with the right leg to return to the starting position and repeat on the opposite side.	3 × 20 per leg
Single-leg foot elevated hip thrust		Lie on the ground. Place your left foot on a bench so that the knee is flexed at 90 degrees. Keeping your right leg in the air, extend your hips and bridge up until they are fully extended. Lower your hips as much as possible without touching the ground. Repeat the bridging motion for prescribed reps. Perform on the right leg.	3 × 15 per leg
Extended range side-lying hip abduction		Lie on a bench or the floor on your right side, resting on your right elbow. With your left hand, hold the bench or floor for support. Bend your right knee at the end of the bench or floor and let your left leg hang over the end of the bench fully extended, your toes pointing to the ground. Abduct your left hip, raising your left foot. Squeeze the left glute at the top of the movement and return to starting position. Repeat and perform to both sides.	3 × 20 per leg
DAY 3			
Spread eagle reverse hyperextension		Kneel in front of a stability ball. Secure your core and upper body over the stability ball, (or substitute with a bench or another secure structure) with your elbows on the ground. Keeping your legs straight, open your legs and externally rotate your feet (feet point out). Extend your hips, raising your legs as high as you can (reverse extension). Lower short of your feet touching the ground and repeat for desired reps.	3 × 20

(continued)

Table 4.8 Her Legs and Hips 2: Bret's At-Home Workout *(continued)*

Exercise	Photo	Description	Sets × reps
DAY 3 (CONTINUED)			
Curtsy lunge		Stand tall, your feet hip-width apart. Hands can be at your waist or in front of you. Keeping your weight on your left foot, take a big step to the left with your right leg, crossing it behind your left leg. Lower your body by bending your knees until your left thigh is parallel to the floor. Return to the starting position and repeat on the opposite side.	3 × 8 per leg
Feet elevated hip thrust		Sit on the ground and rest your upper back on a bench, box, or chair. Place your feet on a bench, box, or chair so that the knees are flexed 90 degrees and your feet are flat on the bench, between hip- and shoulder-width apart. Extend your hips and bridge up until they are fully extended. Lower hips as low as possible without losing your support on the benches, and repeat the bridging motion for prescribed reps.	3 × 20
Fire hydrant (quad-ruped abduction)		Get on your hands and knees. Abduct your left leg to the side until your left thigh is parallel to the ground, slightly externally rotating your foot during your hip abduction. Bring your left leg back down to the starting position and repeat for prescribed reps. Perform with the right leg.	3 × 20 per leg

HER LEGS AND HIPS 3: GLUTES ONLY

This 4-week glutes-only program can be added as an extra day to your existing leg and hip training or can be used if your knees and cervical spine are acting up and you can't do traditional leg exercises such as squats and lunges. Since this workout uses inexpensive equipment that travels well, like a set of JC Predator Jr. and IHP circle bands, it is a great option for a quick workout at home or on the road. Depending on your natural capacity and training history, weeks 1 and 2 can be repeated twice each to reduce the volume and provide more time to adapt. The higher ranges of weeks 3 and 4 are for the advanced trainee.

Equipment

Barbell, dumbbells, circle band, bench, cable machine or band (such as a JC Traveler or Predator Jr.), stability ball

Notes

Weeks 1 and 2: Perform 2 times per week.

Weeks 3 and 4: Perform 1 or 2 times per week.

Table 4.9 Her Legs and Hips 3: Glutes Only

Exercise	Photo	Description	Weeks	Sets × reps
1a. BB/DB Romanian deadlift		Stand in front of a barbell (or hold a dumbbell in each hand), your feet shoulder-width apart and toes pointing forward. Keeping your core tight and your knees slightly bent, flex your hips and knees and grab the bar with your hands hip- to shoulder-width apart (or hold dumbbells in front of your thighs). Use any comfortable grip you prefer. Drive through your heels, extending the legs and hips simultaneously until you are standing fully erect. Reverse the sequence and lower the weight to the starting position. Repeat the lifting motion.	Week 1	2 × 10
			Week 2	3 × 12
			Week 3	4 × 10
			Week 4	5 × 8
1b. Band seated hip abduction		Place band around your legs, below or above the knees, whichever is more comfortable. Sit upright on a bench with your feet slightly wider than shoulder-width apart, your back straight. Abduct your legs and roll to the outside of your feet. Adduct your legs and flatten your feet. Perform prescribed reps.	Week 1	2 × 10
			Week 2	3 × 15
			Week 3	4 × 20
			Week 4	5 × 20
2a. BP staggered stance CLA Romanian deadlift		Stand in a staggered stance, left foot forward. Hold a low cable in your right hand. Keeping your core tight, flex your hips and reach your right hand toward the cable until you feel a comfortable stretch in your left hamstrings. Return to the starting position and repeat, completing successive reps to each side of the body. Repeat.	Week 1	2 × 8 per leg
			Week 2	3 × 10 per leg
			Week 3	4 × 12 per leg
			Week 4	5 × 10 per leg
2b. Band lateral walk		Place band around your legs, below or above the knees, whichever is more comfortable. Stand in a semisquat position with your feet hip-width apart. Keep your back straight. Lean forward slightly. Take a lateral step to the right to a stance slightly wider than shoulder-width apart. Step your left foot toward your right foot until feet are hip-width apart again. Perform prescribed reps to the right, then switch direction and move left.	Week 1	2 × 10 per leg
			Week 2	3 × 10 per leg
			Week 3	4 × 10 per leg
			Week 4	5 × 10 per leg
3a. Frog reverse hyperextension		Kneel in front of a stability ball. Secure your core and upper body over the stability ball, (or substitute with a bench or another secure structure) with your elbows on the ground. Flex your knees and open your legs with the bottoms of your feet together, heels as close to your glutes as possible. Extend your hips, raising your legs as high as you can (reverse extension). Lower your legs short of touching the ground. Repeat for desired reps.	Week 1	2 × 10
			Week 2	3 × 15
			Week 3	4 × 20
			Week 4	5 × 20

(continued)

Table 4.9 Her Legs and Hips 3: Glutes Only *(continued)*

Exercise	Photo	Description	Weeks	Sets × reps
3b. Frog pump		Lie facing up with your knees flexed and legs open, the bottoms of your feet together and your heels as close to your glutes as possible. Tuck in your chin as if you were going to start an abdominal crunch. Raise your hips to perform a short bridge. Lower short of touching the ground. Repeat. I suggest performing this exercise facing a wall away from gym traffic.	Week 1	2 × 20
			Week 2	3 × 30
			Week 3	4 × 40
			Week 4	5 × 50

HER LEGS AND HIPS 4: FUNCTIONAL

This 4-week program is a pure functional training program that will challenge anyone. It's perfect for the female athlete or a woman looking to get in great shape and tone her body without getting big. There is a lot of unilateral training to make sure the lower body is free of possible asymmetric compensations that often lead to injury. This is a perfect home workout since it involves minimal inexpensive yet effective exercise equipment. Depending on your natural capacity and training history, weeks 1 and 2 can be repeated twice to reduce the 4-week volume and provide more time to adapt. The higher-volume ranges of weeks 3 and 4 are for the ladies with very advanced training experience.

Equipment

Medicine ball, dumbbells, gliding disk, stability ball

Notes

Weeks 1 and 2: Perform 2 times per week.

Weeks 3 and 4: Perform 1 or 2 times per week.

Table 4.10 Her Legs and Hips 4: Functional

Exercise	Photo	Description	Weeks	Sets × reps
1a. MB ABC squat		Stand with your feet slightly wider than shoulder-width apart and your knees slightly bent. Hold a medicine ball in front of you. Squat and push the ball to the right, about 45 degrees from center. Return to the starting position. Squat and push the ball to the left, about 45 degrees from center. Return to the starting position. Both directions (i.e., 2 squats) equals 1 rep.	Week 1	2 × 10
			Week 2	3 × 15
			Week 3	4 × 20
			Week 4	5 × 15
1b. MB/DB lateral reaching lunge		Stand with your feet hip-width apart and your knees bent. Hold a medicine ball or dumbbells in your hands. Keeping your core tight, take a big lateral step with your left foot, bending your left leg slightly. Flex the hips and reach toward your left foot until you feel a comfortable stretch in your left hamstrings. Return to the starting position and repeat to the right side.	Week 1	2 × 5 per leg
			Week 2	3 × 7 per leg
			Week 3	4 × 10 per leg
			Week 4	5 × 15 per leg

Exercise	Photo	Description	Weeks	Sets × reps
2a. MB/DB split rear sliding squat		Stand with your feet hip-width apart and your knees bent. Hold a medicine ball or dumbbells in your hands. Keep your left foot on the ground and put your right foot on a gliding disk (or towel if on a wood or tile floor). Keeping your core tight, bend your left knee and slide your right foot back, sinking into a deep split squat; most of the weight remains on your left foot. Straighten your left leg to bring the body to the original position. Repeat for prescribed reps. Repeat with right leg.	Week 1	2 × 10 per leg
			Week 2	3 × 15 per leg
			Week 3	4 × 20 per leg
			Week 4	5 × 25 per leg
2b. MB/DB front reaching lunge		Stand with your feet hip-width apart and your knees bent. Hold a medicine ball or dumbbells in your hands. Keeping your core tight, take a big step to the front with your right leg, bending your right leg slightly. Flex your hips and reach toward your right foot until you feel a comfortable stretch in your right hamstrings. Return to the starting position and repeat to the left side.	Week 1	2 × 5 per leg
			Week 2	3 × 8 per leg
			Week 3	4 × 10 per leg
			Week 4	5 × 15 per leg
3a. 45-degree calf pump		Lean against a wall, with both hands on the wall, both heels up, and your body leaning at about 45-70 degrees. Raise your left knee, keeping your knee and left toes up. Perform quick right ankle pumps using a short range of motion. Repeat the ankle pumps on the left leg.	Week 1	2 × 10 per leg
			Week 2	3 × 20 per leg
			Week 3	4 × 30 per leg
			Week 4	5 × 40-50 per leg
3b. SB triple threat burn		SB bridge (lie supine with your feet on a stability ball; raise and lower hips for reps indicated). SB leg curl (without lowering hips, flex and extend your knees for leg curls). SB hip lift (without lowering hips, walk the ball down until the stability ball is under the balls of your feet; perform short hip lifts).	Week 1	2 × 10 + 10 + 10 with 2 legs
			Week 2	2 × 15 + 15 + 15 with 2 legs
			Week 3	2 × 5-10 + 5-10 + 5-10 with 1 leg
			Week 4	2 × 10-15 + 10-15 + 10-15 with 1 leg

HER LEGS AND HIPS 5: WEIGHTS AND FUNCTIONAL

This 4-week program is a functional training program that focuses on one of the problem areas of women's bodies, the saddlebag area (the upper and outer portion of the thighs). This workout can be tailored to intermediate or advanced trainee, depending on what weeks are completed. It's a perfect home routine since it involves minimal inexpensive yet effective exercise equipment. Depending on your natural capacity and training history, weeks 1 and 2 can be repeated twice to reduce the 4-week volume and provide more time to adapt. The higher-volume ranges of weeks 3 and 4 are for the ladies with very advanced training experience.

Equipment

Medicine ball, dumbbells, low box or step, circle band, bench, stability ball

Notes

Weeks 1 and 2: Perform 2 times per week.

Weeks 3 and 4: Perform 1 or 2 times per week.

Table 4.11 Her Legs and Hips 5: Functional and Weights

Exercise	Photo	Description	Weeks	Sets × reps
1a. MB/DB split squat		Stand in a lunge position (split-squat position) with your left foot forward. Hold a medicine ball in front of you or dumbbells by your sides. Keeping your core tight, bend your left knee and sink into a deep split squat. Straighten your left leg to return to the original position. Repeat for prescribed reps. Repeat with your right foot forward.	Week 1	2 × 10 per leg
			Week 2	3 × 12 per leg
			Week 3	4 × 15 per leg
			Week 4	5 × 10 per leg
1b. MB/DB curtsy lunge		Stand tall with your feet hip-width apart. Hold a medicine ball in front of you or dumbbells at your sides. Keeping your weight on your left foot, take a big step to the left with your right leg, crossing it behind your left leg. Lower your body by bending your knees until your left thigh is parallel to the floor. Return to the starting position and repeat on the opposite side.	Week 1	2 × 5 per leg
			Week 2	3 × 7 per leg
			Week 3	4 × 10 per leg
			Week 4	5 × 12-15 per leg
2a. Single-leg glute bridge (foot elevated)		Lie flat in a supine position. Put your left foot on top of a low box, step, or medicine ball. Keeping your left knee flexed to 90 degrees and your right leg in the air, raise your hips, squeezing your glutes at the top. Lower the hips short of reaching the ground. Repeat with the other leg.	Week 1	2 × 10 per leg
			Week 2	3 × 12 per leg
			Week 3	4 × 15 per leg
			Week 4	5 × 15 per leg

Exercise	Photo	Description	Weeks	Sets × reps
2b. Band seated hip abduction		Place band around your legs, below or above the knees, whichever is more comfortable. Sit on a bench with your feet slightly wider than shoulder-width apart. Keep your back straight. Abduct your legs and roll to the outsides of your feet. Adduct your legs and flatten your feet. Perform prescribed reps.	Week 1	2 × 15
			Week 2	3 × 15
			Week 3	4 × 15-20
			Week 4	5 × 20-30
3a. Single-leg SB bridge		Lie flat in a supine position. Put your right leg on top of a stability ball. Keep your right leg slightly flexed and and your left leg in the air. Raise your hips, squeezing your glutes at the top. Lower your hips short of reaching the ground. Repeat with the other leg.	Week 1	2 × 10 per leg
			Week 2	3 × 10 per leg
			Week 3	4 × 15 per leg
			Week 4	5 × 15 per leg
3b. 45-degree calf pump		Lean against a wall, both hands on the wall, both heels up, and your body leaning forward at about 45-70 degrees. Raise your right knee and keep the toes up. Perform quick left ankle pumps using a short range of motion. Repeat the ankle pumps on your right leg.	Week 1	2 × 10 per leg
			Week 2	3 × 15 per leg
			Week 3	4 × 20 per leg
			Week 4	5 × 30 per leg

HER LEGS AND HIPS 6:
CEM'S FITNESS COMPETITION WORKOUT

This is a 4- to 6-week program performed twice per week. This workout has been used by Cem Eren (www.diamondglutes.com), someone I consider one of the top coaches in the country for female figure competitors. This is a serious workout for women who have access to a well-equipped gym and have the time and energy to devote to developing a great lower body. This kind of workout has been used by figure competitors such as Lauren Irick, who used it to become an IFBB pro and compete in the Olympia.

Equipment

Barbell, bench, dumbbells, power rack, circle band, leg curl machine, kettlebells, medicine ball

Notes

Perform this program 2 times per week for 4 to 6 weeks.

Table 4.12 Her Legs and Hips 6: Cem's Fitness Competition Workout

Exercise	Photo	Description	Sets × reps
1a. Barbell hip thrust (2 sec pause at top)		Sit on the ground and rest your upper back on a bench. Roll a bar over your hips. (You may use a pad between the bar and your hips.) Bend your knees and keep your feet flat on the ground and between hip- and shoulder-width apart. Securing the bar with your hands, extend your hips and bridge up until your hips are fully extended. Pause for 2 sec at the top of the movement. Lower until your glutes almost touch the ground. Repeat.	3 × 12-15
1b. DB split stance deadlift		Stand in a staggered stance, right foot forward. Hold a dumbbell in each hand. Keeping your core tight, flex your hips and reach your hands toward your right foot until you feel a comfortable stretch in your right hamstrings. Return to the starting position and repeat desired reps. Switch sides.	3 × 8-10 per leg
2a. Barbell squat (1 sec pause at bottom)		Using a power rack, safely place a bar on your back, right on the trapezius muscles. Stand with your feet about shoulder-width apart. Keep your core tight and back straight throughout the entire movement. Flex your hips and knees until you reach a sitting position about chair level. Pause for 1 sec at the bottom of the movement. Return to the starting position and repeat.	3 × 10-12
2b. Lateral band walk		Place circle band around your legs, below or above the knees, whichever is more comfortable. Stand in a semisquat position with your feet hip-width apart. Keep your back straight. Lean forward slightly. Take a lateral step to the right so your feet are slightly wider than shoulder-width apart. Step left foot toward right foot until your feet are about hip-width apart again. Perform prescribed reps to the right, then move to the left.	3 × 12 per side
3a. Leg curl (2 sec up, 1 sec down)		Lie facedown on the bench of a leg curl machine and put your feet under the leg pad, keeping the pad behind your ankles. Flex your knees as much as you can without lifting your hips off the bench, taking 2 seconds to complete the flexion. Extend your legs, taking 1 second to complete the extension. Repeat.	3 × 8-10

Exercise	Photo	Description	Sets × reps
3b. Goblet squat		Hold a dumbbell or kettlebell with both hands in front of you at about shoulder level. Stand with your feet about shoulder-width apart and keep your core as tight and vertical as possible throughout the entire movement. Keeping the knees in line with your feet, flex at the knees until you reach a sitting position at about chair level. Return to the starting position and repeat.	3 × 10-12
4a. BB/DB Romanian deadlift (2-3 sec eccentric contraction)		Stand in front of a barbell (or hold a dumbbell in each hand at sides), feet shoulder-width apart and toes pointing forward. Use any comfortable grip you prefer. Keeping your core tight and your knees slightly bent, flex your hips and knees and grab the bar with your hands hip- to shoulder-width apart (or hold your dumbbells in front of thighs). Pause for 2 sec at the bottom of the movement. Drive through your heels, extending your legs and hips simultaneously until you are standing fully erect. Reverse the sequence and lower the weight to the starting position. Repeat the lifting motion.	3 × 8-10
4b. DB/MB lateral reaching lunge		Stand with your feet hip-width apart and your knees bent. Hold a medicine ball or dumbbells in your hands. Keeping your core tight, take a big lateral step with your left leg, bending your left leg slightly. Flex your hips and reach toward your left foot until you feel a comfortable stretch in your left glute hamstrings. Return to the starting position and repeat on right side.	3 × 8-10 per side
5. Frog pump		Lie face up with your knees flexed, your legs open, the bottoms of your feet together, and your heels as close to your glutes as possible. Tuck in your chin as if you were going to start an abdominal crunch. Raise your hips to perform a short bridge. Lower your hips short of touching the ground. Repeat. I suggest performing this exercise facing a wall away from gym traffic.	2 × 50

Summary

I hope you enjoyed the legs and hips workout chapter. Remember, these are just a few of the workouts that will provide excellent results in developing the correct lower body for your needs and preferences. Don't be afraid to mix and match workouts and substitute exercises. The sky is the limit when it comes to creating the right workout for you. For a detailed discussion of the science and practice of program design and periodization, I refer you to *Functional Training*. That text covers periodization and program design and provides full descriptions and progressions for various leg workouts, such as the JC leg crank and triple threat.

CHAPTER 5

Abs and Core

These core workouts are a diverse group of training routines that can sculpt your abs and help you maintain a fit lower back. These workouts are for healthy adults without any past or present back issues and who can perform basic sit-ups and leg raises without negative symptoms or side effects. Just as you wouldn't begin chest training with a 300-pound load for the bench press, you shouldn't start core training with inappropriate loading of the core. Doing so may result in injury. Planned progression is always necessary when training any area of the body, but when it comes to the core, it is extremely important. The spine houses the spinal cord and many critical nerves. One injury anywhere along the spine can result in a debilitating injury, and nobody wants that. Invest in your safety and consult with a certified and insured personal trainer or therapist if you have had back issues in the past, have not worked out in some time, or are simply not very experienced in training and don't know exactly what to do.

Many of the glute workouts from the previous chapter can be used to strengthen the lower back in a more traditional fashion. Although some of the workouts in this chapter include some lower-back training, we will focus on the abdominal region. We will start with the easiest workouts and work up to more intense routines. We start with bodyweight workouts, then throw in stability balls, dumbbells, and bands to make things more interesting. While some of these workouts actually make your core move through a range of motion, others require you to remain stiff while forces are applied, developing core rigidity. I called this "training the invisible" back in 1999. Dr. Stuart McGill has coined the term *super-stiffness* to refer to training core stiffness, which is the foundation of a high-performing core that stays healthy and allows power to be transferred between the hips and shoulders. In many of these workouts, I provide beginner and advanced volume ranges so everyone can safely enjoy the workouts by choosing an appropriate volume to match his or her ability. Always err on the side of caution and be conservative: If in doubt, do less.

Much has been written about the safety or appropriateness of some abdominal exercises. Some exercises, especially those that flex the spine (e.g., sit-ups, leg raises, knee tucks) have been labeled dangerous because they cause unwanted wear on the spine and its discs. Exercises such as sit-ups and leg raises were staples of core training in schools, the military, paramilitary groups, and law enforcement and fire rescue squads. It's likely today's sedentary lifestyle and consequent physical weakness are more to blame for the low-back pain epidemic seen today, not these exercises. It is my humble opinion that none of these exercises are dangerous or undesirable. I point to the generations of athletes and others who have performed them with no deleterious effects on health or function. These exercises simply require a base level of conditioning to be able to perform them without any negative impact, just like any other exercise. Any exercise, if applied incorrectly, with incorrect progression, or with the wrong population, can cause harm. Therefore, the keys to enjoying the workouts in this chapter (or any other chapter) are:

1. Develop a base of training before attempting any workout.
2. Always train without pain and stop at the first sign of pain or other abnormal symptom.
3. Keep your movements under control.
4. Seek the guidance of a certified fitness or strength professional if you are not sure of what you are doing. Even one session with a trainer can save you time and prevent a trip to an orthopedic physician or emergency room.

The *his* and *her* workouts in this chapter are less polarizing than the legs and hips chapter because traditional exercises, such as sit-ups, were traditionally performed by both sexes, as have newer core exercises such as stability ball extensions. Therefore, culturally speaking, these workouts have more carryover across the sexes. Remember, muscles and performance have no bias. Muscles respond to training, and performance is gained by smart, hard work.

Two factors dictate how your core looks: the size of the muscles and the amount of fat covering the muscles. (This will be addressed again in the nutrition chapter.) Of these two factors, when it comes to looks, the more important factor is the amount of fat covering the core. Unfortunately, diet is the most important factor in removing the fat that hides the core muscles, especially the abdominal muscles. Rest assured that some of the muscle-building workouts in this chapter will allow you to build the muscle so it is more visible. And the functional and core-stiffening workouts provide excellent functional performance qualities and tone the core muscles. When combined with a lower percentage of body fat, the muscles will look aesthetically pleasing. Now, let's get to work.

Regardless of the suggestions provided for the sequence and execution of the workouts in this chapter, you can perform these workouts in succession if you need more rest and have more time to train, or you can perform them in sequence if you are in a hurry or want more of a metabolic burn. Each has advantages and disadvantages.

With succession training, you perform all sets of an exercise before going to the next exercise. This type of training is good if you have more time to train, use more rest between sets, and use heavier training loads. The succession method is also preferred if each exercise requires a different load or set-up; changing load and set-up after every set takes time and kills your rhythm.

With the sequence method, you go from one exercise to the next without rest, like you're doing one big circuit. This method is best when you are using the same load with each exercise or have set-ups that can be quickly changed (e.g., a quick change in body positions). However, if you have all exercises (loads and equipment) already set up, you can perform any workout that uses different equipment or loads in a sequence without losing any time. The main benefit of sequence training is its time efficiency. Since you are performing a giant circuit, you use less weight but still get a great pump and tone in a short time. Sequencing (or circuit training) is great when time is tight and you don't want huge muscles.

As always, feel free to mix and match exercises from each of the workouts. Although I added posterior core work in all these workouts, I emphasize the abdominal region

---

Caution: Diastasis Recti

People with a condition called diastasis recti need to be very careful when performing abdominal training. Some abdominal exercises are contraindicated for people with this condition. Diastasis recti, also called abdominal separation, occurs when pressure on the rectus abdominis muscles pushes them apart. Often it is caused by stretching or thinning of the linea alba, the connective tissue that holds the two sides of the rectus abdominis together. Development of the condition may be genetic or may be caused or worsened by pregnancy, overweight, or heavy strength training.

Many exercises in the chapter are not appropriate for people with this condition. Please stay away from the heavy exercises (e.g. sit-ups, leg raises, roll-outs, hanging knee tucks, etc.) and concentrate on more functional exercises that create less abdominal pressure (e.g. standing band and pulley presses and row, rotations, and limited short crunches). Check with your doctor before beginning this or any other exercise program.

---

since there is such a comprehensive selection of workouts for the back of the core in the legs and hips chapter. Therefore, if you are already getting enough posterior core work through other workouts and want to do only abdominal work in these routines, feel free to leave the lower-back work out of these workouts. You can take any workout and split it in half, taking two days to perform the workout. This way, you can work your abs and core a little every day. The abs and core are made up of endurance muscles, so they can take the everyday work unless it becomes excessive, and half of any of these routines is not excessive. Finally, don't be afraid to repeat any week if you feel the workout is progressing too fast for you. If you feel any week is perfect for your capacity, stay there and maintain your core fitness. There is nothing wrong with reaching a level at which you are happy and staying there. So, play conservatively and stay healthy and pain-free.

Base Workout

Although progressions for beginners and advanced trainees are provided in each workout, I strongly recommend everyone finish the two-week workout shown here as a base before attempting any of the workouts in this chapter.

WEEK 1: PERFORM EACH EXERCISE SEPARATELY, IN SUCCESSION

Monday, Wednesday, Friday

Plank (2 × 5-10 sec): Assume a push-up position, balancing on your hands or elbows.

Side plank right (2 × 5-10 sec): Balance on your right hand or elbow and both feet; hold a side position, the right side of your body toward the ground and the left side of your body toward the ceiling.

Side plank left (2 × 5-10 sec): Balance on your left hand or elbow and both feet; hold a side position, the left side of your body toward the ground and the right side of your body toward the ceiling.

Tuesday, Thursday

Contralateral bird dog (2 × 5-10 per side): Assume a four-point position with your hands and knees on the ground. Extend your right arm and left leg until both are parallel to the ground. Alternate sides with each rep.

Crunch (2 × 5-10): Lie on your back with your knees slightly bent, feet flat on ground, and arms across your chest. Crunch your upper torso until your shoulder blades are off the ground. Return to the starting position and repeat.

Single-leg raise (2 × 5-10 per leg): Lie flat on your back with your right knee slightly bent, right foot flat on ground, and arms by your sides. Lift your left leg about a foot (0.3 m) off the ground and then lower until it's just off the ground. Repeat the up-and-down motion of your left foot for desired repetitions, then switch legs. If the single-leg version is too easy, perform with both legs (i.e., simultaneously lifting both legs).

WEEK 2: PERFORM EACH EXERCISE IN SEQUENCE AS A CIRCUIT

Monday, Wednesday, Friday

Side plank right + plank + side plank left (3 × 5-10 sec each): Assume each position and hold the position for the time indicated.

Tuesday, Thursday

Superman + side crunch right + crunch + leg raise + side crunch left (3 × 5-10)

Superman: Lie on your belly and simultaneously lift your arms and legs as if you were flying through the air.

Side crunch right: Lie on your left side. Laterally flex right and lift your upper torso off the ground.

Crunch: Lie on your back with your knees slightly bent, feet flat on ground, and arms across your chest. Crunch your upper torso until your shoulder blades are off the ground. Return to the starting position and repeat.

Leg raise (single- or double-leg) (5-10 per leg, if doing single-leg leg raises): Lie flat on your back with your right knee slightly bent, right foot flat on ground, and arms by your sides. Lift your left leg about a foot off the ground and then lower it until it's just off the ground. Repeat the up-and-down motion of your left foot. If the single-leg version is too easy, simultaneously lift both legs.

Side crunch left: Lie on your right side. Laterally flex left and lift your upper torso off the ground.

HIS ABS AND CORE 1: PLANK AND CRUNCH ABS

This 4-week program is made up of two 2-exercise circuits and a finisher. Since this workout uses plank positions, it may be challenging for people who suffer from wrist issues. If you are one of those people, use push-up handles to help you position your wrists in a more neutral pain-free position. Another option to make the training a little less intense on the wrists and core, but still get good abdominal work, is to use a box or a bar to elevate the push-up position. This workout is an excellent choice for use as a home or travel workout, especially if you don't have too much time to train.

Depending on your natural capacity and training history, weeks 1 and 2 can be repeated twice each to reduce the volume and provide more time to adapt. The higher ranges of weeks 3 and 4 are for the advanced trainee.

Equipment

Bench (optional)

Notes

For added concentration on shoulder stability and abdominal endurance, perform exercises 1a and 2a in a circuit and 1b and 2b in a second circuit. Exhale before every repetition to rid yourself of extra volume in the core and allow a greater contraction.

Weeks 1 and 2: Perform 2 times per week.

Weeks 3 and 4: Perform 1 or 2 times per week.

Table 5.1 His Abs and Core 1: Plank and Crunch Abs

Exercise	Photo	Instructions	Weeks	Sets × reps
1a. Plank with lateral knee tuck		Assume a push-up (plank) position. Bring your right knee to your right elbow. Return to the starting position and perform to the other side.	Week 1	1 × 10 per side
			Week 2	2 × 15 per side
			Week 3	3 × 10 per side
			Week 4	4 × 15 per side
1b. Crunch (use bench to recline and make more difficult)		Lie on your back on the ground or a bench, your knees bent and your feet flat on the ground or bench. Your hands can cup your ears or be crossed across your chest. Flex your core and bring your shoulder blades off the ground or bench. Return to the starting position and repeat.	Week 1	1 × 15
			Week 2	2 × 15
			Week 3	3 × 15
			Week 4	4 × 20
2a. Plank with cross knee tuck		Assume a push-up (plank) position. Bring your right knee to your left elbow. Return to the starting position and perform to the other side.	Week 1	1 × 10 per side
			Week 2	2 × 15 per side
			Week 3	3 × 10 per side
			Week 4	4 × 15 per side

(continued)

Table 5.1 His Abs and Core 1: Plank and Crunch Abs *(continued)*

Exercise	Photo	Instructions	Weeks	Sets × reps
2b. Reverse crunch (use incline bench to make more difficult)		Lie on your back on the ground or a bench, your legs lifted in a vertical position. Hold on to a fixed structure above your head or a partner and lift your hips off the ground or bench toward the ceiling. Lower your hips to the starting position and repeat.	Week 1	1 × 15
			Week 2	2 × 15
			Week 3	3 × 15
			Week 4	4 × 20
Finisher: contralateral bird dog		Assume a four-point position on your hands and knees. Extend your right arm and left leg simultaneously. Return to the starting position and perform on the other side.	Week 1	1 × 10 per side
			Week 2	2 × 15 per side
			Week 3	3 × 10 per side
			Week 4	4 × 15 per side

HIS ABS AND CORE 2: BAND AND CRUNCH ABS

This 4-week program uses body weight and band exercises to create three 2-exercise circuits. The combination of standing and lying positions makes this workout diverse and applicable to a wide array of individuals, from athletes looking to improve function in their sports to individuals looking for a toned and thin midsection. The bands recommended for this workout are the JC Sports Band (4 ft [1.2m] band) or the JC Traveler (2 ft [0.6 m] band). They are the best bands on the market and can really provide a challenge while performing any exercise in this book. Depending on a person's natural capacity and training history, weeks 1 and 2 can be repeated twice each to reduce the volume and provide more time to adapt. The higher ranges of weeks 3 and 4 are for the advanced trainee.

Equipment

Band with handles (such as JC Traveler or sports band), sturdy structure for anchoring the band

Notes

Exhale before every repetition to rid yourself of extra volume in the core and allow a greater contraction.

Weeks 1 and 2: Perform 2 times per week.

Weeks 3 and 4: Perform 1 or 2 times per week.

Table 5.2 His Abs and Core 2: Band and Crunch Abs

Exercise	Photo	Instructions	Weeks	Sets × reps
1a. Band ABC crunch		Attach a band to a high position on a pull-up bar or at the top of a door. Kneel on a soft surface in front of the band. Hold the handles with your palms facing you. Crunch and rotate to the left, bringing your right elbow to your left knee. Return to the starting position and perform to the right side. Return to the starting position and crunch, bringing each hand to the outside of the same side knee. This completes one round trip.	Week 1	2 × 3 round trips
			Week 2	2 × 4 round trips
			Week 3	3 × 5 round trips
			Week 4	4 × 6 round trips

Exercise	Photo	Instructions	Weeks	Sets × reps
1b. Cyclic crunch		Lie flat on your back with your feet about 6 in (15 cm) from the ground. Your hands can cup your ears. Flex your core and hips while rotating, bringing your right elbow toward your left knee. Return to the starting position and perform to the other side.	Week 1	2 × 10 per side
			Week 2	3 × 10 per side
			Week 3	3 × 15 per side
			Week 4	4 × 15 per side
2a. Band ABC extension		Attach a band to a low position on a sturdy object such as a dumbbell rack or below the low hinge of a door. Hold the handles with your palms facing your legs. Extend your arms overhead, rotating to the left to bring both hands high and to the left of your body. Return to the starting position and perform to the right side. Return to the starting position and extend again to bring both hands directly above each shoulder. This completes one round trip.	Week 1	2 × 3 round trips
			Week 2	2 × 4 round trips
			Week 3	3 × 5 round trips
			Week 4	4 × 6 round trips
2b. Contralateral bird dog		Assume a four-point position on your hands and knees. Extend your right arm and left leg simultaneously. Return to the starting position and perform to the other side.	Week 1	2 × 10 per side
			Week 2	3 × 10 per side
			Week 3	3 × 15 per side
			Week 4	4 × 10 per side
3a. BP short rotation (10 to 2 o'clock)		Attach a band to a stable structure (e.g., door) at chest level. Turn sideways so the anchor point is to your right, your feet wider than shoulder-width apart. Hold the handle in both hands in front of you (hands at 12 o'clock). Without moving your hips, move the handle from shoulder to shoulder (from 10 to 2 o'clock). Perform with the other side of the body facing the anchor point.	Week 1	2 × 15 per side
			Week 2	3 × 20 per side
			Week 3	3 × 25 per side
			Week 4	4 × 30 per side
3b. Band lateral bend		Attach a band to a low position (between the knee and ankle) on a sturdy object such as a dumbbell rack or below the low hinge of a door. Turn sideways so the anchor point is to your right, your feet wider than shoulder-width apart. Hold the handle in your right hand to your right side. Without moving your hips, laterally flex (bend) your core to the right, stretching the left side of your core, and return to the starting position. Perform to the other side.	Week 1	2 × 15 per side
			Week 2	3 × 15 per side
			Week 3	3 × 20 per side
			Week 4	4 × 20 per side

HIS ABS AND CORE 3: DUMBBELL ABS

This 4-week program is a straight-up bodybuilding program for the abdominals. If you want big and strong abdominals, this is the one for you. This was one of the first workouts I did more than 40 years ago; it was awesome then, and it's awesome now. For added resistance, you can perform some of these exercises on declined benches or boards. Many people like to perform abdominal exercises on BOSU balls or other padded surfaces, and that's fine too. But keep the surface you are working on as stable as possible so you can use as much weight as possible without dealing with balance issues, which take away from the work done. Perform the exercises as a superset.

Depending on your natural capacity and training history, weeks 1 and 2 can be repeated twice each to reduce the volume and provide more time to adapt. The higher ranges of weeks 3 and 4 are for the advanced trainee.

Equipment

Bench, BOSU (optional), dumbbells or weight plate

Notes

You may use a declined abdominal bench to add difficulty to this workout.

Weeks 1 and 2: Perform 2 times per week.

Weeks 3 and 4: Perform 1 or 2 times per week.

Table 5.3 His Abs and Core 3: Dumbbell Abs

Exercise	Photo	Instructions	Weeks	Sets × reps
1a. DB crunch (on BOSU, floor, or bench)		Lie on your back on the ground, BOSU, or bench, your knees bent and feet flat on ground or bench. Hold a dumbbell in both hands across your chest. Flex your core and bring your shoulder blades off the ground, BOSU, or bench. Return to the starting position and repeat.	Week 1	2 × 10
			Week 2	2 × 15
			Week 3	3 × 10
			Week 4	4 × 15
1b. DB isolation crunch rotation		Lie on your back on the ground or a bench, your knees bent and feet flat on the ground or bench. Assume a crunch position while holding a dumbbell in both hands in front of your core. Rotate from side to side.	Week 1	2 × 10 per side
			Week 2	2 × 15 per side
			Week 3	3 × 10 per side
			Week 4	4 × 15 per side
2a. DB single-arm overhead isometric press with lateral bend		Stand with one dumbbell in your right hand, your right arm extended overhead and your left palm placed on your side pocket. Keeping your right arm extended overhead at all times, laterally bend to your left, sliding your left hand down toward your left knee. Stop when you feel a good stretch on the right side of your core. Return to the starting position. Repeat for desired reps. Perform to the other side.	Week 1	2 × 10 per side
			Week 2	2 × 15 per side
			Week 3	3 × 10 per side
			Week 4	4 × 15 per side

Exercise	Photo	Instructions	Weeks	Sets × reps
2b. DB single-arm side bend		Stand with your hands by your sides. Hold a dumbbell in your right hand. Laterally flex to your right, stretching the left core muscles. Return to the starting position and repeat for the desired reps. Perform to the other side.	Week 1	2 × 10 per side
			Week 2	2 × 15 per side
			Week 3	3 × 10 per side
			Week 4	4 × 15 per side
3. DB reverse hyperextension (use end of bench)		Lie facedown on a bench so your hips and lower body are off the bench. Place a dumbbell or medicine ball near your feet so you can place it between your feet when ready. Grab the dumbbell or medicine ball between your feet. Raise your feet and legs as high as possible, then lower short of touching the ground. Repeat.	Week 1	2 × 10
			Week 2	2 × 15
			Week 3	3 × 10
			Week 4	4 × 15

HIS ABS AND CORE 4: HANGING ABS

This 4-week program is an advanced bodyweight program that depends on grip strength because the body is suspended from your hands. To make this abdominal workout more demanding on your grip, perform exercises 1, 2, and 3 in a circuit fashion without regripping. Talk about an ab and forearm pump! To make this workout even more demanding for the grip, combat athletes not only do the first three exercise without rest but also use oversized grips (e.g., the clamps or lockdowns) instead of a normal bar. If you don't want to be burdened with gripping issues and possible calluses, you can use suspension straps such as the JC Power Slings. Either way, suspending your body weight in midair with your hands or arms and performing these exercises requires strength, so this workout is not for beginners. Exercises should be performed as a superset or in succession.

Depending on your natural capacity and training history, weeks 1 and 2 can be repeated twice each to reduce the volume and provide more time to adapt. The higher ranges of weeks 3 and 4 are for the advanced trainee.

Equipment

Pull-up bar, straps, 45-degree bench with footplate and thigh pads, weight plate or dumbbell, or power slings (optional)

Notes

If your grip allows, perform exercises 1, 2, and 3 as a circuit.

Weeks 1 and 2: Perform 2 times per week.

Weeks 3 and 4: Perform 1 or 2 times per week.

Table 5.4　His Abs and Core 4: Hanging Abs

Exercise	Photo	Instructions	Weeks	Sets × reps
1. Hanging knee tuck		Hang from a pull-up bar with your palms facing out or with your upper arms in hanging straps. Raise your knees to your chest. Lower your legs to the starting position. Repeat.	Week 1	2 × 10
			Week 2	2 × 15
			Week 3	3 × 10
			Week 4	4 × 15

(continued)

Table 5.4 His Abs and Core 4: Hanging Abs *(continued)*

Exercise	Photo	Instructions	Weeks	Sets × reps
2. Hanging side knee tuck		Hang from a pull-up bar with your palms facing out or with your upper arms in hanging straps. Rotate your lower body to the right, then bend your knees and raise your legs toward your chest. Lower your legs as you rotate back to the starting position. Repeat to the left side.	Week 1	2 × 10 per side
			Week 2	2 × 15 per side
			Week 3	3 × 10 per side
			Week 4	4 × 15 per side
3. Hanging windshield wiper		Hang from a pull-up bar with your palms facing out. Raise your straight legs until they are vertical to the ground. Rotate your lower body to the left, then to the right like a windshield wiper, without losing the vertical leg position. Repeat.	Week 1	2 × 5 per side
			Week 2	2 × 7 per side
			Week 3	3 × 10 per side
			Week 4	4 × 12 per side
4. 45-degree bench rotating hyperextension (toes out) (may add weight to increase difficulty)		Place your feet on the footplate of a 45-degree bench, your toes pointing out and the thigh pads set on the thighs below your hip bone. Keeping your back straight, flex at the hips until you feel a comfortable stretch at your glutes and hamstrings. Extend your hips while rotating to the left and return to a flexed position. Repeat to the right side.	Week 1	2 × 5 per side
			Week 2	2 × 7 per side
			Week 3	3 × 10 per side
			Week 4	4 × 12 per side

HIS ABS AND CORE 5: BEYOND THE AB BLAST

This 6-week abdominal program is a heavy-duty version of the ab blast from *Functional Training*. I use this workout with many of my fighters to improve their guard game (i.e., fighting from their backs with an opponent between their legs). Our fighters have strong and great-looking abs because they follow a strict diet and because they do this kind of abdominal work. This advanced routine uses three exercises with a medicine ball. (Instead, you can use a stability ball.) We start by doing this workout resting between exercises. However, the goal is to go through all three exercises back-to-back without rest between each exercise in the circuit. This workout is also a great ab-shredding workout and will help you bring out the abdominals during a fat-burning phase.

Depending on your natural capacity and training history, weeks 1 and 2 can be repeated twice each to reduce the volume and provide more time to adapt. The higher ranges of weeks 4 to 6 are for elite trainees only.

Equipment

Medicine ball: Beginners, use a 2 to 3 lb (1 kg) medicine ball; intermediate athletes, use a 4-6 lb (2-3 kg) medicine ball; and advanced athletes, use a 7-10 lb (3-5 kg) medicine ball.

Notes

Weeks 1 and 2: Perform 2 sets of 10 repetitions of each exercise, resting 1 to 2 min between exercises.

Weeks 3 and 4: Perform 3 sets of 15 repetitions of each exercise, resting 1 min between exercises.

Week 5: Superset the 3 exercises, performing each exercise for 5 to 7 repetitions, with no rest between exercises. Perform 2 supersets, resting 1 min between supersets.

Week 6: Superset the 3 exercises, performing each exercise for 10 to 12 repetitions, with no rest between exercises. Perform 3 supersets, resting 1 to 2 min between supersets.

Table 5.5   His Abs and Core 5: Beyond the Ab Blast

Exercise	Photo	Instructions
1. MB lying knee tuck		Sit on the ground and lean back on your elbows, placing a medicine ball between your knees (or between your feet for more difficulty). Elevate your feet just off the ground and slightly flex your knees, suspending the entire lower body off the ground. Perform a knee tuck and bring your knees and the medicine ball toward your chest. Return to the starting position without allowing your lower body to touch the ground. Repeat.
2. MB short crunch		Lie on the ground with your knees bent or extended and feet off the ground. Hold a medicine ball in your hands, your arms straight toward the ceiling. Push the medicine ball toward the ceiling, performing a crunch and lifting your shoulder blades off the ground. Return to the starting position without allowing your lower body to touch the ground. Repeat.
3. MB ball exchange		Lie on the ground with your legs straight and a medicine ball in your hands right above your head. Simultaneously perform a crunch and a knee tuck (total-body crunch) and place the ball between your legs. Extend the body and repeat the total-body crunch, taking the medicine ball from between your legs and extending the body while bringing the medicine ball overhead. Repeat the ball exchange sequence. Every time the ball is overhead, you have completed a repetition.

HER ABS AND CORE 1: FLOOR ABS

This 4-week program is a quick abdominal training circuit that we used to call around the world because you start on your belly and roll from one position to the other. This workout is a quick circuit burn workout (although it can also be done in succession), making it an excellent choice when time is tight or as a home or travel workout. I love doing this workout on the bed when I travel; the soft mattress acts like sand, cushioning my body and making me work a lot harder. It's also a great way to get a fast burn on the abs when you are done with another body part in the gym.

Depending on your natural capacity and training history, weeks 1 and 2 can be repeated twice each to reduce the volume and provide more time to adapt. The higher ranges of weeks 3 and 4 are for the advanced trainee.

Equipment

None

Notes

Weeks 1 and 2: Perform 2 or 3 times per week.

Weeks 3 and 4: Perform 1 or 2 times per week.

Table 5.6 Her Abs and Core 1: Floor Abs

Exercise	Photo	Instructions	Weeks	Sets × reps
1a. Superman		Lie on your belly, your legs straight and your arms straight and extended over your head. Lift your legs and arms off the ground. Lower your legs and arms without touching the ground. Repeat.	Week 1	2 × 10
			Week 2	2 × 15
			Week 3	3 × 15
			Week 4	4 × 20
1b. Lying side reach V-crunch (left)		Roll to your right side, stabilizing your body with your right arm and your right leg on the floor. Simultaneously lift your left leg and reach your left arm toward your left foot. Lower to the starting position and repeat to other side.	Week 1	2 × 10
			Week 2	2 × 15
			Week 3	3 × 15
			Week 4	4 × 20
1c. V-up		Roll to your back, your legs straight and arms straight and extended over your head. Simultaneously lift your legs and arms off the ground, reaching your hands toward your toes. Lower your legs and arms without touching the ground. Repeat.	Week 1	2 × 10
			Week 2	2 × 15
			Week 3	3 × 15
			Week 4	4 × 20
1d. Lying side reach V-crunch (right)		Roll to your left side, stabilizing your body with your left arm and left leg on the floor. Simultaneously lift your right leg and reach with your right arm toward the right foot. Lower to the starting position and repeat to other side.	Week 1	2 × 10
			Week 2	2 × 15
			Week 3	3 × 15
			Week 4	4 × 20

HER ABS AND CORE 2: STABILITY BALL ABS

This 4-week program uses 2 circuits for the abs and lower back. Feel free to perform just the abdominal section if you are already doing plenty of posterior core work. This routine uses a stability ball and pikes; both are very demanding on balance, stability, and strength so this workout is for intermediate to advanced trainees. The abdominal circuit really targets the abs, from movement to stiffness: It does it all. The exercises flow from one to the other, allowing you to do the entire routine as one continuous circuit if you like to save time or add an additional fitness component.

Depending on your natural capacity and training history, weeks 1 and 2 can be repeated twice each to reduce the volume and provide more time to adapt. The higher ranges of weeks 3 and 4 are for the advanced trainee.

Equipment

Stability ball: 22 in. (55 cm) ball if you are under 5 ft, 4 in. (1.6 m) tall; 26 in. (65 cm) ball if you are 5 ft, 4 in. (1.6 m) or taller

Notes

Weeks 1 and 2: Perform 2 or 3 times per week.

Weeks 3 and 4: Perform 1 or 2 times per week.

Table 5.7 Her Abs and Core 2: Stability Ball Abs

Exercise	Photo	Instructions	Weeks	Sets × reps
1a. SB knee tuck		Assume a plank position, your hands on the floor and a stability ball under your thighs. Tuck your knees toward your chest, allowing the ball to roll down your legs until your knees are on top of the ball. Extend the body to the starting position. Repeat.	Week 1	1 × 10
			Week 2	2 × 15
			Week 3	3 × 15
			Week 4	4 × 20
1b. SB pike		Assume a plank position, your hands on the floor and a stability ball under your thighs. Keeping your legs straight, flex your hips and perform a pike tuck, allowing the ball to roll down your legs until your feet touch the ball. Extend your body to the starting position. Repeat.	Week 1	1 × 5
			Week 2	2 × 10
			Week 3	3 × 10
			Week 4	4 × 10
1c. SB short elbow roll-out pump		Assume a plank position, your elbows on a stability ball and your feet on the ground shoulder-width apart. Extend your arms and roll your elbows forward on the ball. Roll your elbows back to the starting position. Repeat.	Week 1	1 × 10
			Week 2	2 × 15
			Week 3	3 × 15
			Week 4	4 × 20
2a. SB hyperextension		Lie on a stability ball with the ball under your belly, your feet shoulder-width apart and your knees slightly bent. Cup your hands around your ears or cross your arms in front of your chest. Extend your spine until you feel a good contraction of your back muscles, then relax on the ball. Repeat.	Week 1	1 × 10
			Week 2	2 × 15
			Week 3	3 × 15
			Week 4	4 × 20

(continued)

Table 5.7 Her Abs and Core 2: Stability Ball Abs *(continued)*

Exercise	Photo	Instructions	Weeks	Sets × reps
2b. SB reverse hyperextension*		Lie on a stability ball with the ball just below your belly button, your elbows on the floor for stability, your legs and feet together and your feet just off the floor. Extend your hips until your body is fully extended. Lower your feet to the starting position. Repeat.	Week 1	1 × 10
			Week 2	2 × 15
			Week 3	3 × 15
			Week 4	4 × 20

* If your elbows can't touch the floor on the reverse hyperextension, you can use your hands to support yourself.

HER ABS AND CORE 3: CRUNCH PLUS

This 4-week program uses two 2-exercise circuits and a finishing exercise for the anterior and posterior core. Some elements are similar to the Her Abs and Core 1 workout, but this workout increases the position difficulty. You can use medicine balls, dumbbells, and ankle weights to increase the difficulty level of this routine. With light dumbbells (2-5 lb [1-2 kg]), a medicine ball (2-5 lb [1-2 kg]), and ankle weights (2-5 lb [1-2 kg]), this workout is an absolute killer, so don't be fooled by its simplicity.

Depending on your natural capacity and training history, weeks 1 and 2 can be repeated twice each to reduce the volume and provide more time to adapt. The higher ranges of weeks 3 and 4 are for the advanced trainee.

Equipment

Medicine ball, dumbbells, ankle weights, flat or incline bench, sturdy structure for support

Notes

Weeks 1 and 2: Perform 2 times per week.

Weeks 3 and 4: Perform 1 or 2 times per week.

Table 5.8 Her Abs and Core 3: MB Crunch Plus

Exercise	Photo	Instructions	Weeks	Sets × reps
1a. Crunch (can use medicine ball and decline bench for added difficulty)		Lie on your back on the ground or a bench, your knees bent and your feet flat on the ground or bench. You can cup your hands over your ears, cross your arms across your chest, or hold a medicine ball overhead. Flex your core and bring your shoulder blades off the ground or bench. Return to the starting position and repeat.	Week 1	1 × 10
			Week 2	2 × 15
			Week 3	3 × 15
			Week 4	4 × 20
1b. Reverse crunch (can place medicine ball between legs)		Lie on your back on the ground or a bench, your legs lifted in a vertical position. Hold on to a fixed structure above your head. Lift your hips off the ground toward the ceiling. Lower your hips to the starting position and repeat.	Week 1	1 × 10
			Week 2	2 × 15
			Week 3	3 × 15
			Week 4	4 × 20

Exercise	Photo	Instructions	Weeks	Sets × reps
2a. X-up (can hold light dumbbells in hands)		Lie on your back, your arms and legs apart with your toes turned out, forming an *X* with your body. Keep your toes turned out during the entire exercise. Simultaneously lift your left arm and right leg until your left hand touches your right leg as close to your foot as possible. Repeat to the other side, alternating sides for prescribed reps.	Week 1	2 × 10 per side
			Week 2	2 × 15 per side
			Week 3	3 × 10 per side
			Week 4	4 × 15 per side
2b. Side crunch		Lie on your right side with your knees flexed, cupping your hands over your ears. Laterally flex your core to perform a left crunch. Repeat for prescribed reps. Switch sides and perform to the other side.	Week 1	2 × 10 per side
			Week 2	2 × 15 per side
			Week 3	3 × 10 per side
			Week 4	4 × 15 per side
Finisher: cross crunch to contra-lateral bird dog superset (can hold light dumbbells in hands and wear ankle weights)		Assume a four-point position on your hands and knees. Extend your right arm and left leg simultaneously, then bring your right elbow and left knee together underneath you. Repeat for prescribed reps. Perform to the other side.	Week 1	2 × 10 per side
			Week 2	2 × 15 per side
			Week 3	3 × 10 per side
			Week 4	4 × 15 per side

HER ABS AND CORE 4: BAND AND PULLEY ABS

This 4-week band and pulley program consists of two 2-exercise circuits and a finishing exercise for the rotational muscles of the core. This workout uses the standing position, so it's excellent for athletes, such as tennis players, who need a stable core while maintaining good posture in the standing position. Bands, especially the JC Santana line of bands, come in a variety of resistances, and you can use them to tailor this workout to any difficulty needed, from novice to elite.

Depending on your natural capacity and training history, weeks 1 and 2 can be repeated twice each to reduce the volume and provide more time to adapt. The higher ranges of weeks 3 and 4 are for the advanced trainee.

Equipment

Band with handles (such as JC Traveler or Predator Jr.) or cable machine, sturdy structure or door (a band with handles is used in the workout description)

Notes

Weeks 1 and 2: Perform 2 times per week.

Weeks 3 and 4: Perform 1 to 2 times per week.

Table 5.9 Her Abs and Core 4: Band and Pulley Abs

Exercise	Photo	Instructions	Weeks	Sets × reps
1a. BP standing crunch		Attach a band to a high position, such as a pull-up bar or the top of a door. Facing the attachment point, hold the handles with your palms facing you. Crunch and bring your shoulders toward your hips. Return to the starting position and repeat.	Week 1	2 × 10
			Week 2	2 × 15
			Week 3	3 × 20
			Week 4	4 × 20

(continued)

Table 5.9 Her Abs and Core 4: Band and Pulley Abs *(continued)*

Exercise	Photo	Instructions	Weeks	Sets × reps
1b. BP standing single-arm cross crunch		Attach a band to a high position, such as a pull-up bar or the top of a door. Facing the attachment point, hold one handle in your left hand, your palm facing you. Crunch and rotate to the right, bringing your hand to the outside of your right knee. Return to the starting position and repeat for prescribed reps. Perform to the other side.	Week 1	2 × 10 per side
			Week 2	2 × 15 per side
			Week 3	3 × 10 per side
			Week 4	4 × 15 per side
2a. BP diagonal high-to-low chop		Attach a band to a stable structure such as a door as high as possible. Turn sideways so the anchor point is to your right, your feet wider than shoulder-width apart. Hold the handle in both hands high and to your right. Without moving your hips, move the handle diagonally from high right to low left. Return to the starting position and repeat for prescribed reps. Perform to the other side.	Week 1	2 × 10 per side
			Week 2	2 × 15 per side
			Week 3	3 × 10 per side
			Week 4	4 × 15 per side
2b. BP diagonal low-to-high chop		Attach a band to a stable structure such as a door as low as possible. Turn sideways so the anchor point is to your right, your feet wider than shoulder-width apart. Hold the handle in both hands low and to your right. Without moving your hips, move the handle diagonally from low right to high left. Return to the starting position and repeat for prescribed reps. Perform to the other side.	Week 1	2 × 10 per side
			Week 2	2 × 15 per side
			Week 3	3 × 10 per side
			Week 4	4 × 15 per side
Finisher: BP short rotation (10 to 2 o'clock)		Attach a band at chest level to a stable structure such as a door. Turn sideways so the anchor point is to your right, your feet wider than shoulder-width apart. Hold the handle in both hands in front of you (hands at 12 o'clock). Without moving your hips, move the handle from shoulder to shoulder (from 10 to 2 o'clock). Perform the reps indicated, then turn so the anchor point is to your left side and repeat.	Week 1	2 × 10 per side
			Week 2	2 × 15 per side
			Week 3	3 × 20 per side
			Week 4	4 × 20 per side

HER ABS AND CORE 5: HEAVY ABS

This 4-week program is what trainer extraordinaire Cliff Edberg uses with his fitness and bodybuilding competitors. This routine uses two 2-exercise circuits to target the abdominal muscles only. This workout will build and strengthen your abdominals so they will be more visible as you reduce abdominal fat.

Depending on your natural capacity and training history, weeks 1 and 2 can be repeated twice each to reduce the volume and provide more time to adapt. The higher ranges of weeks 3 and 4 are for the advanced trainee.

Equipment

Pull-up bar with straps, cable machine with rope attachment, incline bench, dumbbells

Notes:

Combine these workouts with any of the posterior core (legs and hips) workouts from chapter 4 for complete core training.

Exhale as you perform all abdominal movements.

Use a slow, controlled tempo so you keep constant tension on the abs throughout the movement.

Perform 2 times per week.

Table 5.10 Her Abs and Core 5: Heavy Abs

Exercise	Photo	Instructions	Weeks, sets, and reps
1a. Hanging knee tuck		Hang from a pull-up bar with your palms facing out or with your upper arms in the hanging straps. You can use a power sling if you don't want to use your grip to hold yourself up. Raise your knees to your chest. Lower your legs to the starting position. Repeat.	Weeks 1 and 2: Superset exercises 1a and 1b, performing each exercise for 10 repetitions. Perform 2 supersets, resting 1 min between supersets. Weeks 3 and 4: Superset exercises 1a and 1b, performing each exercise for 10 to 15 repetitions. Perform 3 or 4 supersets, resting 1 min between supersets
1b. Weighted rope crunch		Kneel on a soft surface below a high pulley with a rope attachment. Hold the rope attachment so your hands are next to your head. With your hips stationary, contract your abs so that your elbows travel toward the middle of your thighs. Slowly return to the starting position. Repeat.	
2a. Incline bench reverse crunch		Lie on your back on an incline bench and hold on to the top of the bench with both hands. Start with your low back on the bench and your legs straight. Move your legs toward your torso as you raise your hips off the bench. Lower your hips to the starting position. Repeat.	Weeks 1 and 2: Superset exercises 2a and 2b, performing each exercise for 10 repetitions. Perform 2 supersets, resting 1 min between supersets. Weeks 3 and 4: Superset exercises 2a and 2b, performing each exercise for 10 to 15 repetitions. Perform 3 or 4 supersets, resting 1 min between supersets.
2b. Weighted crunch (use incline bench to make it more difficult)		Lie on your back on the ground or a bench, your knees bent. Hold one dumbbell in both hands across your chest. Flex your core and bring your shoulder blades off the ground or bench. Return to the starting position and repeat.	

Summary

I hope you enjoy the abdominal routines in this chapter. Using these routines, we have built champion athletes. IHP is known for its core training throughout the world. These routines and many more like them have helped develop that reputation. Working with these workouts, you can create workouts of your own as you mix and match your favorite exercises from this and other chapters. For a detailed discussion of the science and practice of program design and periodization, I refer you to my *Functional Training* book.

CHAPTER 6

Arms

This chapter really steps up with a wide array of arm routines that will surely give you the results you are looking for. I have designed functional workouts using bands, suspension equipment, and body weight. I also added dumbbell workouts that can be done at home. For quick burnouts or travel workouts, I included some band-only routines that will volumize and tone your arms quickly. Finally, for people who want to pack on serious muscle, I added some big hypertrophy workouts that use popular machines. In this chapter, we use everything from bands to cables, dumbbells to barbells, body weight to machines.

Each workout provides biceps and triceps work. However, if you want to work only one part of your arm, simply perform the exercises pertaining to that part of the arm only. Obviously, perform the entire workout if you want to train the biceps and triceps in the same workout.

I start with arm training that involves common functional training equipment. Then I proceed to more specialized workouts that use dumbbells, bands, or cables. The chapter finishes with some massive arm workouts that some of the pros I have trained and consulted with have used in the past.

Regardless of the workout you try, there are a couple of issues surrounding the development and sculpting of the arms that everyone should know so there are no unrealistic expectations. First, let's tackle a topic that often makes its way into my email. Many people ask me if they can develop their arms (and other body parts for that matter) with bands as opposed to using free weight or machines. My answer is always the same: "Your muscles respond to tension and volume of work, not necessarily what equipment you use." So, if the right tension and volume are provided, the results will appear but within reason.

The reason for my last "within reason" statement is that there are some things that can't be changed. One of the biggest questions I get is, "If I have a short muscle, such as a short biceps or triceps, is there an exercise I can do to lengthen it?" The answer is no. Personally, I have short biceps. When I started training in my early teens, I was told that a lot of preacher curls would lengthen them. I performed preacher curls for years, and nothing; I still have short biceps. You can see this effect in triceps, calves, quadriceps, and even hamstrings. Short muscles can be made bigger but not longer. The muscle length is set at birth, and no training will change it.

Of all body parts, the most visible are the arms and legs; the rest are usually covered with clothing. I would say the arms are the one body part everyone wants toned. Women want the back of the arms tight, and men usually want bigger arms. The way arms are supposed to look is very much a cultural phenomenon, and it's also a very elastic and changing preference. For this reason, you will see more hypertrophy workouts in the *his* section, while the *her* section has higher-volume toning workouts. As with the other workouts, all these workouts are interchangeable. This means if you are a male athlete and don't want to put on muscle mass due to a weight restriction in your sport or your sport requires your arms to have more muscle endurance than size (e.g., boxing, wrestling), then try the more metabolic routines presented in the *her* section. Likewise, if you are a smaller female who wants to put a little muscle on your arms, try the big hypertrophy workouts in the *his* section. Remember, although men and women may want different things, muscles don't have a sex: They are just muscles and respond to the frequency, volume, and intensity of training.

The usual recommendations for using these workouts apply. More than anything, train pain-free. Mix and match exercises from different workouts to tailor a workout to your specific likes, needs, and environment. For example, if you are like me and have bigger triceps than biceps, reduce or even eliminate the triceps work in any given workout. Also, experiment by changing the order of exercises. For example, if I provide a three-set workout, each with a biceps and triceps exercise, feel free to do all the biceps exercise together (even as a giant set), and then do all the triceps exercises separately as a giant set.

Finally, if you like one workout but feel the daily volume is too much for you (i.e., the soreness and tightness in your arms does not go away), then spread the work over three days or even cut the total volume to a volume you feel allows you to recover. I have found that many clients in their 40s, 50s, and 60s can do the volume of work indicated if they spread the work over three or four workouts over the week. This even means doing back-to-back workouts on consecutive days. At the end of the day, staying pain-free is the name of the game, and anything that helps with that is on the table for consideration.

Note: As a base, although progressions for beginners and advanced trainees are provided in each workout, I strongly recommend that anyone who has been sedentary for three to four weeks finish the two-week program here before attempting any of the other workouts in this chapter.

WEEK 1: DO EACH EXERCISE SEPARATELY

Monday, Wednesday, Friday

EZ bar reverse curl (1-2 sets × 10-15 repetitions): Stand and hold an EZ-bar, your palms facing your body shoulder-width apart. Keeping your upper arms stationary, curl the EZ-bar, flexing at your elbows. Once the elbows are at full flexion, slowly lower the EZ-bar by extending your elbows. Repeat.

BP triceps extension (1-2 sets × 10-15 repetitions): Attach a band such as a JC Traveler to a high position such as a pull-up bar or the top of a door. You may also use a high cable with a small bar or rope attachment. Stand with feet shoulder-width apart. Grasp the handles or the bar in a pronated grip (palms down) and flex your elbows. Keeping the elbows close to the body, extend the elbows until the arms are straight. Flex the elbows to return to the starting position. Repeat.

WEEK 2: DO EACH EXERCISE SEPARATELY

Monday, Wednesday, Friday

DB bent-over triceps extension (2-3 sets × 8-12 repetition): Hold a dumbbell in each hand, your palms facing your torso. Bend your knees slightly and bring your torso forward by bending at the hips. Keep your back flat and your head up. Keeping your upper arms parallel to the ground and close to your body, extend both elbows until your arms are straight and horizontal to the ground. Flex your elbows, bringing the dumbbells back to the starting position. Repeat.

DB biceps curl (2-3 sets × 8-12 repetition): Stand and hold a dumbbell in each hand at arm's length, your elbows close to your body and your palms turned to the front. Flex both elbows, curling the dumbbells toward your shoulders. Extend your elbows, lowering the dumbbells. Repeat.

HIS ARMS 1: FUNCTIONAL ARMS

This 4-week program is a functional training workout for the arms that uses two 3-exercise circuits for maximum training efficiency. However, feel free to rearrange the exercises, such as 1a and 2a, 1b and 2b, and 3a and 3b. This is a perfect workout for people who are interested in getting a considerable amount of core training while also focusing on their arms. If rearranged, this workout can make a great boot camp circuit focusing on the entire upper body; it has plenty of chest and back work in it. Weeks 1 and 2 will be enough for most people, while weeks 3 and 4 should be attempted only by more advanced individuals who have a considerable training base (2 or more years of serious weight training).

Equipment

Pull-up bar, weights, suspension system, superband, parallel bars, medicine ball

Notes

Weeks 1 and 2: Perform 2 times per week.

Weeks 3 and 4: Perform 1 time per week (advanced only).

Table 6.1   His Arms 1: Functional Arms

Exercise	Photo	Instructions	Weeks	Sets × reps
1a. Chin-up (use bands for assistance or weights for additional loading)		Hang with both arms extended from a pull-up bar with your palms facing you (supinated grip) and your hands shoulder-width apart. Pull your body up until the bar is at the collarbone. Lower your body to the starting position. Repeat.	Week 1	2 × 10
			Week 2	3 × 12
			Week 3	4 × 10
			Week 4	5 × 8
1b. Suspension recline curl		Hold each handle of a suspension system, your palms facing up (supinated grip). Recline with your arms and body fully extended. Flex your elbows and curl the handles toward your shoulders. Extend your elbows to the starting position. Repeat.	Week 1	2 × 10
			Week 2	3 × 12
			Week 3	4 × 10
			Week 4	5 × 12

(continued)

Table 6.1 His Arms 1: Functional Arms *(continued)*

Exercise	Photo	Instructions	Weeks	Sets × reps
1c. Superband 3D 60 reverse curl		Step into and on the Superband, your feet hip-width apart. Hold the Superband in a neutral hammer position (palms facing in), your arms extended. Flex your elbows to 90 degrees for the specified reps. Then flex your elbows from 90 degrees to full flexion for the specified reps. Finally, perform full biceps curls for the specified number of reps.	Week 1	2 × 10 + 10 + 10
			Week 2	3 × 15 + 15 + 15
			Week 3	4 × 20 + 20 + 20
			Week 4	5 × 20 + 20 + 20
2a. Dip (use bands for assistance or weights for additional loading)		Balance on the parallel bars, your arms and body fully extended. Flex your elbows to lower your body as far as your range of motion permits and lean forward to accommodate range of motion, or until your elbows are bent 90 degrees. Extend your elbows to push yourself up to the starting position. Repeat.	Week 1	2 × 10
			Week 2	3 × 12
			Week 3	4 × 10
			Week 4	5 × 8
2b. Suspension triceps extension		Hold the handles of a suspension system, arms overhead, facing down, your arms and body fully extended. Flex your elbows until your hands are behind your head and your elbows are next to your ears. Extend your elbows to push your body back to the extended starting position. Repeat.	Week 1	2 × 10
			Week 2	3 × 12
			Week 3	4 × 10
			Week 4	5 × 8
2c. MB hands-on-ball push-up		Assume a push-up (plank) position on a medicine ball with both hands on the ball, your arms and body fully extended. Flex your elbows to lower your body until your elbows are fully flexed (ball is near or touching the chest). Extend your elbows to push your body up to the starting position. Repeat.	Week 1	2 × failure
			Week 2	2 × failure
			Week 3	4 × failure
			Week 4	5 × failure

HIS ARMS 2: SUPERBAND META ARMS

This 4-week program is a metabolic band-only workout that I have been using for more than 20 years now. You can use this program when traveling to get a quick arm pump or toning workout or as a finisher to volumize your arms. This workout is also good for athletes who need muscle endurance in their sports, like combat athletes. Each exercise can be used individually if you are interested in training only one aspect of your arms or you can superset 1a and 1b as indicated. Weeks 1 and 2 will be enough for most people, while weeks 3 and 4 should be attempted only by more advanced individuals who have a considerable training base (2 or more years of serious weight training).

Equipment

Superband (1 in.)

Notes

Weeks 1 and 2: Perform 2 times per week.

Weeks 3 and 4: Perform 1 time per week (advanced only).

Table 6.2   His Arms 2: Superband Meta Arms

Exercise	Photo	Instructions	Weeks	Sets × reps
1a. Superband standing speed curl		Step on a Superband with your feet shoulder-width apart. Hold the ends of the band in a neutral (hammer) grip. Your knees should be slightly flexed, your hands resting on your thighs and your back straight. Perform a speed curl using only your elbows, then lower your hands until they touch the tops of your thighs. Repeat. The speed curls should be performed at a tempo of about 2 repetitions per second.	Week 1	2 × 30 in 15 sec
			Week 2	3 × 40 in 20 sec
			Week 3	4 × 50 in 25 sec
			Week 4	5 × 60 in 30 sec
1b. Superband speed triceps extension		Loop a Superband over a high bar and hold the ends in a neutral (hammer) grip. Your knees should be slightly flexed, your back straight, and your elbows flexed. Extend your elbows until your arms are fully extended and your hands touch your thighs, then flex your elbows to return to the starting position. Repeat.	Week 1	2 × 30 in 15 sec
			Week 2	3 × 40 in 20 sec
			Week 3	4 × 50 in 25 sec
			Week 4	5 × 60 in 30 sec

HIS ARMS 3: DB ARM BLAST

This 4-week program is a specialized dumbbell-only workout for the arms, arranged in three 2-exercise circuits for training efficiency. However, feel free to rearrange the exercises; for example, you could perform giant sets of 1a, 2a, and 3a; 1b, 2b, and 3b; and 1c, 2c, and 3c. This is a perfect workout for people who want to do a specialized workout at home using just dumbbells. Similar workouts have been used by bodybuilding competitors, so don't think just because it uses only dumbbells that this workout is not top-notch. Weeks 1 and 2 will be enough for most people. Week 3 should be attempted only by more advanced individuals, and week 4 is strictly for the pros. Week 4 provides 30 weekly sets for the arms; anybody will tell you that is professional-grade volume.

Equipment

Bench, dumbbells

Notes

Weeks 1 and 2: Perform 2 times per week.

Weeks 3 and 4: Perform 1 time per week (advanced only).

Table 6.3   His Arms 3: DB Arm Blast

Exercise	Photo	Instructions	Weeks	Sets × reps
1a. DB lying triceps extension (hammer-grip skull-crusher)		Lie on your back on the bench, your knees bent and feet flat on the ground. Hold a dumbbell in each hand and keep your elbows in. Extend at your elbows, lifting the dumbbells toward the ceiling. Lower the dumbbells, flexing at your elbows, until they are right above your head. Repeat.	Week 1	2 × 15
			Week 2	3 × 12
			Week 3	4 × 10
			Week 4	5 × 8
1b. DB standing hammer curl		Stand and hold a dumbbell in each hand at arm's length. Your elbows should be close to your body. Flex the left arm, curling the dumbbell toward your shoulder. Lower the left dumbbell. Repeat for prescribed reps, then switch to the other side.	Week 1	2 × 10 per arm
			Week 2	3 × 12 per arm
			Week 3	4 × 10 per arm
			Week 4	5 × 8 per arm
2a. DB double-arm overhead triceps extension		Stand and hold a dumbbell in each hand. Extend your arms over your head. Your palms should face each other with your thumbs around the handles. Keeping your elbows in and upper arms vertical, flex your elbows, lowering the dumbbells behind you. Extend your elbows, pushing the dumbbells back up toward the ceiling. Repeat.	Week 1	2 × 15
			Week 2	3 × 12
			Week 3	4 × 10
			Week 4	5 × 8

Exercise	Photo	Instructions	Weeks	Sets × reps
2b. DB single-arm seated concentration curl		Sit on a flat bench with your knees bent and your feet flat on floor. Hold a dumbbell in your right hand and place the back of the upper arm against your inner thigh. With your palm facing away from your right thigh, flex at your right elbow, curling the dumbbell. Slowly extend your right elbow, lowering the dumbbell. Repeat for prescribed reps, then switch to the other arm.	Week 1	2 × 10 per arm
			Week 2	3 × 12 per arm
			Week 3	4 × 10 per arm
			Week 4	5 × 8 per arm
3a. DB bent-over triceps extension		Hold a dumbbell in each hand, your palms facing your torso. Bend your knees slightly and flex at the hips until your torso is almost parallel to ground. Keep your back flat and your head up. Keeping your upper arms parallel to the ground and close to your body, extend both elbows until your arms are straight and horizontal to the ground. Flex your elbows, bringing the dumbbells back to the starting position. Repeat.	Week 1	2 × 15
			Week 2	3 × 12
			Week 3	4 × 10
			Week 4	5 × 8
3b. DB alternating Zottman curl		Stand holding a dumbbell in each hand, your arms close to your body and your palms facing away from your body. Flex your right elbow to curl the dumbbell. When your right elbow is fully flexed, rotate the dumbbell (pronate hand) and extend your right elbow to lower the dumbbell while initiating a curl with your left hand. Your right arm should be fully extended at the same time your left is fully flexed. Rotate the left dumbbell inward (pronate hand) while rotating the right dumbbell outward (supinating hand). Repeat, alternating the curl and rotating pattern.	Week 1	2 × 10
			Week 2	3 × 12
			Week 3	4 × 10
			Week 4	5 × 8

HIS ARMS 4: ARMS ON A ROPE

This 4-week program is a specialized cable-only workout for the arms using a rope attachment. You can also modify this workout to use a set of bands, such as the JC Traveler or Predator Jr. This workout is arranged in three 2-exercise circuits that use an agonist–antagonist format for an intense volumizing effect. However, feel free to rearrange the exercises in another order, such as separate sets of 1a, 2a, and 3a; 1b, 2b, and 3b. Whether you use a cable and rope attachment or just use a set of bands, this workout provides a ton of volume and has been used by physique competitors to get in contest shape. Feel free to combine exercises from this workout and workout 5. The combination of the equipment used in both workouts offers unlimited possibilities for excellent arm training. Weeks 1 and 2 will be enough for most people. Week 3 should be attempted only by more advanced individuals, and week 4 is strictly for the pros.

Equipment

Double cable machine or bands, rope attachment, handle attachment (optional), dumbbells

Notes

Weeks 1 and 2: Perform 2 times per week.

Weeks 3 and 4: Perform 1 time per week (advanced only).

Table 6.4 His Arms 4: Arms on a Rope

Exercise	Photo	Instructions	Weeks	Sets × reps
1a. Cable rope triceps push-down		Attach a rope attachment to a high pulley. Stand with your feet shoulder-width apart. Grasp the rope in a neutral grip (palms in) and flex your elbows. Keeping your elbows close to the body, extend them until your arms are straight. Flex your elbows and return to the starting position. Repeat.	Week 1	2 × 15
			Week 2	3 × 12
			Week 3	4 × 10
			Week 4	5 × 8
1b. Cable rope curl with neutral grip		Attach a rope attachment to a low pulley. Grasp the rope with both hands in a neutral (palms in) grip. Keeping your elbows tucked in and upper arms stabilized, flex your elbows to curl the rope up as far as possible. Once your elbows are fully flexed, slowly lower the rope back down. Repeat.	Week 1	2 × 10
			Week 2	3 × 12
			Week 3	4 × 10
			Week 4	5 × 8
2a. Cable single-arm bent-over triceps extension		Attach a rope attachment to a low pulley. Grasp both ends with your right hand using a neutral (palms in) grip. Facing the anchor point, bend over while keeping your right elbow tucked, upper arms stabilized and parallel to the ground, and right elbow fully flexed. Extend your right elbow until your right arm is fully extended and parallel to the ground. Once your right elbow is fully flexed, slowly lower the rope back to the starting position. Complete repetitions with your right arm then repeat with the left side.	Week 1	2 × 15 per arm
			Week 2	3 × 12 per arm
			Week 3	4 × 10 per arm
			Week 4	5 × 8 per arm
2b. Cable single-arm rear pull curl		Attach a handle to a low pulley. Facing away from the machine, grasp the handle behind your back with one hand, your palm facing forward. Keeping the arm angled back toward the cable, flex your elbow and curl the handle up toward the shoulders. Extend your elbow, slowly lowering the handle. Repeat for prescribed repetitions, then switch to the other side.	Week 1	2 × 10 per arm
			Week 2	3 × 12 per arm
			Week 3	4 × 10 per arm
			Week 4	5 × 8 per arm
3a. Cable staggered stance forward rope triceps extension		Attach a rope attachment to a pulley position at eye level. Grasp the rope with a neutral grip, turn away from the pulley, and assume a staggered stance. Start with your elbows fully flexed and pointing straight ahead. Keeping your upper arms stabilized, extend your elbows until both arms are fully extended. Slowly flex your elbows to allow the rope to go backward to starting position. Repeat for the prescribed number of repetitions. Switch the position of your feet and repeat.	Week 1	2 × 10
			Week 2	3 × 12
			Week 3	4 × 10
			Week 4	5 × 8

Exercise	Photo	Instructions	Weeks	Sets × reps
3b. Cable double-arm high curl		Stand between 2 high pulleys. Hold a handle in each hand. Make sure your arms are extended and parallel to the floor with your palms to the ceiling. Curl the cable toward your ears while flexing your elbows, keeping your upper arms stabilized. Slowly extend your elbows, lowering the cable. Repeat.	Week 1	2 × 10
			Week 2	3 × 12
			Week 3	4 × 10
			Week 4	5 × 8

HIS ARMS 5: BIG PAPA PUMP ARMS

This 4-week program is a professional bodybuilder arm routine. Similar routines have been used by the top bodybuilders competing at the Olympia. It is arranged into two 3-exercise groups. However, if you want to work fast and volumize your arms to the max, rearrange the order and perform one biceps exercise immediately followed by a triceps exercise. For example, perform supersets of 1a and 2a; 1b and 2b; 1c and 3c. Also, consider combining exercises from this workout and workout 4; the combination of cables, ropes, dumbbells, and barbells delivers the optimal training environment for blasting the arms. Weeks 1 and 2 will be enough for most people. Week 3 should be attempted only by more advanced individuals, and week 4 is strictly for the pros.

Equipment

EZ-bar, weight plates, dumbbells, incline bench, parallel bars, bench, cable machine or bands, handle attachment

Notes

Weeks 1 and 2: Perform 2 times per week.

Weeks 3 and 4: Perform 1 time per week (advanced only).

Table 6.5 His Arms 5: Big Papa Pump Arms

Exercise	Photo	Instructions	Weeks	Sets × reps
1a. EZ-bar reverse curl		Stand and hold an EZ-bar, your palms facing your body and shoulder-width apart. Keeping your upper arms stationary, curl the EZ-bar, flexing at your elbows. Once the EZ-bar is at full flexion, slowly lower the EZ-bar by extending your elbows. Repeat.	Week 1	2 × 15
			Week 2	3 × 12
			Week 3	4 × 10
			Week 4	5 × 8
1b. DB single-arm cross hammer curl		Stand holding a dumbbell in each hand, your palms facing your body. Keeping your palms in, curl the right dumbbell up toward your left chest, close to your torso. Once the dumbbell reaches your left chest, slowly lower the dumbbell, extending your elbow. Repeat, bringing the left dumbbell to your right chest.	Week 1	2 × 5 per arm
			Week 2	3 × 12 per arm
			Week 3	4 × 10 per arm
			Week 4	5 × 8 per arm

(continued)

Table 6.5 His Arms 5: Big Papa Pump Arms *(continued)*

Exercise	Photo	Instructions	Weeks	Sets × reps
1c. DB incline bench curl		Sit back on an incline bench, your feet flat on the floor. Hold a dumbbell in each hand. Let your arms by your sides with your palms facing forward. Keeping your upper arms stationary, curl both dumbbells by flexing your elbows. Slowly lower the dumbbells by extending your elbows to the starting point. Repeat.	Week 1	2 × 5
			Week 2	3 × 12
			Week 3	4 × 10
			Week 4	5 × 8
2a. Dip (upright on parallel bars or bench)		Stand between parallel bars and place a hand on each bar. Start with your arms extended and your body upright. Lower your body by flexing your elbows until they reach 90 degrees. Return to the extended position. Repeat.	Week 1	2 × 10-12
			Week 2	3 × 8-10
			Week 3	4 × 6-8
			Week 4	5 × 8
2b. DB lying crossover triceps extension		Lie on a bench and hold a dumbbell in your left hand with your arm extended. Keeping your left arm stabilized and elbow pointed to the ceiling, flex your left elbow and bring the dumbbell across the body to the right side of your head. Extend your left arm to the starting position. Repeat for prescribed repetitions on your left arm, then repeat with your right side.	Week 1	2 × 15 per arm
			Week 2	3 × 12 per arm
			Week 3	4 × 10 per arm
			Week 4	5 × 8 per arm
2c. Cable bent-over triceps extension		Attach a handle to a low pulley. Stand with the pulley to your left side. Hold the handle in your right hand, and your palm facing the pulley. Bend your knees slightly. Bend at the waist to bring your torso forward. Make sure your back is straight and parallel to the floor. Keeping your right upper arm stabilized, fully extend your right elbow until your right arm is parallel to the floor, your palm facing the floor. Slowly bring your right elbow to a fully flexed position. Repeat for prescribed repetitions on your right arm, then switch to the left.	Week 1	2 × 5 per arm
			Week 2	3 × 12 per arm
			Week 3	4 × 10 per arm
			Week 4	5 × 8 per arm

HER ARMS 1: FUNCTIONAL TONING

This 4-week program is a specialized functional workout for the arms but with a bodybuilding format. It is arranged in three 2-exercise supercircuits that target the biceps and triceps in a superset fashion. This volumizing format will bring excellent blood flow to the entire arm, while giving you the benefits of functional training. Feel free to combine this functional workout with the more traditional workouts offered later in this chapter. Weeks 1 and 2 will be enough for most people. Weeks 3 and 4 should be attempted only by more advanced individuals (2 or more years of serious weight training).

Equipment

Suspension system, barbell, bench, cable machine, handle attachment, bands (such as the JC Traveler or Predator Jr.), medicine ball

Notes

Weeks 1 and 2: Perform 2 times per week.

Weeks 3 and 4: Perform 1 time per week.

Table 6.6 Her Arms 1: Functional Toning

Exercise	Photo	Instructions	Weeks	Sets × reps
1a. Reclined curl (use suspension equipment or barbell)		Place barbell or suspension handles between your chest and belly button. Hold the bar or handles with extended arms, your hands shoulder-width apart and your palms facing up. Recline so your body is straight and at an angle. Return to the starting position. Flex your elbows and curl your body up until your elbows are fully flexed. Repeat.	Week 1	2 × 15
			Week 2	3 × 12
			Week 3	4 × 10
			Week 4	5 × 8-12
1b. Bench dip		Sit on the edge of a bench and place your hands on each side of you on the bench. Walk your legs out until your hips are off the bench. Flex your elbows to lower your body (dip). Extend your elbows to return to the starting position. Repeat.	Week 1	2 × 10
			Week 2	3 × 12
			Week 3	4 × 10
			Week 4	5 × 8-12
2a. BP single-arm side curl		Position a band or pulley at about shoulder height. Hold the handle in your right hand. Turn sideways so the band is to your right side. Extend your right arm to point to the anchor point, keeping your right palm turned up. Perform an arm curl with your right arm. Return to the starting position and repeat for prescribed repetitions. Turn around, switch to your left arm, and repeat the curl motion.	Week 1	2 × 15 per arm
			Week 2	3 × 20 per arm
			Week 3	4 × 15 per arm
			Week 4	5 × 15 per arm

(continued)

Table 6.6 Her Arms 1: Functional Toning *(continued)*

Exercise	Photo	Instructions	Weeks	Sets × reps
2b. MB crossover push-up		Assume a plank position with a hard medicine ball under your right hand. Perform a push-up, then bring your left hand to the ball after placing your right hand on the floor to the right. Perform a push-up. Repeat.	Week 1	2 × 4 per side
			Week 2	3 × 6 per side
			Week 3	4 × 8 per side
			Week 4	5 × 8-10 per side
3a. Band hammer curl		Attach a resistance band to a low position or step on the nylon strap to secure it under your right foot. Stand with your feet staggered and shoulder-width apart and hold one end of the band in each hand, your palms facing each other (hammer grip). Without moving your upper arms, flex your elbows and curl the band toward your shoulders. Extend your arms to the starting position. Repeat.	Week 1	2 × 15
			Week 2	3 × 15
			Week 3	4 × 20
			Week 4	3 × 20 + 2 to failure
3b. Band bent-over triceps extension		Attach a resistance band to a secure object at about chest level. Hold the handles and stand with your feet shoulder-width apart while flexing at the hips to assume a bent-over position. Keep your torso bent over and your back flat, your elbows flexed as much as possible. Extend your elbows so they are in line with your torso and parallel to the ground. Flex your elbows to return to the starting position. Repeat.	Week 1	2 × 10
			Week 2	3 × 15
			Week 3	4 × 20
			Week 4	3 × 20 + 2 to failure

HER ARMS 2: META ARM SCULPTING

This 4-week program is similar to the *his* metabolic band-only workout, and you can follow the same recommendations outlined there. This workout isolates the arms a bit more than the *his* workout due to the challenge and support offered by the stability ball (i.e., using it as a preacher curl bench and as a body stabilizer). Additionally, you can superset the biceps and triceps exercises by simply changing body position on the stability ball. Weeks 1 and 2 will be enough for most people. Weeks 3 and 4 should be attempted only by more advanced individuals who have a considerable training base (2 or more years of serious weight training).

Equipment

Stability ball, Superband or JC Traveler or sports band

Notes

Weeks 1 and 2: Perform 2 times per week.

Weeks 3 and 4: Perform 1 time per week (advanced only).

Table 6.7 Her Arms 2: Meta Arm Sculpting

Exercise	Photo	Instructions	Weeks	Sets × reps
1a. SB band speed preacher curl		Anchor a band to a low position, about a foot (30 cm) off the ground. Facing the band and at a distance that provides the right amount of resistance, kneel on the floor and place a stability ball between you and the band. Using the ball as a preacher curl bench, place your upper arms on the stability ball and hold the bands with your arms extended and palms facing up. Perform simultaneous arm curls.	Week 1	2 × 30 in 15 sec
			Week 2	3 × 40 in 20 sec
			Week 3	4 × 50 in 25 sec
			Week 4	5 × 50 in 30 sec
1b. SB band lying prone speed triceps extension		Anchor a band to a low position, about a foot (30 cm) off the ground. Facing the band and at a distance that provides the right amount of resistance, position a stability ball under your core so your body is parallel to the ground. You may balance on your feet or go to your knees for added stability. Place your extended arms by your sides with your palms facing the ceiling. Flex your elbows and extend them to perform a triceps extension while supporting your torso on the stability ball. Repeat.	Week 1	2 × 30 in 15 sec
			Week 2	3 × 40 in 20 sec
			Week 3	4 × 50 in 25 sec
			Week 4	5 × 60 in 30 sec

HER ARMS 3: DB ARM SHAPING

This 4-week program is a dumbbell-only workout. For this reason, it is perfect for home training or the gym. It is arranged in an agonist–antagonist format consisting of three 2-exercise circuits for training efficiency and maximum volumizing of the arms. If you want to spend more time on arm training, rest more between sets and use greater loads. Consider rearranging the order of the exercises so that all biceps training is done in succession, followed by all triceps training in succession. For example, you can perform the routine in this order: 1a, 2a, and 3a; 1b, 2b, and 3b; 1c, 2c, and 3c. You can also add the biceps portion to a back day and the triceps portion to a chest day to save time and train more efficiently. Don't let the dumbbell format fool you; this is serious training, providing 30 sets for the arms in a week. That is serious volume and not for beginners. Weeks 1 and 2 will be enough for most people. Week 3 should be attempted only by more advanced individuals, and week 4 is strictly for the pros.

Equipment

Adjustable bench, dumbbells

Notes

Weeks 1 and 2: Perform 2 times per week.

Weeks 3 and 4: Perform 1 time per week (advanced only).

Table 6.8 Her Arms 3: DB Arm Shaping

Exercise	Photo	Instructions	Weeks	Sets × reps
1a. DB lying double-arm triceps extension		Lie on a flat bench, your knees bent and your feet flat on the ground. Hold dumbbells in both hands, your arms fully extended and pointing to the ceiling. Flex your elbows and lower the dumbbells behind your head. Extend your elbows to return to the starting position. Repeat.	Week 1	2 × 15
			Week 2	3 × 15
			Week 3	4 × 12
			Week 4	5 × 12

(continued)

Table 6.8 Her Arms 3: DB Arm Shaping *(continued)*

Exercise	Photo	Instructions	Weeks	Sets × reps
1b. DB simultaneous curl		Stand straight, feet together, dumbbells by your sides with your palms facing forward. Flex your elbows to curl the dumbbells up until your elbows are fully flexed. Slowly extend your elbows to return to the starting position. Repeat.	Week 1	2 × 15
			Week 2	3 × 20
			Week 3	4 × 15
			Week 4	5 × 12
2a. DB overhead single-arm triceps extension		Stand straight, your feet together. Hold a dumbbell in your right hand. Fully extend your right arm and point it to the ceiling. Flex your right elbow to lower the dumbbell behind your head until your right elbow is fully flexed. Slowly extend your elbow to return to the starting position. Repeat for prescribed repetitions with your right arm, then switch to your left arm.	Week 1	2 × 15 per arm
			Week 2	3 × 15 per arm
			Week 3	4 × 12 per arm
			Week 4	5 × 12 per arm
2b. DB standing alternating cross hammer curl		Stand straight and hold a dumbbell in each hand, your palms facing the body. Flex your right elbow to curl the dumbbell toward your left chest until your right elbow is fully flexed. As you extend your right elbow and lower the dumbbell, flex your left elbow to curl the dumbbell toward your right chest. Repeat.	Week 1	2 × 15 per arm
			Week 2	3 × 12 per arm
			Week 3	4 × 10 per arm
			Week 4	5 × 10 per arm
3a. DB single-arm bent-over triceps extension		Hold a dumbbell in your right hand, your palm facing your torso. Bend your knees slightly and bring your torso forward by bending at the waist. Keep your back flat and head up. You may use your left arm to stabilize your body by placing your hand on your thigh or a bench. Keeping your right upper arm parallel to the ground and close to your body, flex your right elbow so your forearm is perpendicular to the ground. Extend your right elbow until your right arm is straight and horizontal to the ground. Flex your right elbow to return to the starting position. Repeat for prescribed repetitions on your right arm, then switch to your left arm.	Week 1	2 × 15 per arm
			Week 2	3 × 15 per arm
			Week 3	4 × 12 per arm
			Week 4	5 × 12 per arm
3b. DB incline bench alternating curl		Sit back on an incline bench, your feet flat on the floor. Hold a dumbbell in each hand with your arms hanging down and your palms facing forward. Keeping your upper arm stationary, flex your right elbow and curl the dumbbell until your elbow is fully flexed. As you extend your elbow to bring the right dumbbell back to the starting position, flex your left elbow to curl the left dumbbell. Repeat.	Week 1	2 × 12 per arm
			Week 2	3 × 15 per arm
			Week 3	4 × 12 per arm
			Week 4	5 × 10 per arm

HER ARMS 4: CABLE TIGHT ARMS

This 4-week program is a cable and band workout for the arms. You can use various handles and accessories, such as ropes, V-bars, straight bars, and EZ-bars to give the muscles a different angle of work during the cable exercises. Feel free to experiment with the cable exercises. It is arranged in three 2-exercise circuits for training efficiency. You can also consider rearranging this routine by performing giant sets for each body part, such as 1a, 2a, and 3a; 1b, 2b, and 3b; 1c, 2c, and 3c. This giant set approach is advanced work and only for those training at a very high level. Exercises from this workout can be mixed with the previous dumbbell-only workout to create very efficient and comprehensive arm training routines. Weeks 1 and 2 will be enough for most people. Week 3 should be attempted only by more advanced individuals (2 or more years of serious weight training), and week 4 is strictly for the pros.

Equipment

Cable machine or bands, rope attachment, handle attachment, bench, stability ball

Notes

Weeks 1 and 2: Perform 2 times per week.

Weeks 3 and 4: Perform 1 time per week (advanced only).

Table 6.9 Her Arms 4: Cable Tight Arm

Exercise	Photo	Instructions	Weeks	Sets × reps
1a. Cable lying rope triceps extension (hammer grip)		Attach a rope to a low pulley about 2 ft off the ground. Lie on a flat bench facing away from the pulley, your knees bent and your feet flat on the ground. Hold the ends of the rope attachment in both hands, your arms fully extended and pointing to the ceiling. Flex your elbows to lower the rope ends behind your head. Extend your elbows to return to the starting position. Repeat.	Week 1	2 × 15
			Week 2	3 × 20
			Week 3	4 × 15
			Week 4	5 × 12
1b. SB rope preacher curl		Place a stability ball between you and a low pulley with a rope attachment at the end of it. Holding the rope ends in a neutral grip, kneel and lay your chest over the ball, resting your upper arms on the ball. Flex your elbows and curl the rope until your elbows are fully flexed. Extend your elbows to the starting position. Repeat.	Week 1	2 × 15
			Week 2	3 × 20
			Week 3	4 × 12
			Week 4	5 × 12
2a. Cable single-arm overhead triceps extension		Hold a handle attached to a low pulley in your right hand. Face away from the pulley and extend your right arm so it is pointing toward the ceiling, your palm facing away from the pulley. Flex your right elbow to lower the handle until your arm is fully flexed. Extend your right arm to the starting position. Repeat for prescribed repetitions on your right arm, then switch to the left.	Week 1	2 × 10 per arm
			Week 2	3 × 12 per arm
			Week 3	4 × 10 per arm
			Week 4	5 × 12 per arm

(continued)

Table 6.9 Her Arms 4: Cable Tight Arm *(continued)*

Exercise	Photo	Instructions	Weeks	Sets × reps
2b. Cable single-arm high curl		Stand facing the pulley with a handle attachment set at about eye level. Hold the handle in your left hand, your arm fully extended, parallel to the ground. Your palm should be facing up. Flex your left elbow to bring the handle toward your head until the left elbow is fully flexed. Extend your left elbow to return to the starting position. Repeat for prescribed repetitions on your left arm, then switch to the right .	Week 1	2 × 15 per arm
			Week 2	3 × 15 per arm
			Week 3	4 × 12 per arm
			Week 4	5 × 12 per arm
3a. Cable single-arm supinated triceps extension		Stand in front of a high pulley with a handle attachment. Hold the handle with your right hand and your arm fully extended and perpendicular to the ground, your palm facing the pulley. Flex your elbow until it is fully flexed. Extend your elbow to return to the starting position. Repeat for prescribed repetitions with your right arm, then switch to your left arm.	Week 1	2 × 10 per arm
			Week 2	3 × 12 per arm
			Week 3	4 × 10 per arm
			Week 4	5 × 12 per arm
3b. Cable single-arm rear pull curl		Stand with your back to a low cable pulley. Hold the handle in your right hand, your palm facing the front. Keep your arm straight behind your body and hold your upper arm still while you flex your elbow to curl the handle toward your shoulder. Slowly extend your arm to return to the starting position. Repeat for prescribed repetitions on your right arm, then switch to the left.	Week 1	2 × 10 per arm
			Week 2	3 × 12 per arm
			Week 3	4 × 10 per arm
			Week 4	5 × 12 per arm

HER ARMS 5: PROFESSIONAL PHYSIQUE ARMS

This 4-week program is one of our professional fitness competitor routines for the arms. It is arranged in three 2-exercise circuits for training efficiency. Believe it or not, this is a very similar routine to ones I learned in the 1970s from my professional bodybuilding friends, such as Mr. America, Jorge Navarrete, and Mr. Southeastern U.S., George Prince. Since then, many of our professional fitness competitors, ladies and men, have used this workout. Like some of the other workouts, it is arranged in an agonist–antagonist format to volumize the arms quickly. But you can also rearrange this workout to blast the biceps or triceps independently, such as performing giants sets of 1a, 2a, and 3a; 1b, 2b, and 3b; 1c, 2c, and 3c. Weeks 1 and 2 will be enough for most people. Week 3 should be attempted only by more advanced individuals (2 or more years of serious weight training), and week 4 is strictly for the pros.

Equipment

EZ-bar, dumbbells, cable machine or bands, handle attachment, rope attachment, adjustable weight bench, barbell

Notes

Weeks 1 and 2: Perform 2 times per week.

Weeks 3 and 4: Perform 1 time per week (advanced only).

Table 6.10 Her Arms 5: Professional Physique Arms

Exercise	Photo	Instructions	Weeks	Sets × reps
1a. EZ-bar curl		Hold an EZ curl bar with your hands about shoulder-width apart, your palms facing away from your body (supinated grip). Keeping your elbows tucked and upper arms stable, flex your elbows to curl the bar up until they are fully flexed. Extend your elbows to return to the starting position. Repeat.	Week 1	2 × 15
			Week 2	3 × 20
			Week 3	4 × 15
			Week 4	5 × 12
1b. DB alternating Zottman curl		Stand upright and hold a dumbbell in each hand. Keep your arms close to the body, your palms facing your body. Curl the left dumbbell while rotating your palm so it's facing the ceiling (supinated) when the dumbbell gets to shoulder level. As you lower the dumbbell, rotate your palm so it faces the floor (pronated) as the arm extends. Repeat with the other arm.	Week 1	2 × 10 per arm
			Week 2	3 × 12 per arm
			Week 3	4 × 10 per arm
			Week 4	5 × 12 per arm
1c. Cable single-arm bent-over lateral biceps curl		Attach a handle to a low pulley. Stand with the pulley to your right and the handle in your right hand using a pronated grip (palms turned down). Bend your knees slightly and bend at the waist to bring your torso forward and parallel to the ground. Keeping your right upper arm stable, flex your elbow and curl the handle in toward your chest. Slowly fully extend your elbow. Repeat for prescribed repetitions on your right arm, then switch to your left arm.	Week 1	2 × 15 per arm
			Week 2	3 × 12 per arm
			Week 3	4 × 10 per arm
			Week 4	5 × 12 per arm
2a. EZ-bar lying triceps extension		Using a pronated grip (palms turned down), grab the EZ-bar at the inner handles and lie on a flat bench. Extend your arms in front of you so that they are perpendicular to the floor. Keeping your upper arms stable, bend at your elbows to lower the weight toward your forehead. Use your triceps to return the weight to the starting position. Repeat for prescribed reps.	Week 1	2 × 10
			Week 2	3 × 12
			Week 3	4 × 10
			Week 4	5 × 12
2b. Cable incline bench rope triceps extension		Lie on an incline bench facing away from a pulley with a high rope attachment. Grasp the rope and keep your elbows tucked to your sides. Keeping your upper arms stable, pull the rope forward until your arms are fully extended. Slowly return to the starting position. Repeat for prescribed reps.	Week 1	2 × 10
			Week 2	3 × 12
			Week 3	4 × 10
			Week 4	5 × 12
2c. Close-grip barbell bench press		Lie on a flat bench. Grab the barbell with a close grip, your hands a little inside shoulder-width. Slowly lower the barbell toward the middle of your chest, keeping your elbows close to your body. Press the bar back up to the starting position. Repeat.	Week 1	2 × 10
			Week 2	3 × 12
			Week 3	4 × 10
			Week 4	5 × 12

BONUS WORKOUT: 21S ARM SALUTE

Here is the famous 21-rep arm burnout. This is more of a protocol and a strategy than it is a workout. Many of you have heard about it because it has stood the test of time. The 21-rep protocol begins with 7 partial repetitions from the starting position to the halfway point of the complete contraction. Next, you perform 7 partial repetitions from the halfway point to the end point of the full contraction. Finally, the protocol ends with 7 full contractions, spanning the complete range of motion. The concept of combining partial repetitions that cover various ranges of an exercise to create a huge metabolic demand and mechanical load is as old as lifting itself. We now use different repetition schemes and combine a wide array of ranges to create killer protocols. However, all our new protocols that involve partials were born out of the 21-rep protocol I learned in the early 1970s, and it was not new then by any stretch!

Here are some exercises you can use with the 21-rep protocol. Obviously, the biceps curl with a barbell or dumbbells is the most popular, but any other exercise can be done using the 21-rep protocol.

BICEPS CURL 21S

Perform the biceps curl while standing or sitting, using a barbell, dumbbells, or cables.

1. Perform 7 curls, from arms extended to 90 degrees of elbow flexion.
2. Perform 7 curls, from 90 degrees of elbow flexion to full flexion (about 135 degrees of flexion).
3. Perform 7 curls through the full range of motion.

TRICEPS EXTENSION 21S

Perform the triceps extension while standing, sitting, or lying down, using a barbell, dumbbells, or cables.

1. Perform 7 extensions, from arms extended to 90 degrees of elbow flexion.
2. Perform 7 extensions, from 90 degrees of elbow flexion to full extension.
3. Perform 7 extensions through the full range of motion.

Also try the protocol with bench presses, rows, and flys using this approach. You can do 2 to 4 sets and you are done—instant pump! Give them a shot.

Summary

I certainly hope this chapter offered some new ideas for training your arms. Hitting your arm training from a different angle may not only provide a different training stimulus but also reinvigorate your interest in training—a great bonus to any training approach. Remember to play with the volume throughout the week and spread out your program if you feel you are not recovering well from a workout that loads all arm work in one day. Also remember that when you train your back, chest, and shoulders, you also work your arms. Realizing this may reduce the amount of specialized arm work you perform, saving you time as well as wear and tear on your joints.

CHAPTER 7

Shoulders

This chapter offers a wide spectrum of shoulder workouts, from shoulder health to shoulder-building workouts. You'll find workouts with equipment that travels or stores easily and routines that bodybuilders perform in the local gym. I also provide a progression scheme that will allow most people to start the workouts with low volumes and slowly progress to the higher-volume weeks.

Some workouts provide general conditioning, others focus on metabolic shoulder endurance, and others attack each aspect of shoulder development individually. However, if you want to work on only one aspect of your shoulders, you can simply perform only the exercises pertaining to the part of the shoulders you want to emphasize. For example, if you want to train the front of the shoulders (anterior or front deltoids) on the day you train chest, you can take a few of the front deltoid exercises and combine them with your chest routine. Likewise, you can take some of the posterior deltoid work provided in this chapter and combine it with your back work. This approach takes advantage of the synergy between adjacent body parts, thereby enhancing training efficiency.

Another way to use these exercises and routines, especially the metabolic routines, is to incorporate them as flush protocols after your traditional shoulder training. This means that you can use one to three flush sets of a metabolic routine (high volume of fast repetitions) to volumize the shoulders after you complete 12 to 20 total sets of traditional shoulder strength training. By *volumize,* I mean to bring a lot of blood volume into an area quickly. This approach is standard practice in bodybuilding and finishes the pump; often these protocols are called *finishers.* Volumizing an area not only feels good by providing an incredible pump, it also provides a host of hypertrophic stimuli that trigger muscle growth.

Of all body parts, the shoulders frame the body, and this is especially true for men. From the front, and even the back, the shoulders provide the perception of width of the upper body. Combining this with a small waist results in the V shape every man wants. The V the shoulders provide is also the top of the hourglass shape every woman is looking for. This is especially true today, when women are increasingly looking for a toned and muscular body.

From a performance perspective, the shoulder attaches the body to its most used and skilled limbs, the arms. From picking up kids to serving a tennis ball and from swinging a golf club to carrying groceries, the shoulders connect the arms to the body. The shoulders have to accelerate and decelerate the arms during throwing motions, cover big ranges of motion in activities such as swimming, and absorb high forces during punching or when breaking falls. The shoulders serve as the attachment point of the arms and body during swinging, transferring enormous torque from the hips to the club or bat. Finally, the shoulders also have to keep the arms in place during heavy lifting and holding, such in wrestling and while carrying heavy objects. Therefore, few body parts are as complex and as involved in so many important movements as the shoulders. It would be wise to give the same importance to the shoulders as to other body parts such as the chest, legs, arms, and abs.

The shoulders are as complex and temperamental as any structure in the body. Therefore, training and staying pain-free is of paramount importance. If you are going to consider slowing the tempo and working on partial ranges of motion with any body part, the shoulders are a great candidate for both. The time-under-tension approach allows you to effectively overload a muscle while using a lighter weight without overloading the joint with a heavier load. The partial training approach also allows you to train the shoulder in ranges that don't hurt, instead of avoiding an exercise altogether. I have been specifically effective with high-volume, partial-range-of-motion lateral raises when faced with an impinged supraspinatus. This approach allowed time for me to rehabilitate the impingement while I maintained excellent muscular development in my deltoids.

The deltoids lend themselves to performing higher and lighter volume over the week, instead of banging 20 to 30 sets in one day. I found that I could better handle 30 sets over three days (e.g., Tuesday, Thursday, and Saturday) rather than doing 20 sets in one day. Yes, if I spread out the volume, I can actually get more work in without overtraining my shoulders. Therefore, if you are not recovering from your weekly volume on one day, split the weekly volume over a few days. Your shoulders will thank you for it.

I have suggested progressions for beginner and advanced trainees in almost all workouts. However, if you have not trained in more than a month and feel like you need to establish a base or you are inexperienced in training, I strongly recommend you finish this two-week program before attempting any of the workouts in this chapter.

WEEK 1: DO EACH EXERCISE SEPARATELY.

Monday, Wednesday, Friday

DB overhead press (1-2 sets × 10-15 repetitions)

DB upright row (1-2 sets × 10-15 repetitions)

WEEK 2: DO EACH EXERCISE SEPARATELY.

Monday, Wednesday, Friday

DB overhead press (2-3 sets × 8-12 repetitions)

DB upright row (2-3 sets × 8-12 repetitions)

DB lateral raise (2-3 sets × 10-12 repetitions)

Due to our excessive sitting and structural flexing to the pull of gravity, the shoulders and the hips are extremely susceptible to postural and functional issues. Although these workouts provide excellent work and address the postural muscles, it's always a great idea to have some kind of warm-up to prepare the shoulders for work and to restore some of the postural deficiencies. Tables 7.1 and 7.2 provide two examples. I've added these warm-up routines in the shoulder chapter because in my experience, shoulders are complicated joints and may be temperamental, often requiring a longer warm-up compared to other body parts. However, these warm-up routines can be used before any upper-body workout.

Table 7.1 Superset With 5-24 Lb (3-11 Kg) Plate

Exercise	Photo	Description	Sets × reps
Short halo with weight plate (elbows flexed)		Stand upright, holding a weight plate in both hands above your head. Make a small circle (i.e., halo) around your head with the plate. Repeat for desired repetitions, then reverse direction.	2 × 10 each direction
Pressed halo with weight plate (elbows extended)		Stand upright, holding a weight plate in both hands high above your head, arms fully extended. Make a big circle (i.e., halo) above your head with the plate. Repeat for prescribed repetitions, then reverse direction.	2 × 10 each direction
Push–pull with weight plate		Stand upright, holding a weight plate with both hands in front of you at chest level. Extend your arms forward, then flex your elbows to bring the plate back to your chest. Repeat.	2 × 10
Short chop		Stand upright, holding a weight plate with your arms fully extended and level with your head. Keeping your arms straight, lower the plate to waist height, then back to starting position. Repeat.	2 × 10

Table 7.2 Superset With Stability Ball and JC Traveler or Sports Bands

Exercise	Photo	Description	Sets × reps
SB roll-out		Stand tall in front of a wall. Hold the stability ball between your hands and the wall at chest height. With your arms fully extended, roll the ball up the wall until your entire body is extended and the ball is right above your head. Pull your arms and roll the ball to return to the starting position. Repeat.	2 × 10
SB single-arm pitcher's roll-out		Stand tall in front of a wall with the stability ball between your right hand and the wall at chest height. With your arm fully extended, step with your left leg and roll the ball up the wall until you are in a lunge position, with your right arm in a throwing motion and supported by the stability ball. Step back and roll your right arm to the starting position. Repeat to the other side.	2 × 10 per side
SB arm through (cross reach)		Face the wall with a stability ball between your chest and the wall. Slide your right hand across your body, between the stability ball and your chest. Slide your arm across and rotate left until the stability ball is behind your right shoulder. Rotate right and slide your left hand between the stability ball and your chest, rotating right until the stability ball is behind your left shoulder. Repeat.	2 × 10 per side
BP Y		Stand facing a set of bands at chest to shoulder height, your feet shoulder-width apart. Hold the handles with your arms extended in a neutral grip (palms facing each other and thumbs pointing up) at shoulder height. Keeping your arms extended and your shoulder blades back and down (retracted and depressed), raise your arms overhead to create a Y. Lower your arms to shoulder height. Repeat.	2 × 10
BP T		Stand facing a set of bands at chest to shoulder height, your feet shoulder-width apart. Hold the handles with your arms extended in a supinated grip (palms facing up and thumbs pointing out) at shoulder height. Keeping your arms fully extended and your shoulder blades back and down (retracted and depressed), open your arms laterally to create a T. Bring your arms back to the starting position. Repeat.	2 × 10

Exercise	Photo	Description	Sets × reps
BP I		Stand facing a set of bands at chest to shoulder height, your feet shoulder-width apart. Hold the handles with your arms extended in a supinated grip (palms facing up and thumbs pointing out) at shoulder height. Keeping your arms fully extended and your shoulder blades back and down (retracted and depressed), pull your arms by your sides, thumbs pointing behind you. Bring your arms back to the starting position. Repeat.	2 × 10

HIS SHOULDERS 1: ROTATOR CUFF WORKOUT

This shoulder rehabilitation program can help your recovery from a shoulder injury, but it can also be a maintenance program for athletes who perform overhead throwing motions. It is arranged in three 2-exercise circuits for maximum training efficiency. However, feel free to rearrange the exercises, such as mixing up internal and external rotation exercises in a 1a, 2a, and 3a circuit, then 1b, 2b, and 3b.

Equipment

Band such as JC Traveler or sports band, sturdy object, dumbbells, bench

Notes

Perform 2 or 3 times per week.

Table 7.3 His Shoulders 1: Rotator Cuff Workout

Exercise	Photo	Instructions	Weeks	Sets × reps
1a. Isometric IR (up) band walk		Face away from a band placed at shoulder height. Hold the handle in your right hand, your arm raised by your side and your elbow flexed at 90 degrees. Keeping your right arm in place, slowly take 2 or 3 steps forward or until you reach maximum tension. When you have reached maximum tension, hold for 2 sec and walk back to the starting position. Repeat for prescribed repetitions, then switch to the other side.	Week 1	2 × 2 walks
			Week 2	2 × 3 walks
			Week 3	3 × 2 walks
			Week 4	4 × 3 walks
1b. Isometric IR (down) band walk		Stand with the band to your right and at elbow height. Hold the handle in your right hand, your right upper arm tight against your right side and your elbow flexed at 90 degrees. Keeping your right arm in place, slowly take 2 or 3 steps to your left or until you reach maximum tension. When you have reached maximum tension, hold for 2 sec, then walk back to the starting position. Repeat for prescribed repetitions, then switch to the other side.	Week 1	2 × 2 walks
			Week 2	2 × 3 walks
			Week 3	3 × 2 walks
			Week 4	4 × 3 walks

(continued)

Table 7.3 His Shoulders 1: Rotator Cuff Workout *(continued)*

Exercise	Photo	Instructions	Weeks	Sets × reps
2a. Isometric ER (up) band walk		Face a band placed at shoulder height, the handle in your right hand, your arm raised by your side, and your elbow flexed at 90 degrees. Keeping your right arm in place, slowly take 2 or 3 steps back or until you reach maximum tension. When you have reached maximum tension, hold for 2 sec, then walk back to the starting position. Repeat for prescribed repetitions, then switch to the other side.	Week 1 Week 2 Week 3 Week 4	2 × 2 walks 2 × 3 walks 3 × 2 walks 4 × 3 walks
2b. Isometric ER (down) band walk		Stand with the band to your left and at elbow height, the handle in your right hand, right upper arm tight against your right side, and your elbow flexed at 90 degrees. Keeping your right arm in place, slowly take 2 or 3 steps to the right or until you reach maximum tension. When you have reached maximum tension, hold for 2 sec, then walk back to the starting position. Repeat for prescribed repetitions, then switch to the other side.	Week 1 Week 2 Week 3 Week 4	2 × 2 walks 2 × 3 walks 3 × 2 walks 4 × 3 walks
3a. DB isometric IR (supine)		Lie flat on your back on a bench and hold a dumbbell in your right hand. Keep your upper right arm parallel to the ground and your right elbow flexed at 90 degrees (like at the bottom of the bench press). Allow your right arm to externally rotate until the right forearm is parallel to the ground. Hold for 3 sec, then return to the starting position. Repeat for prescribed repetitions, then switch to the other side.	Week 1 Week 2 Week 3 Week 4	2 × 2 2 × 3 3 × 2 4 × 3
3b. DB isometric ER (prone)		Lie flat on your belly on a bench, your feet shoulder-width apart. Hold a dumbbell in your right hand. Keep your right elbow flexed at 90 degrees and your right forearm perpendicular to the ground. Externally rotate the right shoulder until your right forearm is parallel to the ground. Hold for 3 sec, then return to the starting position. Repeat for prescribed repetitions, then switch to the other side.	Week 1 Week 2 Week 3 Week 4	2 × 2 2 × 3 3 × 2 4 × 3

HIS SHOULDERS 2: FUNCTIONAL SHOULDERS

This 4-week program is a functional training program for the shoulders. It is arranged in two 2-exercise circuits, with a band finisher for maximum training efficiency. However, you can rearrange the exercises in another order, such as 1a and 2a, 1b and 2b, and finish with the band routine. This is a perfect workout for people interested in getting a considerable amount of core training while also focusing on their shoulders. Weeks 1 and 2 will be enough for most people, while weeks 3 and 4 should be attempted only by more advanced individuals who have a considerable training base.

Equipment

Stability ball, dumbbells, suspension system, double cable machine with handle attachments or bands such as JC Travelers or Sports Bands, Superband

Notes

Weeks 1 and 2: Perform 2 times per week.

Weeks 3 and 4: Perform 1 time per week (for advanced trainees only).

Table 7.4 His Shoulders 2: Functional Shoulder

Exercise	Photo	Instructions	Weeks	Sets × reps
1a. SB pike press		From a plank position (prone), place your hands on the floor and extend your elbows, the tops of your feet on the stability ball. Contracting your core, roll the stability ball toward you, hinging your hips up into an inverted position. Roll the stability ball away from you until you are back in plank position. Perform a push-up. Repeat.	Week 1	2 × 6
			Week 2	3 × 8
			Week 3	4 × 10
			Week 4	4 × 10
1b. DB muscle snatch		Hold a dumbbell in each hand. Squat, lowering the dumbbells in front of your thighs with your arms straight. Pull the dumbbells up by extending your hips and knees. Shrug your shoulders and pull up aggressively as you pull your body under the dumbbells. Catch the dumbbells at arm's length with legs fully extended. Lower the dumbbells to the front of your thighs. Repeat.	Week 1	2 × 6 per arm
			Week 2	3 × 8 per arm
			Week 3	4 × 10 per arm
			Week 4	4 × 10 per arm
2a. Suspension rear delt high row		Grab the suspension handles in a pronated grip, keeping your arms extended. Step forward until your body reclines, keeping your legs and body straight. Pull your body up until your elbows are directly lateral to each side without allowing your elbows to drop. Return to the reclined position until your arms are fully extended. Repeat.	Week 1	2 × 6
			Week 2	3 × 8
			Week 3	4 × 10
			Week 4	4 × 10

(continued)

Table 7.4 His Shoulders 2: Functional Shoulder *(continued)*

Exercise	Photo	Instructions	Weeks	Sets × reps
2b. BP double-arm 3D 60 lateral raise		Stand between 2 low bands or 2 cables set at the lowest level. Hold the handles in a pronated grip and let the bands or cables create an X in front of you. Split a lateral raise into 3 ranges: the lower third, the middle third, and the highest third. Keeping your arms straight, laterally raise your arms, then return to the starting position. Repeat. Perform the indicated repetitions at each range: lower, mid, and high.	Week 1	2 × 10 + 10 + 10
			Week 2	3 × 15 + 15 + 15
			Week 3	4 × 20 + 20 + 20
			Week 4	4 × 20 + 20 + 20
BAND FINISHER: PERFORM AS A SUPERSET. STAND IN FRONT OF A CABLE MACHINE OR SET OF LOW BANDS OR STEP ON A SUPERBAND FOR THIS SUPERSET.				
3a. BP front raise		Hold the band, palms down. Raise your arms to the front to shoulder height and lower to starting position. Repeat.	Week 1	2 × 10
			Week 2	3 × 15
			Week 3	4 × 20
			Week 4	4 × 20
3b. BP wide upright row		Hold the band, palms down. Initiating the pull with your elbows, pull the band until your hands are wider than shoulder-width and shoulder height. Lower to starting position. Repeat.	Week 1	2 × 10
			Week 2	3 × 15
			Week 3	4 × 20
			Week 4	4 × 20
3c. BP close upright row		Hold the bands with your arms straight and in front of your thighs with palms facing the body. Initiating the pull with your elbows, pull the band until the hands are chest-width and shoulder height. Lower to starting position. Repeat.	Week 1	2 × 10
			Week 2	3 × 15
			Week 3	4 × 20
			Week 4	4 × 20

HIS SHOULDERS 3: IRON-PLATED SHOULDERS

This is a 4-week killer plate program for the shoulders. I first learned of this workout from a 1990s bootleg video of the Cuban wrestling and weightlifting teams warming up and conditioning. When you don't have any money to train, you come up with ingenious ways to train, and this is one of them. Although each exercise can be performed by itself as a strengthening move, I first saw it as a conditioning circuit, so this is how it's presented here. The plates are 10-45 lb (5-20 kg), depending on how many repetitions are being completed and your strength and conditioning level. I have done each of these circuits with a 45 lb (20 kg) plate, and one set crushed me! So, be ready if you decide to go for it with the big 45! Weeks 1 and 2 will be enough for most people, while weeks 3 and 4 should be attempted only by more advanced individuals with a considerable training base.

Equipment

Weight plates

Notes

Perform exercises 1a, 1b, and 1c as a superset without resting or putting down the plate. Then after 1-3 min of rest, perform exercises 2a, 2b, and 2c as a superset without resting or putting down the plate. Very elite athletes can try 20-rep sets.

Weeks 1 and 2: Perform 2 times per week.

Weeks 3 and 4: Perform 1-2 time per week (very advanced trainees only).

Table 7.5 His Shoulders 3: Iron-Plated Shoulders

Exercise	Photo	Instructions	Weeks	Sets × reps
1a. Short halo with weight plate (elbows flexed)		Stand upright, holding a weight plate in both hands above your head. Make a small circle (i.e., halo) around your head with the plate. Repeat for prescribed repetitions, then reverse direction.	Week 1	2 × 6 per side
			Week 2	3 × 8 per side
			Week 3	3 × 10 per side
			Week 4	4 × 12 per side
1b. Push–pull with weight plate		Stand upright, holding a weight plate with both hands in front of you at chest level. Extend your arms forward, then flex your elbows to bring the plate back to your chest. Repeat.	Week 1	2 × 6
			Week 2	3 × 8
			Week 3	3 × 10
			Week 4	4 × 12
1c. Infinity		Stand upright, holding a weight plate with both hands in front of you at chest level with arms fully extended forward. Move the plate in an infinity sign or a sideways number 8. Repeat for prescribed repetitions, then reverse direction.	Week 1	2 × 6 per side
			Week 2	3 × 8 per side
			Week 3	3 × 10 per side
			Week 4	4 × 12 per side

(continued)

Table 7.5 His Shoulders 3: Iron-Plated Shoulders *(continued)*

Exercise	Photo	Instructions	Weeks	Sets × reps
1d. Steering wheel		Stand upright, holding a weight plate with both hands in front of you at chest level with your arms fully extended forward. Rotate the plate to the right and then to the left, like driving a car. Repeat for prescribed repetitions.	Week 1	2 × 6 per side
			Week 2	3 × 8 per side
			Week 3	3 × 10 per side
			Week 4	4 × 12 per side
2a. Overhead press with weight plate		Stand upright, holding a weight plate with both hands above your head with your arms fully extended. Lower the plate to just above your head. Push the plate up toward the ceiling until your arms are fully extended. Repeat.	Week 1	2 × 6
			Week 2	3 × 8
			Week 3	3 × 10
			Week 4	4 × 12
2b. Pressed halo with weight plate		Stand upright, holding a weight plate in both hands high above your head, your arms fully extended. Make a big circle (i.e., halo) above your head with the plate. Repeat for prescribed repetitions, then reverse direction.	Week 1	2 × 6 per side
			Week 2	3 × 8 per side
			Week 3	3 × 10 per side
			Week 4	4 × 12 per side
2c. Clock		Stand upright, holding a weight plate with both hands above your head with your arms fully extended. Keeping your arms straight, move the plate in a large circle, like a giant clock; 12 is arms over the head, and 6 is at waist height. Repeat for prescribed repetitions, then reverse direction.	Week 1	2 × 6 per side
			Week 2	3 × 8 per side
			Week 3	3 × 10 per side
			Week 4	4 × 12 per side
2d. Full (long) chop		Stand upright, holding a weight plate with both hands overhead with your arms fully extended. Keeping your arms straight, lower the plate to waist height, then return to starting position. Repeat.	Week 1	2 × 6
			Week 2	3 × 8
			Week 3	3 × 10
			Week 4	4 × 12

HIS SHOULDERS 4: DB AND CABLE SHOULDER WORKOUT

This 4-week program is a dumbbell and cable workout that can easily pack on some muscle. It is arranged in three 2-exercise circuits for maximum training efficiency. Some of our big athletes like to go slowly, do each exercise in succession, and rest a little more between sets. This takes well over an hour and a half to do the higher volumes of week 3 and 4, especially week 4. This added time allows them to use more weight, which they feel provides better hypertrophy. However, with this two-movement superset format, weeks 1 and 2 will be enough for most people who don't have too much time to train and want to train at a faster pace. Weeks 3 and 4 should be attempted only by more advanced individuals who have a considerable training base.

Equipment

Adjustable weight bench, dumbbells, dual cable machine with rope, bar, and single-handle attachments, JC Bands

Notes

Weeks 1 and 2: Perform 2 times per week.

Weeks 3 and 4: Perform 1 time per week (for advanced trainees only).

Table 7.6   His Shoulders 4: DB and Cable Shoulder Workout

Exercise	Photo	Instructions	Weeks	Sets × reps
1a. Seated dumbbell press		Sit upright on a bench with a back support. Keep your feet flat on the floor and shoulder-width apart. Hold a dumbbell in each hand. Bring the dumbbells up, outside of shoulder-width, palms facing forward. Press the dumbbells overhead until your arms are fully extended. Lower the dumbbells to the starting position. Repeat.	Week 1	2 × 10
			Week 2	3 × 12
			Week 3	4 × 10
			Week 4	5 × 8
1b. Low rope face pull		Stand in front of a pulley machine with a rope attachment attached in a low position, about knee height, your feet shoulder-width apart and knees slightly bent. (You may also use a seated cable row machine.) Hold the ends of the rope in a pronated grip. Pull the weight toward the neck until your hands are at shoulder height inside of shoulder-width. Extend your elbows to return to the starting position. Repeat.	Week 1	2 × 10
			Week 2	3 × 12
			Week 3	4 × 12
			Week 4	5 × 15
2a. Seated wide and high pull-down		Sit upright at a cable pull-down machine with a bar attachment. Hold the bar with extended arms, using a neutral or pronated grip, depending on the bar used, your hands wider than shoulder-width. Keeping your elbows high, lean back slightly and squeeze the backs of your shoulders, pulling the bar toward your clavicle. Extend the arms back to the starting position. Repeat.	Week 1	2 × 10
			Week 2	3 × 12
			Week 3	4 × 10
			Week 4	5 × 10

(continued)

Table 7.6 His Shoulders 4: DB and Cable Shoulder Workout *(continued)*

Exercise	Photo	Instructions	Weeks	Sets × reps
2b. Lean away cable lateral raise		Stand with a low pulley to the right of you. Hold the handle with your left hand in a pronated grip (palm down). Hold on to the cable column with your right arm and lean your entire body to the left about 60 degrees. Keeping a consistent lean, laterally raise your left arm until your left hand is at shoulder height. Lower the cable and repeat for prescribed repetitions, then switch to the other side.	Week 1	2 × 10 per side
			Week 2	3 × 12 per side
			Week 3	4 × 10 per side
			Week 4	5 × 12 per side
3a. Wide-grip supinated cable row		Sit upright at a seated cable rowing machine, feet flat on the platform. Hold the bar with extended arms using a supinated grip with hands wider than shoulder-width. Keeping your elbows high, squeeze the backs of your shoulders and pulling the bar high to the chest. Extend the arms back to the starting position. Repeat.	Week 1	2 × 10
			Week 2	3 × 12
			Week 3	4 × 10
			Week 4	5 × 8
3b. BP pronated short T		Stand in front of a dual cable or JC band, your feet shoulder-width apart. With one handle in each hand at shoulder height, extend your arms in front of you in a pronated grip (palms down). Keeping your arms extended and palms facing down, squeeze the backs of your shoulders to open your arms laterally to create a T, contracting your back. Return 1/2 of the way to the starting position and open your arms again, staying in the zone where the rear delts don't have time to rest. Repeat through that short range of motion.	Week 1	2 × 15
			Week 2	3 × 20
			Week 3	4 × 25
			Week 4	5 × 30

HIS SHOULDERS 5: PRO BURN SHOULDERS

This 4-week program is a monster, professional-grade shoulder workout. It is performed on 2 separate days with a customary 2-exercise superset. However, our pros often like to complete each exercise in succession before going to the next exercise during their mass-building periods (non-competition phase), then they switch to this fast superset format during their precontest phase. Some pros who claimed their shoulders were weak areas in their physiques have even added a third day of lighter training to this program. Weeks 1 and 2 will be enough for most people, while weeks 3 and 4 should be attempted only by more advanced individuals who have a considerable training base.

Equipment

Shoulder press machine, cable machine with handle attachment, dumbbells, Smith machine, barbell, JC Sports Bands, Superband, adjustable weight bench, rear delt machine

Notes

Weeks 1 and 2: Perform 2 times per week.

Weeks 3 and 4: Perform 1 time per week (for advanced trainees only).

Table 7.7 His Shoulders 5: Pro Burn Shoulders

Exercise	Photo	Instructions	Weeks	Sets × reps
		DAY 1		
1a. Machine shoulder press		Sit at a shoulder press machine, feet flat on the floor and shoulder-width apart, your back against the backrest. Hold the handles at shoulder height, keeping your elbows flexed and in line with your torso. Extend your elbows, pressing the handles overhead. After your arms are fully extended, lower the handles to the starting position. Repeat.	Week 1	2 × 10
			Week 2	3 × 12
			Week 3	4 × 10
			Week 4	5 × 8
1b. Cable single-arm cross upright row		Stand with a low pulley to the left of you, your feet shoulder-width apart, your knees slightly bent, and use a pronated grip (palm facing you) to hold the cable handle in your right hand. Keep your body rigid and laterally raise your right elbow to pull the handle diagonally across your body to the right chest. Lower the handle to the starting position. Repeat for prescribed repetitions, then switch to the other side.	Week 1	2 × 10 per side
			Week 2	3 × 12 per side
			Week 3	4 × 10 per side
			Week 4	5 × 12 per side
2a. DB front raise (neutral grip)		Stand upright with your feet shoulder-width apart. Hold a dumbbell in each hand. Keeping a neutral grip (palms facing each other) and your elbows extended, raise the dumbbells in front of you to shoulder height. Lower the dumbbells to the starting position. Repeat.	Week 1	2 × 10
			Week 2	3 × 12
			Week 3	4 × 12
			Week 4	5 × 15
2b. BB behind-the-back grip shrug		Stand with a barbell behind you, racked at arm's length, and your feet shoulder-width apart. Holding the barbell behind your back, palms away from you (pronated grip), unrack the bar and raise your shoulders. Squeeze your trapezius muscles at the top and lower to the starting position. Repeat.	Week 1	2 × 10
			Week 2	3 × 12
			Week 3	4 × 15
			Week 4	5 × 15
		BAND FINISHER: CAN PERFORM AS A SUPERSET		
3a. BP Y (pulse at top end of movement)		Stand facing a set of bands at chest to shoulder height, your feet shoulder-width apart. Hold the handles with your arms extended in a neutral grip at shoulder height (palms facing each other and thumbs pointing up). Keeping your arms extended and your shoulder blades back and down (retracted and depressed), raise your arms overhead to create a Y. Lower your arms halfway to shoulder height. Repeat.	Week 1	2 × 15
			Week 2	3 × 20
			Week 3	4 × 15
			Week 4	5 × 20

(continued)

Table 7.7 His Shoulders 5: Pro Burn Shoulders *(continued)*

Exercise	Photo	Instructions	Weeks	Sets × reps
3b. BP pronated short T		Stand in front of a dual cable or JC band, your feet shoulder-width apart. With a handle in each hand at shoulder height, extend your arms in front of you in a pronated grip (palms down). Keeping your arms extended and palms facing down, squeeze the backs of your shoulders to open your arms laterally to create a T, contracting your back. Return 1/2 of the way to the starting position and open your arms again, staying in the zone where the rear delts don't have time to rest. Repeat through that short range of motion.	Week 1	2 × 15
			Week 2	3 × 20
			Week 3	4 × 15
			Week 4	5 × 20
DAY 2				
1a. Arnold press		Sit on a bench, your feet flat on the floor and shoulder-width apart. Hold a dumb-bell in each hand. Lift the dumbbells to chest level, your elbows flexed and side by side, palms facing your chest. Extend your elbows, pressing the dumbbells up, while rotating your palms out so the arms are fully extended above your head and your palms face away from you. Lower the dumbbells to the starting position. Repeat.	Week 1	2 × 10
			Week 2	3 × 12
			Week 3	4 × 10
			Week 4	5 × 8
1b. Lean away DB lateral raise		Stand with a sturdy column to your right. Hold a dumbbell in a neutral grip with your left hand. Hold on to the column with your right arm and lean your entire body to the left about 60 degrees. Keeping a consis-tent lean, laterally raise the dumbbell until your left hand is at shoulder height. Lower the dumbbell and repeat for prescribed repetitions, then switch to the other side.	Week 1	2 × 10 per side
			Week 2	3 × 12 per side
			Week 3	4 × 12 per side
			Week 4	5 × 15 per side
2a. Machine rear delt lift		Sit at the rear delt machine, your feet flat on the floor and shoulder-width apart and your chest against the chest pad. Hold on to the handles in front of you in a pronated grip and with your elbows slightly bent. Pull the handles laterally out to your sides and back, contracting your rear delts. Slowly return the handles to the starting position. Repeat.	Week 1	2 × 10
			Week 2	3 × 12
			Week 3	4 × 12
			Week 4	5 × 15

Exercise	Photo	Instructions	Weeks	Sets × reps
2b. DB shrug		Stand upright with your feet shoulder-width apart. Hold a dumbbell in each hand. Keeping your palms facing your body, raise your shoulders, contracting your trapezius muscles. Slowly lower your shoulders to the starting position. Repeat.	Week 1	2 × 10
			Week 2	3 × 12
			Week 3	4 × 15
			Week 4	5 × 15
BAND FINISHER: CAN PERFORM AS A SUPERSET				
3a. BP Y (pulse at top end of movement)		Stand facing a set of bands at chest to shoulder height, your feet shoulder-width apart. Hold the handles in a neutral grip (palms facing each other and thumbs pointing up) with your arms extended at shoulder height. Keeping your arms extended and your shoulder blades back and down (retracted and depressed), raise your arms overhead to create a Y. Lower your arms a quarter of the way to shoulder height. Repeat.	Week 1	2 × 15
			Week 2	3 × 20
			Week 3	4 × 15
			Week 4	5 × 20
3b. BP pronated short T		Stand in front of a dual cable or JC band, your feet shoulder-width apart. Hold a handle in each hand at shoulder height, your arms extended in front of you in a pronated grip (palms down). Keeping your arms extended and palms facing down, squeeze the backs of your shoulder to open your arms laterally to create a T, contracting your back. Come back 1/2 of the way to the starting position and open the arms again, staying in the zone where the rear delts don't have time to rest. Repeat through that short range of motion.	Week 1	2 × 15
			Week 2	3 × 20
			Week 3	4 × 15
			Week 4	5 × 20

HER SHOULDERS 1: HEALTHY SHOULDERS WORKOUT

This 4-week program is a standard rehab/prehab workout for the shoulders. These are the remedial exercises I used to help rehab a SLAP tear, 4 weeks before the 1997 U.S. Open weightlifting competition. Since then, we have used these exercises to warm up, get a little pump, and keep your shoulders healthy. They are not the most functional exercises, but they are certainly useful enough to make it into this book. We like to use the pink JC Sports Bands for most applications, but stronger people can use the orange JC Sports Bands. Weeks 1 and 2 will be enough for most people, while weeks 3 and 4 should be attempted only by more advanced individuals who have a considerable training base.

Equipment

Bands with handles such as JC Sports Bands or JC Traveler

Notes

Weeks 1 and 2: Perform 2 times per week.

Weeks 3 and 4: Perform 1 time per week (for advanced trainees only).

Table 7.8 Her Shoulders 1: Healthy Shoulders Workout

Exercise	Photo	Instructions	Weeks	Sets × reps
1a. BP Y		Stand facing a set of bands at chest to shoulder height, your feet shoulder-width apart. Hold the handles with your arms extended in a neutral grip (palms facing each other and thumbs pointing up) at shoulder height. Keeping your arms extended and your shoulder blades back and down (retracted and depressed), raise your arms overhead to create a Y. Lower your arms to shoulder height. Repeat.	Week 1	2 × 10
			Week 2	3 × 15
			Week 3	4 × 15
			Week 4	5 × 20
1b. BP T		Stand facing a set of bands at chest to shoulder height, your feet shoulder-width apart. Hold the handles with your arms extended in a supinated grip (palms facing up and thumbs pointing out) at shoulder height. Keeping your arms fully extended and your shoulder blades back and down (retracted and depressed), open your arms laterally to create a T. Bring your arms back to the starting position. Repeat.	Week 1	2 × 10
			Week 2	3 × 15
			Week 3	4 × 15
			Week 4	5 × 20
1c. BP I		Stand facing a set of bands at chest to shoulder height, your feet shoulder-width apart. Hold the handles with your arms extended in a supinated grip (palms facing up and thumbs pointing out) at shoulder height. Keeping your arms fully extended and your shoulder blades back and down (retracted and depressed), pull your arms down as close as you can to the sides of your hips, thumbs pointing behind you. Bring your arms back to the starting position. Repeat.	Week 1	2 × 10
			Week 2	3 × 15
			Week 3	4 × 15
			Week 4	5 × 20

HER SHOULDERS 2: FUNCTIONAL SHOULDERS

This 4-week program is a functional training program for the shoulders. It is arranged in two 3-exercise circuits for maximum training efficiency. You can also rearrange the exercise into 3 circuits, such as 1a and 2a, 1b and 2b, and 1c and 2c. This is a functional workout for people interested in getting a considerable amount of core training while also developing nice tone in their shoulders. If rearranged, this workout can make a great boot camp circuit that targets upper-body endurance. Weeks 1 and 2 will be enough for most people, while weeks 3 and 4 should be attempted only by more advanced individuals who have a considerable training base.

Equipment

Dumbbells, cable machine with handle attachment or bands with handles (such as JC Sports Band or a JC Traveler), battle rope, weight plate

Notes

Weeks 1 and 2: Perform 2 times per week.

Weeks 3 and 4: Perform 1 time per week (for advanced trainees only).

Table 7.9 Her Shoulders 2: Functional Shoulders

Exercise	Photo	Instructions	Weeks	Sets × reps
1a. DB overhead press		Stand with your feet shoulder-width apart. Hold a dumbbell in each hand at shoulder height, palms facing away from you. Press both dumbbells overhead until arms are fully extended and dumbbells are in line with your shoulders. Lower the dumbbells to the starting position and repeat.	Week 1	2 × 10 per side
			Week 2	3 × 12 per side
			Week 3	4 × 10 per side
			Week 4	5 × 8 per side
1b. Low band alternating upright row		Attach a band to a low attachment point (can use a low cable set) or stand on the nylon strap. Stand facing the band, holding a handle in each hand. Keeping your hands shoulder-width apart, pull straight up with your right arm, raising your elbow until it's at chest level. Lower the right handle and simultaneously upright row to chest level with your left arm. Repeat for prescribed repetitions.	Week 1	2 × 10 per side
			Week 2	3 × 12 per side
			Week 3	4 × 12 per side
			Week 4	5 × 15 per side
1c. Bent-over rope circles (in-out)		Stand with a secured battle rope in front of you, your feet shoulder-width apart. Hold the ends of the rope at arm's length in front of you. Bend over at the waist. Hold this position while creating clockwise circles with your right hand and counterclockwise circles with your left hand. Repeat for prescribed repetitions, then switch directions.	Week 1	2 × 15 per direction
			Week 2	3 × 20 per direction
			Week 3	4 × 20 per direction
			Week 4	5 × 25 per direction

(continued)

Table 7.9 Her Shoulders 2: Functional Shoulders *(continued)*

Exercise	Photo	Instructions	Weeks	Sets × reps
2a. DB cross uppercut		Stand with your feet shoulder-width apart. Hold a dumbbell in each hand using a supinated grip (palms up), elbows flexed to 90 degrees. Using your right hand, uppercut across your body toward your left shoulder, allowing a slight body rotation to the left. As you bring your right arm back to the starting position, perform a cross uppercut with your left hand, bringing it across your body toward the right shoulder. Repeat.	Week 1	2 × 10 per side
			Week 2	3 × 12 per side
			Week 3	4 × 10 per side
			Week 4	5 × 8 per side
2b. Figure eight with weight plate		Stand upright, holding a weight plate in front of you at chest level, your arms fully extended. Paint a figure eight with the weight plate, from the top of your head to your waist. Perform in both directions.	Week 1	2 × 6 each direction
			Week 2	3 × 8 each direction
			Week 3	4 × 10 each direction
			Week 4	5 × 8 each direction
2c. Bent-over rope wave (up-down)		Stand with a secured battle rope in front of you, your feet shoulder-width apart. Hold the ends of the rope at arm's length in front of you. Bend over at the waist. Hold this position while bringing your right hand up as your left hand goes down and vice versa. You should create vertical waves in the rope. Repeat for prescribed number of repetitions.	Week 1	2 × 15 per side
			Week 2	3 × 20 per side
			Week 3	4 × 20 per side
			Week 4	5 × 25 per side

HER SHOULDERS 3: DB AND ROPE SHOULDERS

This 4-week program is a dumbbell and battle rope metabolic protocol for the shoulders. It is arranged in three 2-exercise circuits for maximum muscular endurance in a time-efficient manner. The dumbbell exercise strengthens, tones, and prefatigues the shoulders, while the ropes provide endurance and volumize the entire shoulder area. These exercises also can be used in a group circuit with the goal to provide a lot of upper-body toning and killer cardio. Weeks 1 and 2 will be enough for most people, while weeks 3 and 4 should be attempted only by more advanced individuals who have a considerable training base.

Equipment

Dumbbells, battle rope

Notes

Weeks 1 and 2: Perform 2 times per week.

Weeks 3 and 4: Perform 1 time per week (advanced trainees only).

Table 7.10 Her Shoulders 3: Dumbbell and Rope Shoulders

Exercise	Photo	Instructions	Weeks	Sets × reps
1a. Running curl		Stand upright, holding a dumbbell in each hand. Keeping your hands shoulder-width apart, bend your elbows 90 degrees. Rapidly pump one arm forward and the other backward, as if you were running. One repetition is a full arm-swing cycle (i.e., forward and back). Repeat.	Week 1	2 × 10 per side
			Week 2	3 × 12 per side
			Week 3	4 × 10 per side
			Week 4	5 × 8 per side
1b. Rope up and down		Stand with a secured battle rope in front of you, feet shoulder-width apart. Hold the ends of the rope at arm's length in front of you. Keeping your body rigid, simultaneously bring both hands up and then down to create symmetrical and identical waves in the rope.	Week 1	2 × 10
			Week 2	3 × 15
			Week 3	4 × 20
			Week 4	5 × 25
2a. DB alternating upright row		Stand upright, holding a dumbbell in each hand with palms facing the body (pronated). Keeping your hands shoulder-width apart, use your right arm to pull the dumbbell up to chest level, raising your elbow until it's at shoulder level. Lower the right dumbbell and simultaneously upright row the left dumbbell. Repeat.	Week 1	2 × 10 per side
			Week 2	3 × 12 per side
			Week 3	4 × 10 per side
			Week 4	5 × 8 per side
2b. Rope circles (clockwise and counterclockwise)		Stand with a secured battle rope in front of you, your feet shoulder-width apart. Hold the ends of the rope at arm's length in front of you. Keeping your body rigid, simultaneously create clockwise circles with your right hand and counterclockwise circles with your left hand. Perform repetitions indicated and reverse direction.	Week 1	2 × 10 per direction
			Week 2	3 × 15 per direction
			Week 3	4 × 20 per direction
			Week 4	5 × 25 per direction
3a. DB lateral 3D 60 raise		Stand upright, holding a dumbbell in each hand by your sides, your palms facing in. Separate a lateral raise into 3 sections: lower third, middle third, and top third. For the first movement, keeping a slight bend in your elbow, perform short and fast lateral pumps through the first third of the range. For the second movement, keeping a slight bend in your elbow, perform short and fast lateral pumps through the middle third of the range. For the third movement, keeping a slight bend in your elbow, perform short and fast lateral pumps through the top third of the range. Repeat for prescribed repetitions in each of the 3 ranges.	Week 1	2 × 15 + 15 + 15
			Week 2	3 × 10 + 10 + 10
			Week 3	4 × 15 + 15 + 15
			Week 4	5 × 10 + 10 + 10

(continued)

Table 7.10   Her Shoulders 3: Dumbbell and Rope Shoulders *(continued)*

Exercise	Photo	Instructions	Weeks	Sets × reps
3b. Rope circles (counterclockwise and clockwise)		Stand with a secured battle rope in front of you, your feet shoulder-width apart. Hold the ends of the rope at arm's length in front of you. Keeping your body rigid, simultaneously create counterclockwise circles with your right hand and clockwise circles with your left hand. Perform the repetitions indicated and reverse direction.	Week 1	2 × 10 per direction
			Week 2	3 × 15 per direction
			Week 3	4 × 20 per direction
			Week 4	5 × 25 per direction

HER SHOULDERS 4: DB AND CABLES/BANDS SHOULDERS

This 4-week program is a dumbbell and cable program that can easily pack on or tone the entire shoulder musculature. You can use bands instead of pulleys and make this a great home workout. It is arranged in three 2-exercise circuits for maximum training efficiency. Some of our big athletes go at a slower pace and perform each exercise in succession, using dumbbells and resting a little more between sets. This approach takes well over an hour and a half to do the higher volumes of weeks 3 and 4, especially week 4. The added rest time allows more weight to be used in each exercise, which in turn provides better muscular development. However, with this two-movement superset format, weeks 1 and 2 will be enough for most people who don't have too much time to train and want to train at a faster pace. Weeks 3 and 4 should be attempted only by more advanced individuals who have a considerable training base (more than two years of steady training).

Equipment

Dumbbells, dual cable machine with two single-handle attachments (or a JC Traveler or Predator Jr.), adjustable weight bench

Notes

Weeks 1 and 2: Perform 2 times per week.

Weeks 3 and 4: Perform 1 time per week (for advanced trainees only).

Table 7.11   Her Shoulders 4: Dumbbell and Cables/Bands Shoulders

Exercise	Photo	Instructions	Weeks	Sets × reps
1a. DB overhead press		Stand upright with your feet shoulder-width apart. Hold a dumbbell in each hand at shoulder height, just outside of shoulder width, with your palms facing to the front. Press the dumbbells overhead until your arms are fully extended. Lower the dumbbells to the starting position. Repeat.	Week 1	2 × 10
			Week 2	3 × 12
			Week 3	4 × 10
			Week 4	5 × 8

Exercise	Photo	Instructions	Weeks	Sets × reps
1b. DB double-arm upright row		Stand upright with your feet shoulder-width apart. Hold a pair of dumbbells in each hand in front of your thighs, your palms facing you. Simultaneously pull both dumbbells up to your chest, laterally raising your elbows to shoulder height. Lower the dumbbells to the starting position. Repeat.	Week 1	2 × 10
			Week 2	3 × 12
			Week 3	4 × 10
			Week 4	5 × 12
2a. DB lateral raise		Stand upright with your feet shoulder-width apart. Hold a dumbbell in each hand, palms facing your body. Keeping your elbows slightly flexed, laterally raise your arms to shoulder height. Lower the dumbbells to the starting position. Repeat.	Week 1	2 × 10
			Week 2	3 × 12
			Week 3	4 × 12
			Week 4	5 × 15
2b. Cable single-arm bent-over lateral raise		Stand with a low pulley or band to the left of you, your feet shoulder-width apart and your knees slightly bent. Hold the cable in your right hand with a neutral grip (palm facing the cable). Bend over at the hips, keeping your torso rigid. Raise your right elbow to shoulder height. Lower the handle to the starting position. Repeat for prescribed repetitions, then switch to the other side.	Week 1	2 × 10 per side
			Week 2	3 × 12 per side
			Week 3	4 × 10 per side
			Week 4	5 × 10 per side
3a. DB single-arm bent-over wide row (neutral to supinated)		Stand in front of a weight bench, your feet shoulder-width apart. Flex at the hips and place your left hand on the bench for support. Hold a dumbbell in your right hand in a neutral grip (palm facing in). Row the dumbbell wide while turning it clockwise so that the palm faces the bench when at the top of the row. Lower the dumbbell to the starting position. Repeat for prescribed repetitions, then switch to the other side.	Week 1	2 × 10 per side
			Week 2	3 × 12 per side
			Week 3	4 × 10 per side
			Week 4	5 × 10 per side
3b. Reverse cross cable fly (mid-height)		Stand with your feet shoulder-width apart between 2 pulleys at shoulder height (or use bands). Hold the left cable in your right hand and the right cable in your left hand. (You don't need handles; you can hold on to the knobs that hold the carabiners.) Keeping your elbows slightly flexed, start with your arms crossed so your right hand is in front of your left shoulder and your left hand is in front of your right shoulder. Laterally open your arms until they are in line with your shoulders and your body forms a T. Bring your arms to the starting crossed position. Repeat.	Week 1	2 × 10
			Week 2	3 × 12
			Week 3	4 × 12
			Week 4	5 × 15

HER SHOULDERS 5: PRO PHYSIQUE SHOULDERS

This 4-week program is a hard core shoulder program for professional fitness competitors. It is arranged in three 2-exercise circuits for maximum training efficiency. However, many professional physique competitors perform each exercise in succession during their muscle-building phase then go to the circuit format when they are ready to diet and cut down. Also you can rearrange the order of the exercises, such as 1a and 2a, 1b and 2b, and then the finisher, to create different circuits. Weeks 1 and 2 will be enough for most people, while weeks 3 and 4 should be attempted only by more advanced individuals who have a considerable training base.

Equipment

Landmine machine, barbell, dumbbells, dual cable machine (with rope and single-handle attachments), weight bench with back support or adjustable incline bench

Notes

Weeks 1 and 2: Perform 2 times per week.

Weeks 3 and 4: Perform 1 time per week (for advanced trainees only).

Table 7.12   Her Shoulders 5: Pro Physique Shoulders

Exercise	Photo	Instructions	Weeks	Sets × reps
DAY 1				
1a. Landmine press		Stand in front of the end of a barbell that has the opposite end secured in a landmine machine, your feet shoulder-with apart. Hold the end of the barbell in your right hand, to the right of your right shoulder. Press the end of the barbell up until your right arm is fully extended. Lower the barbell to the starting position. Repeat for prescribed repetitions, then switch to the other side.	Week 1	2 × 10 per side
			Week 2	3 × 12 per side
			Week 3	4 × 10 per side
			Week 4	5 × 8 per side
1b. 45-degree lateral raise		Stand upright with your feet shoulder-width apart. Hold a dumbbell in each hand, your palms facing your body (neutral grip). Keeping your elbows slightly flexed, raise your arms diagonally 45 degrees until at shoulder height. Lower the dumbbells to the starting position. Repeat.	Week 1	2 × 10
			Week 2	3 × 12
			Week 3	4 × 15
			Week 4	5 × 12
2a. DB full overhead lateral raise		Stand upright with your feet shoulder-width apart. Hold a dumbbell in each hand, your palms facing the front (supinated grip). Keeping your elbows slightly flexed, raise your arms laterally in a big semi-circle until the dumbbells are overhead. Lower the dumbbells to the starting position. Repeat.	Week 1	2 × 10
			Week 2	3 × 12
			Week 3	4 × 10
			Week 4	5 × 10

Exercise	Photo	Instructions	Weeks	Sets × reps
2b. Bent-over cross cable rear delt fly		Stand with your feet shoulder-width apart between 2 pulleys set at shoulder height. Hold the left cable in your right hand and the right cable in your left hand. (You don't need handles; you can hold on to the knobs that hold the carabiners). Bend at your hips, keeping your back straight and your elbows slightly flexed. Start with your arms crossed so your right hand is in front of your left shoulder and your left hand is in front of your right shoulder. Laterally open your arms until they are in line with your shoulders. Lower your arms to the starting crossed position. Repeat.	Week 1	2 × 10
			Week 2	3 × 12
			Week 3	4 × 12
			Week 4	5 × 15
DB FINISHER: USE DUMBBELLS THAT ALLOW YOU TO PERFORM BENT-OVER LATERAL RAISES FOR 12 REPETITIONS. PERFORM 3A FOR 12 REPETITIONS (WEEKS 1 AND 2) OR 10 REPETITIONS (WEEKS 3 AND 4) AND ALL OTHERS TO FAILURE.				
3a. DB bent-over lateral raise		Stand upright with your feet shoulder-width apart. Hold a dumbbell in each hand, your palms facing each other (in). Bend at the hips, keeping your back straight and your elbows slightly flexed. Laterally raise your arms to shoulder height. Lower the dumbbells to the starting position. Repeat.	Week 1	1 × 12
			Week 2	1 × 12
			Week 3	2 × 10
			Week 4	2 or 3 × 10
3b. DB lateral raise		Stand upright with your feet shoulder-width apart. Hold a dumbbell in each hand, your palms facing your body. Keeping your elbows slightly flexed, laterally raise your arms to shoulder height. Lower the dumbbells to the starting position. Repeat.	Week 1	1 × failure
			Week 2	1 × failure
			Week 3	2 × failure
			Week 4	2 or 3 × failure
3c. DB front raise		Stand upright with your feet shoulder-width apart. Hold a dumbbell in each hand. Keeping a neutral grip (palms facing each other) and elbows extended, raise the dumbbells in front of you to shoulder height. Lower the dumbbells to the starting position. Repeat.	Week 1	1 × failure
			Week 2	1 × failure
			Week 3	2 × failure
			Week 4	2 or 3 × failure

(continued)

Table 7.12 Her Shoulders 5: Pro Physique Shoulders *(continued)*

Exercise	Photo	Instructions	Weeks	Sets × reps
3d. DB overhead press		Stand upright with your feet shoulder-width apart. Hold a dumbbell in each hand at shoulder height, just outside of shoulder width, your palms facing to the front. Press the dumbbells overhead until your arms are fully extended. Lower the dumbbells to the starting position. Repeat.	Week 1	1 × failure
			Week 2	1 × failure
			Week 3	2 × failure
			Week 4	2 or 3 × failure
DAY 2				
1a. DB elbow in seated shoulder press		Sit on a bench with a back support (shoulder press bench or adjustable bench). Keep your feet flat on the floor and shoulder-width apart. Hold a dumbbell in each hand. Lift the dumbbells inside shoulder width, your palms facing each other and your elbows resting on your ribs. Keeping your forearms and elbows less than shoulder width and press dumbbells up well above head level. Lower the dumbbells to the starting position. Repeat.	Week 1	2 × 10
			Week 2	3 × 12
			Week 3	4 × 10
			Week 4	5 × 8
1b. Behind-the-back DB lateral raise		Stand slightly leaning back with your feet shoulder-width apart. Hold a dumbbell in each hand behind your rear pockets, your palms facing your body. Keep your elbows slightly flexed and laterally raise your arms, keeping your thumbs up until the dumbbells are at shoulder height. Lower the dumbbells to the starting position. Repeat.	Week 1	2 × 10
			Week 2	3 × 12
			Week 3	4 × 15
			Week 4	5 × 12
2a. Head rope pull		Sit upright with your feet flat on the floor and shoulder-width apart on a rowing machine (or cable machine with a middle pulley) with a rope attachment. Holding the ends of the rope in a pronated grip, pull the rope back toward your face until your hands are on each side of your head (as if you were showing your arm muscles to someone). Extend your arms forward to the starting position. Repeat.	Week 1	2 × 10
			Week 2	3 × 12
			Week 3	4 × 10
			Week 4	5 × 8
2b. Bent-over single-arm cable rear delt raise		Stand with a low pulley to your left. Hold the handle in your right hand with a pronated grip. Bend at the waist, keeping your back parallel to the ground and your right arm hanging straight down (cable in hand). Keeping a slight bend in your right elbow, laterally raise your right hand until it is at shoulder height and your arm is parallel to the floor. Slowly return your right hand to the starting position. Repeat for prescribed repetitions, then switch to the other side.	Week 1	2 × 10 per side
			Week 2	3 × 12 per side
			Week 3	4 × 12 per side
			Week 4	5 × 15 per side

Exercise	Photo	Instructions	Weeks	Sets × reps
DB FINISHER: USE DUMBBELLS THAT ALLOW YOU TO PERFORM BENT-OVER LATERAL RAISES FOR 12 REPETITIONS. PERFORM 3A FOR 12 REPETITIONS (WEEKS 1 AND 2) OR 10 REPETITIONS (WEEKS 3 AND 4) THEN ALL OTHERS TO FAILURE.				
3a. DB bent-over lateral raise		Stand upright with your feet shoulder-width apart. Hold a dumbbell in each hand, your palms facing each other. Bend at the hips, keeping your back straight and your elbows slightly flexed. Laterally raise your arms to shoulder height. Lower the dumbbells to the starting position. Repeat.	Week 1	1 × 12
			Week 2	1 × 12
			Week 3	2 × 10
			Week 4	2 or 3 × 10
3b. DB lateral raise		Stand upright with your feet shoulder-width apart. Hold a dumbbell in each hand, your palms facing your body. Keeping your elbows slightly flexed, laterally raise your arms to shoulder height. Lower the dumbbells to the starting position. Repeat.	Week 1	1 × failure
			Week 2	1 × failure
			Week 3	2 × failure
			Week 4	2 or 3 × failure
3c. DB front raise		Stand upright with your feet shoulder-width apart. Hold a dumbbell in each hand. Keeping a neutral grip (palms facing each other) and your elbows extended, raise the dumbbells in front of you to shoulder height. Lower the dumbbells to the starting position. Repeat.	Week 1	1 × failure
			Week 2	1 × failure
			Week 3	2 × failure
			Week 4	2 or 3 × failure
3d. DB overhead press		Stand upright with your feet shoulder-width apart. Hold a dumbbell in each hand at shoulder height, just outside of shoulder width, your palms facing to the front. Press the dumbbells overhead until your arms are fully extended. Lower the dumbbells to the starting position. Repeat.	Week 1	1 × failure
			Week 2	1 × failure
			Week 3	2 × failure
			Week 4	2 or 3 × failure

Summary

The shoulders are a complex joint, and training them can be a challenge, but they also provide an opportunity for diverse programming. The shoulders certainly are one of my favorite body parts to train and program. I know you have found a couple of new exercises and some exciting workouts in this chapter. If you put in the work, the result can be extremely dramatic in aesthetics as well as performance. If your shoulders are temperamental, use a longer warm-up, spread the volume over more days in a week, and use partial ranges of motion that are pain free. I can't emphasize enough that muscles are muscles and respond to the same stimulus in both men and women. Therefore, don't be afraid to mix and match these workouts to create your own unique workout.

Also, don't be afraid to spread the volume over three sessions in a week. The training of a body part only one time a week is effective, but I've seen professionals spread the volume over two or three training sessions. This is especially effective with the shoulders since the shoulders can handle volume a lot easier than they can handle load.

CHAPTER 8

Chest

This chapter focuses on an area that men especially are interested in developing: the chest. I offer everything here from bodyweight and park-type workouts to monster bodybuilding workouts. I incorporate various pieces of equipment so you can train your chest at home, when you travel, or when at a well-equipped gym. As with all the other workouts, I provide a progression schedule so that beginners and advanced trainees can select the appropriate training volume.

Like the shoulders, the chest is right there in your face: Everyone looks at it, and depending on what they see, they form an opinion. Men are especially in tune to chest development for many reasons. The most often asked question of a muscular man is, "What do you bench press?" The muscle group required for the bench press is the chest, so the question is understandable. The workouts in this chapter will build the chest and improve your bench press as well. Additionally, the chest is the first big muscle group that protrudes from the body. It almost serves as a "hedge" for the body, establishing a boundary as well as making a statement of power and focus of attention in both sexes. Although many women don't necessarily want big pecs, they do want a toned chest, shoulders, and triceps, which are all part of chest work. Working the chest is important for both men and women.

Although push-ups and bench presses are the most popular exercises for the chest, I provide other exercises to add some spice to your training. However, regardless of the type of training you do, the biceps (especially the long head) are involved in many of the straight pressing movements, even chest flys. Often the biceps take a beating during chest work. Therefore, I have developed a few ways to minimize overuse symptoms and pain that can affect the biceps tendon due to excessive pressing motions. Biceps tendonitis, which can occur when you train your chest heavy, can be caused by a variety of issues, from weak rotator cuff muscles to other muscular imbalances. A few principles have helped me work through this condition. Here are some of the important strategies I have used successfully to deal with anterior shoulder pain due to biceps tendonitis. These strategies will help you avoid what hurts, rest the joints or tissues, and work around and on the opposite side of the injury.

The first time I suffered a serious bout of biceps tendonitis (right in the anterior shoulder), I took a break from all bench pressing. Instead, I focused on pulling and external rotation exercises. I did band flys and focused on ranges of motions that did not hurt the shoulder or biceps. I did that for about six weeks to rest the inflamed tissues, and the results were awesome. Although I don't understand the exact mechanism of recovery, and I'm fine with that, this approach helped me get around the issue and allow healing while getting stronger. In this chapter, I include some band and fly workouts in case you have biceps tendonitis and want to rest your biceps while working the chest and core.

Muscular development is about muscle tension and repair due to the cellular disruption caused by the tension the muscles experience. The amount of tension and disruption has always been associated with the load and volume of an exercise. After many years of constantly using more loads, the joints can take a beating, and conditions such as arthritis can develop. Using lighter loads, slower tempos, and better mind-to-muscle connection puts tension on a muscle using less weight and fewer sets and reps. This strategy is especially good for individuals in their 40s, 50s, and 60s who may have joint issues. It can also be used by younger individuals who want to be strong, fit, and healthy but avoid the overuse issues seen in athletes who push for maximum loads. Obviously, some of these strategies may not apply to athletes who require extreme levels of strength and conditioning, but they are certainly worth considering by those who are looking for health, fitness, and body transformation and those in sports that don't require insane strength.

With this in mind, feel free to alter the volume of these workouts if you are training at a slower tempo. For example, if you are using a three-second eccentric, two-second hold, and three-second concentric, feel free to cut the reps in half. I'm not a huge fan of very slow training, but I do occasionally use it when I don't feel like training heavy but I want to get a good pump. As a former combat athlete, I have a bias toward hard and fast strength training, and that has led me to many injuries. Due to necessity, I'm now open to other methods and use slower training (time under tension) to get results with less weight. Try this approach with these chest workouts, and I guarantee you fewer shoulder issues and better chest development.

I have suggested progressions for beginner and advanced trainees in almost all workouts. However, if you have not trained in more than two months and feel like you need to build a base or you are inexperienced in training, I strongly recommend you finish this two-week program before attempting any of the workouts in this chapter.

WEEK 1: DO EACH EXERCISE SEPARATELY

Monday, Wednesday, Friday
Bodyweight push-up (1-2 sets × 10-15 repetitions)
Diamond push-up (1-2 sets × 10-15 repetitions)

WEEK 2: DO EACH EXERCISE SEPARATELY

Monday, Wednesday, Friday
Bodyweight push-up (2-3 sets × 15-20 repetitions)
Lateral shuffle push-up (2-3 sets × 15-20 repetitions)
Diamond push-up (2-3 sets × 15-20 repetitions)

HIS CHEST 1: CHEST TRAINING IN THE PARK

This 4-week bodyweight training program for the chest can be done at a park just as easily as at the gym. During my high school days, many of us lived on these types of workouts, spending hours talking, kidding around, and doing pull-ups, dips, push-ups, squats, lunges, stairs, and sprints. Sometimes we would hit just one body part; this workout represents that approach. It's arranged so each exercise is done in succession with a little more rest between sets for maximum training efficiency. However feel free to rearrange the exercises, such as starting with dips ending with a diamond push-up flush. This is a perfect workout for people who are interested in chiseling the chest while also focusing on the triceps. Weeks 1 and 2 will be enough for most people, while weeks 3 and 4 should be attempted only by more advanced individuals who have a considerable training base.

Equipment

Parallel bars, bench, or elevated platform

Notes

Weeks 1 and 2: Perform 2 times per week.

Weeks 3 and 4: Perform 1 time per week (for very advanced trainees only).

Table 8.1 His Chest 1: Chest Training in the Park

Exercise	Photo	Instructions	Weeks	Sets × reps
1. Dip		Stand between 2 parallel bars. Holding on to the bars, lift your body, elbows extended. Lower your body until you feel a good stretch in your upper chest and shoulders. Extend your elbows to lift your body, contracting the triceps. Repeat.	Week 1	2 × 10
			Week 2	3 × 12
			Week 3	4 × 20
			Week 4	5 × 25
2. Decline push-up		Stand facing away from a bench or elevated platform. Place your feet on the edge of the bench or platform and put your hands on the ground, shoulder-width apart. Keeping your body straight, flex your elbows and lower your body until the chest is 4-5 inches (12 cm) from the ground. Extend your elbows to return to the starting position. Repeat.	Week 1	2 × 10
			Week 2	3 × 12
			Week 3	4 × 15
			Week 4	5 × 20
3. Parallel bar push-up		Place your hands and feet on 2 parallel bars, with your body in a push-up position. Flex your elbows to lower your chest to the level of the bars. Extend your elbows to return to the starting position. Repeat.	Week 1	2 × 10
			Week 2	3 × 12
			Week 3	4 × 20
			Week 4	5 × 25

(continued)

Table 8.1 His Chest 1: Chest Training in the Park *(continued)*

Exercise	Photo	Instructions	Weeks	Sets × reps
4. Diamond push-up		Get into a push-up position with your index fingers and thumbs touching, forming a diamond shape. Your hands can be on the ground or elevated. Flex your elbows to lower your chest until it's just above your fingers. Extend your elbows to return to the starting position. Repeat.	Week 1	2 × 10
			Week 2	3 × 12
			Week 3	4 × 15
			Week 4	5 × 15

HIS CHEST 2: FUNCTIONAL CHEST

This 4-week program is a functional training program for the chest that uses body weight, medicine balls, and cables or bands. Although this is a functional workout, don't think for an instant that it's not hard and it won't get you strong. I recommend you approach this workout as a normal strength program and perform the exercises in succession, with plenty of rest between each set and total concentration and effort. This way, you will be able to put maximum effort into each exercise and hit the repetition ranges. Weeks 1 and 2 will be enough for most people, while weeks 3 and 4 should be attempted only by more advanced individuals who have a considerable training base.

Equipment

Medicine ball, band with handles (such as the JC Sports Band, Traveler, or Predator)

Notes

Weeks 1 and 2: Perform 2 times per week.

Weeks 3 and 4: Perform 1 time per week (for very advanced trainees only).

Table 8.2 His Chest 2: Functional Chest

Exercise	Photo	Instructions	Weeks	Sets × reps
1. MB single-arm push-off		Get into a push-up position, with the left hand on the ground and the right hand on a medicine ball. Put your hands shoulder-width apart. Flex your elbows to lower your chest to about an inch (3 cm) above the ground. Extend your elbows to lift your body back to the starting position. As your elbows reach full extension, the hand on the ground should push up, aggressively coming off the ground. As that hand lands, lower back into a push-up. Repeat. After completing the desired repetitions, switch to the other side.	Week 1	2 × 6-10 per side
			Week 2	3 × 8-12 per side
			Week 3	4 × 12-15 per side
			Week 4	5 × 15 per side
2. T push-up		Get into a push-up position. Flex your elbows to lower your chest. Once your chest reaches an inch (3 cm) above the ground, extend your elbows to lift your body back to the starting position. As your elbows reach full extension, lift your right arm, rotating your chest as you come into a side plank. Lower your right arm back to push-up position. Repeat. After completing the desired repetitions, switch to the other side.	Week 1	2 × 10 per side
			Week 2	3 × 12 per side
			Week 3	4 × 10 per side
			Week 4	5 × 10 per side

Exercise	Photo	Instructions	Weeks	Sets × reps
3. MB crossover push-up		Get into a push-up position, with one hand on the ground and the other on a medicine ball. Put your hands shoulder-width apart. Flex your elbows to lower your chest until it is an inch (3 cm) above the ground. Extend your elbows to lift your body. As your elbows reach full extension, roll the medicine ball to the other hand and perform another push-up. Repeat.	Week 1	2 × 8-10 per side
			Week 2	3 × 10-12 per side
			Week 3	4 × 8-10 per side
			Week 4	5 × 10 per side
4. MB hands-on-ball push-up		Get into a push-up position with both hands on a medicine ball. Flex your elbows to lower your chest to an inch (3 cm) above the ball. Extend your elbows to lift your body. Repeat.	Week 1	2 × 8-10
			Week 2	3 × 10-12
			Week 3	4 × 12-15
			Week 4	5 × 12-15
5. BP single-arm fly		Stand with a band attached to a point at chest height and to the right of you. Hold the handle in your right hand, your palm facing forward. Keeping your elbow slightly flexed and torso stable, bring your arm out and up to shoulder height, keeping your torso stable. Return your arm to the starting position. Repeat. After completing the desired repetitions, switch to the other side.	Week 1	2 × 10 per side
			Week 2	3 × 12 per side
			Week 3	4 × 15 per side
			Week 4	5 × 20 per side

HIS CHEST 3: DB AND CABLE CHEST

This 4-week program is a heavy-duty dumbbell and cable program for the chest. If you don't have a cable machine, you can use heavy-duty bands like the JC Predator Jr. You can also consider substituting any dumbbell exercise for a barbell or even a machine exercise to change the workout. This is a high-volume workout perfect for gaining mass while using lighter loads and less time under tension. You can cut the repetitions to 5-8 if you are spending 5-7 seconds per rep. The volume of the flys also allows for good sculpting and separation of the chest muscles. Weeks 1 and 2 will be enough for most people, while weeks 3 and 4 should be attempted only by more advanced individuals who have a considerable training base.

Equipment

Incline bench, dumbbells, flat bench, double cable machine with attachments or bands, decline bench

Notes

Weeks 1 and 2: Perform 2 times per week.

Weeks 3 and 4: Perform 1 time per week (for very advanced trainees only).

Table 8.3 His Chest 3: Dumbbell and Cable Chest

Exercise	Photo	Instructions	Weeks	Sets × reps
1a. DB incline bench press		Lie on an incline bench. Hold a dumbbell in each hand, your arms extended and palms facing forward. Flex your elbows and lower the dumbbells until you feel a good stretch in your upper chest. Extend your elbows to return to the starting position. Repeat.	Week 1	2 × 10
			Week 2	3 × 12
			Week 3	4 × 10
			Week 4	5 × 8
1b. Cable incline fly		Lie on an incline bench with a cable machine or bands anchored low on each side of you. Hold a handle in each hand, arms extended above your chest, palms facing one another. Keeping your elbows slightly flexed, lower the cables laterally until they are in a T position. Keeping your elbows slightly flexed, bring the cables back to the original position above your shoulders. Repeat.	Week 1	2 × 10
			Week 2	3 × 12
			Week 3	4 × 12
			Week 4	5 × 15
2a. DB bench press		Lie on a flat bench. Hold a dumbbell in each hand, your arms extended and palms facing forward. Flex your elbows and lower the dumbbells until you feel a good stretch in your chest. Extend your elbows, pushing the dumbbells to the ceiling. Repeat.	Week 1	2 × 10
			Week 2	3 × 12
			Week 3	4 × 10
			Week 4	5 × 8
2b. Cable fly		Stand between 2 cable machines or anchored bands and hold a handle in each hand. Extend your arms from your sides in a T position, palms facing the front. Keeping your elbows slightly flexed, bring the cables together in front of you at chest level. Once your hands touch in front of you, return to the starting position. Repeat.	Week 1	2 × 10
			Week 2	3 × 12
			Week 3	4 × 12
			Week 4	5 × 15
3a. DB decline bench press		Lie on a decline bench. Hold a dumbbell in each hand, arms extended and palms facing forward. Flex your elbows and lower the dumbbells until you feel a good stretch in your upper chest. Extend your elbows to return to the starting position. Repeat.	Week 1	2 × 10
			Week 2	3 × 12
			Week 3	4 × 10
			Week 4	5 × 8

Exercise	Photo	Instructions	Weeks	Sets × reps
3b. Cable decline fly		Stand between 2 high cable columns or anchored bands. Hold a cable handle in each hand, arms extended out from your sides in a Y position and palms facing the front. Keeping your elbows slightly flexed, bring the cables together in front of you at hip level. Once your hands touch in front of you, return to the starting position. Repeat.	Week 1	2 × 10
			Week 2	3 × 12
			Week 3	4 × 12
			Week 4	5 × 15

HIS CHEST 4: OLD-SCHOOL SUPERSET CHEST

This workout comes from the old Nautilus, Arthur Jones, and Mike Mentzer days of the 1970s. It is arranged into what was called *pre-exhaust pairs,* going from the isolation exercise to the compound exercise with no rest. The last 2 weeks of this program are so exhausting, I use either week singularly once in a while just to kill the chest. I never use weeks 3 or 4 for more than 2 straight weeks, and never twice in one week. The idea is to pre-exhaust the muscles with a single-joint movement, then crush it with a compound movement (the opposite of the traditional bodybuilding volumizing approach of compound to isolation). I prefer to use machines for as many exercises as possible so no energy is required to balance or stabilize the weight: All the energy goes to challenging the muscle to grow. Weeks 1 and 2 will be enough for most people, while weeks 3 and 4 should be attempted only by more advanced individuals who have a considerable training base.

Equipment

Pec deck machine, chest press machine, adjustable incline bench, dumbbells, elevated items for deep partial push-up (e.g., hex dumbbells, boxes, benches, push-up handles), cable machine (optional), Smith machine (optional)

Notes

Weeks 1 and 2: Perform 2 times per week.

Weeks 3 and 4: Perform 1 time per week (for very advanced trainees only).

Table 8.4   His Chest 4: Old-School Superset Chest

Exercise	Photo	Instructions	Weeks	Sets × reps
1a. Pec deck machine chest fly (can use cables or bands instead)		Sit in the pec deck machine with your arms open and elbows slightly bent. Squeeze your chest and bring the handles together. Return to the starting position. After completing the desired repetitions, go straight to the compound exercise with no rest.	Week 1	2 × 12-15
			Week 2	3 × 10-12
			Week 3	4 × 12-15
			Week 4	5 × 10-15

(continued)

Table 8.4 His Chest 4: Old-School Superset Chest *(continued)*

Exercise	Photo	Instructions	Weeks	Sets × reps
1b. Machine chest press (can use Smith machine instead)		For this exercise, use a weight that allows you to complete 20-25 repetitions when fresh. Sit in the chest press machine with your elbows bent, feeling a good stretch in your chest. Press the weight away from you until your arms are fully extended, then return to the starting position. Repeat. After completing the desired repetitions, rest 2-3 min and start the 1a–1b sequence again.	Week 1	2 × 10-12
			Week 2	3 × 10-12
			Week 3	4 × 8-12
			Week 4	5 × 8-12
5-10 MIN REST				
2a. DB incline chest fly (can use cables instead)		Lie on an incline bench and hold a dumbbell in each hand. Extend your arms above your chest, palms facing one another. Keeping your elbows slightly flexed, lower the dumbbells laterally until they are in a T position and you feel a good stretch in your upper chest. Keeping your elbows slightly flexed, bring the dumbbells back to the original position above your shoulders. Repeat.	Week 1	2 × 12-15
			Week 2	3 × 10-12
			Week 3	4 × 12-15
			Week 4	5 × 10-15
2b. Barbell incline bench press (can use Smith machine instead)		For this exercise, use a weight that allows you to complete 20-25 repetitions when fresh. Lie on an incline bench holding a barbell in both hands. Lie on an incline bench holding a barbell with your hands shoulder-width apart and extend your arms. Lower the barbell toward your upper chest until you feel a good stretch on your upper chest. Extend your elbows, pushing the barbell to the starting position. Repeat. After completing the desired repetitions, rest 2-3 min and start the 2a–2b sequence again.	Week 1	2 × 10-12
			Week 2	3 × 10-12
			Week 3	4 × 8-12
			Week 4	5 × 8-12
Finisher: deep partial push-up flush		Place 2 items (e.g., hex dumbbells, boxes, benches, push-up handles) on the ground a little wider than shoulder-width apart. Assume a push-up position with your hands resting on the items. Perform a deep push-up to get a good stretch in the chest muscles. Extend your elbows to come up about halfway, then lower your body into the deep push-up. Repeat.	Weeks 1 to 4	2-3 sets to failure

HIS CHEST 5: TRADITIONAL BODYBUILDING CHEST

This 4-week program is a traditional old-school chest program. Back in the day, when we wanted to get strong and big, this is the kind of workout we did. This workout has the benefit of the strength gains one gets from the heavy loads and low reps, but it also has the volumizing effects of the high rep range shaping and flushing protocols. People who want to grind a simple, yet effective workout will love this one—it's a no-brainer! This is not a short, intense workout; doing the sets in succession, with good weight and getting plenty of rest, takes time. When I perform this workout, it takes me about 2 hours to get ample rest to hit big numbers. At my age, I start feeling a little overtrained at weeks 3 to 4, so monitor your volumes and aches and pains. Weeks 1 and 2 will be enough for most people, while weeks 3 and 4 should be attempted only by more advanced individuals who have a considerable training base.

Equipment

Incline bench, barbell, weight bench, dumbbells, parallel bars, weight belt and weight plates, double cable machine or bands, chest press machine (optional)

Notes

Weeks 1 and 2: Perform 2 times per week.

Weeks 3 and 4: Perform 1 time per week (for very advanced trainees only).

Table 8.5 His Chest 5: Traditional Bodybuilding Chest

Exercise	Photo	Instructions	Weeks	Sets × reps
1. Barbell incline bench press (or machine incline chest press)		Lie on an incline bench holding a barbell in both hands. Lie on an incline bench holding a barbell with your hands shoulder-width apart and extend your arms. Lower the barbell toward your upper chest until you feel a good stretch on your upper chest. Extend your elbows, pushing the barbell to the starting position. Repeat.	Week 1	2 × 10
			Week 2	3 × 8
			Week 3	4 × 8
			Week 4	5 × 4-6
2. DB bench press (or machine chest press)		Lie on a bench and hold a dumbbell in each hand. Extend your arms, palms facing forward. Lower the dumbbells until your elbows reach 90 degrees. Extend your elbows, pushing the dumbbells toward the ceiling. Repeat.	Week 1	2 × 10
			Week 2	3 × 8
			Week 3	4 × 8
			Week 4	5 × 4-6
3. Weighted dip (or machine equivalent)		Stand between 2 parallel bars. Attach a belt with chains and weight plates to add the appropriate intensity. Holding on to the handles, lift your body with your elbows extended. Lower your body until you feel a good stretch in your upper chest and shoulders. Extend your elbows to lift your body, contracting the triceps. Repeat.	Week 1	2 × 10
			Week 2	3 × 12
			Week 3	4 × 10
			Week 4	5 × 8

(continued)

Table 8.5 His Chest 5: Traditional Bodybuilding Chest *(continued)*

Exercise	Photo	Instructions	Weeks	Sets × reps
4. DB incline chest fly		Lie on an incline bench. Hold a dumbbell in each hand, your arms extended out from your chest and palms facing one another. Lower the dumbbells laterally into a T position until you feel a good stretch in your upper chest and shoulders. Return the dumbbells to the starting position. Repeat.	Weeks 1-2	2 × 10
			Weeks 3-4	3 × 12
Finisher: cable chest 3D 21 fly		Stand between 2 cable machines set at chest height. Hold a handle in each hand, your arms extended to your sides in a T position, your palms facing the front. Split a chest fly into 3 ranges: the upper half (arms apart) to the halfway point, the lower half (to the halfway point until the arms come together), and the full range. Keeping your elbows slightly bent, squeeze your chest and bring the handles halfway. Return to the upper half, with your arms apart, and perform 7 reps. Perform 7 reps from halfway until your hands touch. Finish with 7 full-range chest flys. That's one set.	Weeks 1-2	2 × 21
			Weeks 3-4	3 × 21

HER CHEST 1: BAND CHEST TONING

This is a 4-week band-only training program for the chest. It is arranged in three 2-exercise circuits for maximum efficiency chest training. However feel free to rearrange the exercises and perform them in succession if you have more time to train and want to use heavier loads and focus on strength. This workout is perfect for focusing on the chest while also getting excellent core training. Weeks 1 and 2 will be enough for most people, while weeks 3 and 4 should be attempted only by more advanced individuals who have a considerable training base.

Equipment

Bands with handles (such as JC Sport or JC Predator)

Notes

Alternate the forward leg with each set.

Weeks 1 and 2: Perform 2 times per week.

Weeks 3 and 4: Perform 1 time per week (for very advanced trainees only).

Table 8.6   Her Chest 1: Band Chest Toning

Exercise	Photo	Instructions	Weeks	Sets × reps
1a. BP staggered stance incline press		Stand facing away from 2 low-anchored bands or cables. Hold the handles by your chest (palms down) so you feel a comfortable stretch in your chest. Assume a staggered stance or a split-squat position. Extend your elbows up and out in front of you at about 45 degrees until your arms are fully extended, then return to the starting position. Repeat. Alternate legs with each set.	Week 1	2 × 10
			Week 2	2 × 15
			Week 3	4 × 10
			Week 4	4 × 15
1b. BP staggered stance incline fly		Stand facing away from 2 low-anchored bands or cables. Hold the handles and open your arms in a T position. Slightly flex your elbows (palms to the front) so you feel a comfortable stretch in your chest. Assume a staggered stance or a split-squat position. Keeping your elbows slightly flexed, bring the handles up and out in front of you at about 45 degrees until your hands touch, then return to the starting position. Repeat. Alternate legs with each set.	Week 1	2 × 10
			Week 2	4 × 12
			Week 3	4 × 15
			Week 4	4 × 20
2a. BP staggered stance press		Stand facing away from 2 bands or cables set at chest height. Hold handles by your chest (palms down) so you feel a comfortable stretch in your chest. Assume a staggered stance or a split-squat position. Extend your elbows out in front of you until your arms are fully extended, then return to the starting position. Repeat. Alternate legs with each set.	Week 1	2 × 10
			Week 2	2 × 15
			Week 3	4 × 10
			Week 4	4 × 15

(continued)

121

Table 8.6 Her Chest 1: Band Chest Toning *(continued)*

Exercise	Photo	Instructions	Weeks	Sets × reps
2b. BP staggered stance fly		Stand between 2 bands set at chest height. Hold the handles and open your arms in a T position. Slightly flex your elbows (palms to the front) so you feel a comfortable stretch in your chest. Assume a staggered stance or a split-squat position. Keeping your elbows slightly flexed, bring the handles together until your hands touch, then return to the starting position. Repeat. Alternate legs with each set.	Week 1	2 × 10
			Week 2	4 × 12
			Week 3	4 × 15
			Week 4	4 × 20
FINISHER				
1a. BP alternating decline fly		Stand facing away from two bands or cables secured in a position well above your head. Hold the handles with your arms in an open T position, elbows slightly flexed (palms to the front). Assume a staggered stance or split-squat position. Bring your right arm forward and perform a single-arm fly. As the right arm returns to the starting position, bring the left arm forward to perform a single-arm fly. Repeat. Alternate legs with each set.	Week 1	2 × 10 per side
			Week 2	2 × 15 per side
			Week 3	4 × 10 per side
			Week 4	4 × 15 per side
1b. BP staggered stance decline fly		Stand facing away from 2 bands or cables set as high as possible. Hold handles with your arms open in a T position. Slightly flex your elbows (palms to the front) so you feel a comfortable stretch in your chest. Assume a staggered stance or a split-squat position. Keeping your elbows slightly flexed, bring the handles out in front of you and down at about 45 degrees until your hands touch, then return to the starting position. Repeat. Alternate legs with each set.	Week 1	2 × 10
			Week 2	4 × 12
			Week 3	4 × 15
			Week 4	4 × 20
1c. Partial dive bomber (cobra) push-up		Begin in a push-up position, your hands and feet both shoulder-width apart. Push your hips up so they are higher than your shoulders. Flex your elbows to perform a push-up so your chest gently grazes the floor. Keep your legs straight. Arch your back and extend your arms as your hips lower to the floor. Reverse the movement to come back to the elevated hip position. Repeat.	Week 1	2 × 10
			Week 2	4 × 12
			Week 3	4 × 15
			Week 4	4 × 20

HER CHEST 2: FUNCTIONAL CHEST

This 4-week program is a functional training program for anyone looking to tone and acquire excellent function and core strength. Although it is presented in a succession format, you can certainly try it as a circuit, but don't be surprised if you can't finish the prescribed number of reps at the end. Weeks 1 and 2 will be enough for most people, while weeks 3 and 4 should be attempted only by more advanced individuals who have a considerable training base.

Equipment

Bands with handles, stability ball, suspension system

Notes

Weeks 1 and 2: Perform 2 times per week.

Weeks 3 and 4: Perform 1 time per week (for very advanced trainees only).

Table 8.7   Her Chest 2: Functional Chest

Exercise	Photo	Instructions	Weeks	Sets × reps
1. BP staggered stance alternating press (alternate legs each set)		Stand between 2 bands set at chest height, handles in hands and by your chest (palms down) so you feel a comfortable stretch in your chest. Assume a staggered stance or a split-squat position. Extend your right elbow and keep the left by the chest. Extend your left elbow, while your right hand comes back to the side of the chest. Repeat alternating presses. Alternate legs with each set.	Week 1	2 × 10 per side
			Week 2	2 × 15 per side
			Week 3	4 × 12 per side
			Week 4	4 × 15 per side
2. SB hands-on-ball push-up		Get into a push-up position with your hands on the sides of the stability ball, your fingers pointing toward the floor. Flex your elbows to lower your chest to the stability ball. Once your chest reaches the stability ball, extend your elbows to push yourself back up. Repeat.	Week 1	2 × 10
			Week 2	2 × 15
			Week 3	4 × 10
			Week 4	4 × 12
3. Suspension fly		Using a suspension system (e.g., SBT), hold on to both handles and get into an inclined, suspended push-up position. Keeping your elbows slightly flexed, pull the handles laterally out to your sides in a T position. Once the handles are at your sides, contract your pecs, keeping your elbows slightly flexed and bring the handles back medially in front. Repeat.	Week 1	2 × 8
			Week 2	2 × 10
			Week 3	4 × 8
			Week 4	4 × 10
4. Dive-bomber (cobra) push-up		Begin in a push-up position, your hands and feet both shoulder-width apart. Push your hips up so you resemble an inverted V. Flex your elbows to perform a push-up so your chest gently grazes the floor. Keep your legs straight. Arch your back and extend your arms as your hips lower to the floor. Reverse the movement to come back to an inverted V. Repeat.	Week 1	2 × 10
			Week 2	2 × 15
			Week 3	4 × 12
			Week 4	4 × 15

Table 8.7 Her Chest 2: Functional Chest *(continued)*

Exercise	Photo	Instructions	Weeks	Sets × reps
Diamond push-up (elevate if needed to complete the rep range prescribed)		Get into a push-up position, with your hands underneath your chest so your index fingers and thumbs touch, forming a diamond. Flex your elbows to lower the chest. Once your chest is an inch (3 cm) above the floor, extend your elbows to lift your body. Repeat.	Week 1	2 × 10
			Week 2	2 × 12
			Week 3	4 × 10
			Week 4	4 × 12

HER CHEST 3: UNILATERAL DB AND CABLE CHEST

This 4-week specialized program with some of my Tri Fitness competitors. It focuses on the upper chest and shoulders, using the more popular compound-to-isolation prefatigue format, a reverse of the traditional prefatigue format. I also have used a version of this workout workout with some of my male fitness clients who want to really focus on chest development for their modeling shoots. This workout uses two-arm training and supersets 2 exercises without rest, but even then, it does take a little time since you are finishing each superset with your right hand before going on to your left hand. The second superset is a simple two-arm grind that sets you up for the 3D finisher. Although the single arm work slows you down for a bit, if you keep your focus without getting distracted, you can complete this one in well under 60 min. Weeks 1 and 2 will be enough for most people, while weeks 3 and 4 should be attempted only by more advanced individuals who have a considerable training base.

Equipment

Incline bench, dumbbells, cable machine with handle attachment or bands

Notes

Weeks 1 and 2: Perform 2 times per week.

Weeks 3 and 4: Perform 1 time per week (for very advanced trainees only).

Table 8.8 Her Chest 3: Unilateral DB and Cable Chest

Exercise	Photo	Instructions	Weeks	Sets × reps
1a. DB incline single-arm press (can use incline chest machine)		Lie on an incline bench. Hold a dumbbell in your right hand, your arm extended and your palm facing forward. Lower the dumbbell until you feel a good stretch in the right chest area. Extend your elbow to press the dumbbell up. Repeat. After completing the desired reps with your right hand, begin the 1b exercise with your right hand with no rest.	Week 1	2 × 10 per side
			Week 2	3 × 12 per side
			Week 3	4 × 10 per side
			Week 4	5 × 12 per side
1b. Cable incline single-arm fly		Sit on an incline bench with a low pulley or band to your right, holding the handle in you right hand, your palm facing forward. Keeping your elbow slightly flexed and your torso stable, bring your arm out and up to shoulder height. Bring your arm back to the starting position. Repeat. After completing the desired reps with your right hand, rest 2-3 min and repeat the 1a–1b sequence with your left hand.	Week 1	2 × 12 per side
			Week 2	3 × 15 per side
			Week 3	4 × 12 per side
			Week 4	5 × 15 per side

Exercise	Photo	Instructions	Weeks	Sets × reps
REST 5 MIN				
2a: DB two-arm incline bench press (can use chest machine)		Lie on an incline bench. Hold a dumbbell in each hand with your arms extended and your palms facing forward. Lower the dumbbells until you feel a good stretch in the chest area. Extend your elbows to press the dumbbells up. Repeat. After completing the desired reps, begin the 2b exercise with no rest in between 2a and 2b.	Week 1	2 × 10 per side
			Week 2	3 × 12 per side
			Week 3	4 × 10 per side
			Week 4	5 × 12 per side
2b: Cable two-arm incline fly		Stand with a low pulley set of JC Bands behind you at about shin height. Hold the handles in your hands with your arms open and palms facing forward at hip height. Keeping your elbows slightly flexed and torso stable, bring your arms up and in front of you to shoulder height, hinging only at the shoulders. Bring your arms back to the starting position. Repeat. Rest 2-3 minutes before starting the 2a, 2b superset again.	Week 1	2 × 12 per side
			Week 2	3 × 15 per side
			Week 3	4 × 12 per side
			Week 4	5 × 15 per side
Finisher: DB incline press 3D 21		Lie on an incline bench and hold a dumbbell in each hand, your arms extended out from your chest and your palms facing one another. Split an incline chest press into 3 ranges: the lower half (arms apart in the low position to halfway point), the upper half (halfway point until arms are extended), and the full range. Lower the dumbbells laterally until you feel a good stretch in your upper chest and shoulders. Squeeze your chest and bring the dumbbells halfway up, repeating for 7 reps. Then perform 7 reps from halfway until your arms are fully extended. Finish with 7 full-range incline chest presses. That's one set.	Weeks 1 to 4	2-3 sets of 21

HER CHEST 4: PREFATIGUED HYBRID CHEST

This 4-week program uses a hybrid format with some isolation-to-compound and compound-to-isolation prefatigue. As if that was not enough, I threw in an oldie but goodie as a finisher with a pullover flush. I used this workout about 19 years ago with female bodybuilders and male professional wrestlers. This workout really has it all, from a bodybuilding backbone to a functional training overtone. My personal training clients love this workout for the chest, even if we do no more than week 2, a great addition to training for other body parts. As usual, weeks 1 and 2 will be enough for most people, while weeks 3 and 4 should be attempted only by more advanced individuals who have a considerable training base.

Equipment

Chest press machine, suspension system, double cable machine, medicine ball, bench, dumbbell

Notes

Weeks 1 and 2: Perform 2 times per week.

Table 8.9 Her Chest 4: Prefatigued Hybrid Chest

Exercise	Photo	Instructions	Weeks	Sets × reps
1a. Machine chest press		Sit upright on the chest press machine with a handle in each hand at the sides of your chest. Extend your elbows and press the weight forward until your elbows reach full extension. Flex your elbows, bringing the weight back until you feel a good stretch in your chest. Repeat.	Week 1	2 × 10
			Week 2	2 × 8
			Week 3	4 × 6
			Week 4	5 × 6
1b. Suspension fly to push-up superset		Using a suspension system (e.g., SBT), hold on to both handles and get into an inclined, suspended T position. Keep your arms out and your elbows slightly flexed. Bring your hands together in front of you to perform the chest fly movement. Open your arms to the original T position and repeat for the desired reps. Once done with the fly, go right to a push-up, extending and flexing your elbows for the desired number of push-ups. Repeat.	Week 1	2 × 8 + 10
			Week 2	2 × 8 + 12
			Week 3	4 × 8-10 + 12-15
			Week 4	5 × 10 + 15
2a. Cable fly		Stand between 2 cable machines. Hold a cable handle in each hand. Extend your arms to your sides, palms facing the front in a T-position. Keeping your elbows slightly flexed, bring the cables together in front of you at chest level. Once your hands touch in front of you, bring them back to the starting position. Repeat.	Week 1	2 × 10
			Week 2	2 × 12
			Week 3	4 × 15
			Week 4	5 × 12

Exercise	Photo	Instructions	Weeks	Sets × reps
2b. MB hands-on-ball push-up		Assume a plank position, both hands on a firm medicine ball and feet shoulder-width apart. Flex your elbows and lower your chest to the ball. Extend your elbows to return to the starting position. Repeat.	Week 1	2 × 8
			Week 2	2 × 8
			Week 3	4 × 10
			Week 4	5 × 12
Finisher: DB pullover		Lie perpendicularly on a flat bench and hold the ends of a dumbbell in your hands. Position the dumbbell over your chest, with your elbows slightly bent. Keeping your elbows slightly bent, lower the dumbbell over and beyond the head until the upper arms are in line with the torso. Pull the dumbbell up and over the chest to the starting position. Repeat. Rest 2-3 min between sets.	Weeks 1 to 4	3 sets to failure (10-20 rep range)

Weeks 3 and 4: Perform 1 time per week (for very advanced trainees only).

HER CHEST 5: BREAKDOWN CHEST

This insane workout is used as a shocker to bring your chest out of a funk or plateau. A professional female fitness competitor shared this workout with me. This is another workout I've used it with both men and women. Normally it is used as a one-time workout, perhaps performed twice 7-10 days apart. This workout will leave you spent for days; even if you feel recovered 3 or 4 days after, you are not. Give yourself another 2 or 3 days. I cannot emphasize *complete recovery* enough—don't repeat this workout until you've waited 7-10 days and don't do more than 2 of these in a 3- or 4-week span. The *50* is in the name because that is the total number of reps you are aiming for in each breakdown set, and you have 9 of those! It takes a few attempts to get it right, but once you do, this is an insane workout. Depending on what machine you use and how the plates are arranged, you may need to move the pin up four to six times, reducing the weight each time to complete more than the 50 reps.

Equipment

Smith machine, chest press machine, pec deck machine, bench, dumbbell

Notes

Beginners should rest 7-10 days after this program before resuming chest training. Advanced athletes should rest 7-10 days after this program, repeat it, rest another 7-10 days, and then

Table 8.10 Her Chest 5: Breakdown Chest

Exercise	Photo	Instructions	Sets × reps
Smith machine incline chest press breakdown 50		Sit on an incline bench set up inside a Smith machine. Set the weight so your arms are extended and aligned vertically with your upper chest. Flex your elbows, bringing the weight back until you feel a good stretch in your chest. Repeat. Start with a weight you can do about 15 times and perform to failure. Drop the weight 15%-20% and rep out to failure. Continue to drop the weight 15%-20% and rep out to failure until you complete more than 50 reps. Rest 3-5 min between each set.	3 × 50 total

(continued)

Table 8.10 Her Chest 5: Breakdown Chest *(continued)*

Exercise	Photo	Instructions	Sets × reps
REST 5 MIN			
Machine chest press breakdown 50		Sit upright on the chest press machine with a handle in each hand at the sides of your chest. Extend your elbows and press the weight forward until your elbows reach full extension. Flex your elbows, bringing the weight back until you feel a good stretch in your chest. Repeat. Start with a weight you can do about 15 times and perform to failure. Drop the weight 15%-20% and rep out to failure. Continue to drop the weight 15%-20% and rep out to failure until you complete more than 50 reps. Rest 3-5 min between each set.	3 × 50 total
REST 5 MIN			
Pec deck machine chest fly breakdown 50		Sit upright on the pec deck machine with your elbows flexed at 90 degrees and resting on the elbow pads. Squeeze your elbows together until they touch or you feel a maximum squeeze in your chest. Open your arms until you feel a comfortable stretch in your chest and repeat. Start with a weight you can do about 15 times and perform to failure. Drop the weight 15%-20% and rep out to failure. Continue to drop the weight 15%-20% and rep out to failure until you complete more than 50 reps. Rest 3-5 min between each set.	3 × 50 total
REST 5 MIN			
Finisher: DB pullover		Lie perpendicularly on a flat bench and hold the ends of a dumbbell in your hands. Position the dumbbell over your chest with your elbows slightly bent. Keeping your elbows slightly bent, lower the dumbbell over and beyond your head until your upper arms are in line with the torso. Pull the dumbbell up and over the chest to the starting position. Repeat. Rest 3 min between each set.	3 sets to failure (10-20 rep range)

resume chest training.

Summary

Remember that this big volume does not have to come with gut-wrenching intensity that will mess up your joints. You can take your time, slow down the movement, squeeze your muscles, and spare your joints. This is especially true if you are not in a sport that requires insane strength and power. If you just want to be healthy and look great, work on form and the mind-muscle connection, get your pump, and get out of the gym. Don't stay in the gym just to do junk volume. That's not the way to get results, and it's a direct route to injuries. Trust me, the crazy high volume and high intensity catch up to you when you are 40 or 50, and then it's too late. Train your chest, spare the shoulders, and be happy.

CHAPTER **9**

Back

This chapter is last in the body transformation section because it is the most unique. Although the back is the biggest region of the body and has some of the largest musculature, it often is neglected in training, taking a back seat to the chest, abs, arms, and quads. Because of this neglect, the back, especially the lower and mid back, also is one of the areas most prone to injury, even as it protects and stabilizes one of the most important neurological systems of the body. The back supports the core and creates the biggest bridge of force transfer in the body. During the transfer of force between the hips and shoulders, the back and anterior core muscles assume much of the heavy lifting. The back serves as the anchor point for the body's limbs. The diagonal orientation of the latissimus dorsi make the back a key player in generating rotational power. This chapter covers the IHP way to train this important muscle system.

In terms of visual appeal, the shoulders frame the upper body and give the illusion of width, but the back provides the V-shaped physique all men are looking for as well as the hourglass shape women are looking for. However, width is not enough when it comes to the back. A wide back without depth does not look complete, yet few will actually know what is missing. Therefore, paying attention to the V without looking at the other parts also leaves you short of the optimal-looking back. Women may not be looking for the width men are, but they are looking for a muscularly toned and lean back, free of obvious fat around the bra strap. It's difficult to see your own back, so unless you have special mirrors, it's hard to analyze and critique it. Therefore, from an aesthetic perspective, the back is important, yet it is undervalued and misunderstood.

In terms of size, the major muscle in the back is the big latissimus dorsi. However, the trapezius and paraspinals are big and important muscles as well. The traditional, simplistic way to look at back training is to do a lot of full-range-of-motion pull-downs, pull-ups, and rows. Although this approach will yield results, contemporary bodybuilders use a more specialized approach to back training. The workouts in this chapter take into account the old tried-and-true approaches but also bring a new perspective to back training. Let's go over a few approaches that are trending in the world of bodybuilding today.

For years, the traditional rule all bodybuilders followed was full-range-of-motion training. Recently, I'm seeing more partial-range-of-motion training. Although I see this approach applied to all body parts, back training brings it to center stage in exercises such as bent-over rows, in which many bodybuilders stabilize their back positions at about 45 degrees instead of 90 degrees and row to the belly instead of the chest. The back is also being separated into more sections than any other body part and tied in with other muscle systems. For example, the posterior deltoid is worked during back and shoulder workouts; therefore, the back gets a double dip when the shoulders are trained. The same thing goes for the trapezius muscle (or traps), which is also part of shoulder training and technically part of the back as well (the lower fibers of the traps go below the middle of the back). The lower back is also part of back training but is worked with the hips during exercises such as deadlifts and extensions as well as bent-over rows. The development of the lower back is important to the aesthetic quality of the back because it ties the lower back to the lower fibers of the lats. This is also a huge factor in the rehabilitation and prehabilitation of lumbar injuries.

Finally, the entire paraspinal musculature provides a huge amount of depth to the back and is one of the reasons we see so much spinal flexion and big movements of the scapulae during rowing motions and partial deadlifts.

These are some general observations that illustrate just how complex the back is, how much training it can take, how we incorporate it into the training of other body parts, and why we are seeing some of these trends in training. This chapter encompasses all these factors into the workouts so you don't have to worry about them.

These workouts are snapshots of three to four weeks, and the possibilities and permutations are endless. You can change the rep range, combine workouts, and mix and match different workouts on different days to create unique programs that better fit your likes and needs. You can change the intensity by simply manipulating reps and time under tension. For example, keep the load of an exercise the same, cut the reps in half, but slow the movement to a two-second contraction (up), two-second hold (peak contraction), and three-second eccentric (lower the weight). As mentioned in chapter 2 and at the beginning of part II (transformation workouts), this time under tension will give you great muscular development and minimize the wear and tear on the joints due to the lighter loads. Other than for intense athletic performance for which high strength levels have to be developed and displayed, muscular development does not have to come at the high cost of tearing up joints. If you just want to look good and be fit and strong, you don't have to tear up your body!

I have suggested progressions for beginners and advanced trainees in all workouts. However, if you have not trained in more than a month and feel like you need to develop a base or are inexperienced in training, I strongly recommend you finish the two-week program here before attempting any of the workouts in this chapter.

WEEK 1: DO EACH EXERCISE SEPARATELY

Monday, Wednesday, Friday
Perform each exercise separately.

Dumbbell bent-over row (use a dumbbell that weighs 15%-25% of your body weight: 1-2 sets × 10-15 repetitions

Cable single-arm high row (use about 25%-35% of your body weight): 1-2 sets × 10-15 repetitions

WEEK 2: DO EACH EXERCISE SEPARATELY

Monday, Wednesday, Friday
Dumbbell bent-over row: 2-3 sets × 15-20 repetitions

Cable single-arm high row: 2-3 sets × 15-20 repetitions

Pull-down (use 40%-60% of your body weight): 2-3 sets × 15-20 repetitions

HIS BACK 1: BACK TRAINING IN THE PARK

This 4-week program can be done in a park and will get you super strong. This is the kind of workout my friends and I did in our younger days. Gymnasts thrive with this kind of movement, and look at the width of their backs and the size of their arms. If you are not strong on pull-ups, don't worry; this workout will make you strong. With just a portable pull-up bar on a door in your house, you can develop a very strong set of arms and a wide and strong back. Weeks 1 and 2 will be enough for most people, while weeks 3 and 4 should be attempted only by more advanced individuals who have a considerable training base.

Equipment

Pull-up bar

Notes

Weeks 1 and 2: Perform 2 times per week.

Weeks 3 and 4: Perform 1 time per week (for very advanced trainees only).

Table 9.1 His Back 1: Back Training in the Park

Exercise	Photo	Instructions	Weeks	Sets × reps
1. Pull-up (medium grip) (you may use a band or partner to assist you)		Hang on a pull-up bar with your hands shoulder-width apart and palms facing forward with both elbows extended. Flex your elbows and pull your body up until your chin is above the bar. Lower your body to the starting position. Repeat.	Week 1	2 × 8-12
			Week 2	3 × 8-12
			Week 3	4 × 8-10
			Week 4	5 × 8-10
2. Isometric at top (chin above bar) (medium grip)		Hang on a pull-up bar with your hands shoulder-width apart and palms facing forward with both elbows extended. Flex your elbows and pull your body up until your chin is above the bar. Hold that position for the time indicated. Lower your body to the starting position. Repeat.	Week 1	2 × 5 sec.
			Week 2	3 × 8-10 sec.
			Week 3	4 × 12-15 sec.
			Week 4	5 × 15-20 sec.
3. Isometric at midway (halfway down) (medium grip)		Hang on a pull-up bar with your hands shoulder-width apart and palms facing forward with both elbows extended. Flex your elbows and pull your body up until your elbows are at 90 degrees. Hold that position for the time indicated. Lower your body to the starting position. Repeat.	Week 1	2 × 5 sec.
			Week 2	3 × 8-10 sec.
			Week 3	4 × 12-15 sec.
			Week 4	5 × 15-20 sec.

(continued)

Table 9.1   His Back 1: Back Training in the Park *(continued)*

Exercise	Photo	Instructions	Weeks	Sets × reps
4. Wide-grip eccentric pull-up		Hang on a pull-up bar with your hands wider than shoulder-width apart and palms facing forward with both elbows extended. Flex your elbows and pull your body up until your chin is above the bar. Hold that position for the time indicated. Lower your body to the starting position. Repeat.	Week 1	2 × 3 sec.
			Week 2	3 × 5 sec.
			Week 3	4 × 5 sec.
			Week 4	5 × 5 sec.

HIS BACK 2: BAND-ONLY BACK WORKOUT

This is a 4-week band-only program. I recommend using a set of heavy-duty exercise bands, such as the JC Predator or Predator Jr. The workout is arranged in two 2-exercise circuits for maximum training efficiency. However, you can perform this workout in succession if you want to rest more between exercises and increase your loading intensity. This is a perfect workout for home or while traveling. It's also a great exercise for a young person who wants to start strength training at home. Treat these exercises with the same intensity you treat any machine exercises, and the results will be the same: great tone and strength. Weeks 1 and 2 will be enough for most people, while weeks 3 and 4 should be attempted only by more advanced individuals who have a considerable training base.

Equipment

Heavy-duty exercise bands with handles (such as JC Predator or Predator Jr.), stable object to anchor bands

Notes

Weeks 1 and 2: Perform 2 times per week.

Weeks 3 and 4: Perform 1 time per week (for very advanced trainees only).

Table 9.2   His Back 2: Band-Only Back Workout

Exercise	Photo	Instructions	Weeks	Sets × reps
1a. BP staggered stance single-arm compound row		Stand in a staggered stance, your left leg forward. Hold the handle of a band secured at knee level in your right hand. Use a neutral grip. Hinge at the hips and move your shoulders forward until your torso is parallel to the ground, and you feel a good stretch in your hamstrings. Simultaneously extend the hips and row with your right arm until your right hand is next to the right side of your ribs. Repeat for the desired number of repetitions, then switch to the other arm.	Week 1	2 × 8 per arm
			Week 2	3 × 10 per arm
			Week 3	4 × 12 per arm
			Week 4	5 × 10 per arm

Exercise	Photo	Instructions	Weeks	Sets × reps
1b. BP parallel stance bent-over mid row		Stand in a parallel stance, your feet shoulder-width apart and knees slightly bent. Hold the handles of a band secured at waist level. Use a pronated grip. Hinge at the hips and lean your shoulders forward until your torso is parallel to the ground, your arms are straight overhead, and you feel a good stretch in your hamstrings. Holding the bent-over position, pull the handles with your elbows out by your sides (same upper-body motion as a pull-up) until your elbows are fully flexed and by your sides. Extend your elbows, straightening your arms in front. Repeat.	Week 1	2 × 10
			Week 2	3 × 12
			Week 3	4 × 15
			Week 4	5 × 12
2a. BP staggered stance single-arm high-to-low row		Stand in a staggered stance, left leg forward. Hold the handle of a band secured at a high position in your right hand. Use a neutral grip. With your right arm extended, flex your elbows and row the band to the right side of your ribs. Extend your arm to the starting position. Repeat for the desired number of repetitions, then switch to the other side.	Week 1	2 × 8
			Week 2	3 × 10
			Week 3	4 × 12
			Week 4	5 × 10
2b. Band swim		Stand in a parallel stance, your feet shoulder-width apart and knees slightly bent. Hold the handles of a band secured at a high point above your head. Use a pronated grip. Keeping your arms fully extended through the entire motion, pull the bands down while flexing your torso until your hands are near your back pockets and the bands are touching the shoulders. Return to the starting position. Repeat.	Week 1	2 × 10
			Week 2	3 × 12
			Week 3	4 × 15
			Week 4	5 × 15

HIS BACK 3: HYBRID BACK STRENGTH

This 4-week program integrates the best of the best—function and pure strength. This is a great workout for those interested in getting good muscle and great core strength they can transfer into sports. Although this workout can be done in a circuit format, I recommend you treat this like a typical strength workout and take your time between each set. This approach will allow you to really develop the strength and size this workout can deliver. Weeks 1 and 2 will be enough for most people, while weeks 3 and 4 should be attempted only by more advanced individuals who have a considerable training base.

Equipment

Pull-up bar, wheel, suspension system, cable machine or band with handles, dumbbells

Notes

Weeks 1 and 2: Perform 2 times per week.

Weeks 3 and 4: Perform 1 time per week (for very advanced trainees only).

Table 9.3 His Back 3: Hybrid Back Strength

Exercise	Photo	Instructions	Weeks	Sets × reps
1. Wide-grip V-pull-up		Hang on a pull-up bar with your hands just outside of shoulder-width apart, your palms facing forward and both elbows extended. Flex your elbows and pull your body up and to the right until your chin is above your right hand. Return to the hanging position and pull your body up and to the left until your chin is above your left hand. That's one repetition. Repeat to both sides.	Week 1	2 × 2
			Week 2	3 × 3
			Week 3	4 × 4
			Week 4	5 × 5
2. Wheel roll-out from knees		Hold the wheel with both hands while balancing in a plank position on your knees. Keep your abs tight and arms straight during the entire motion. Roll the wheel out in front of you until your arms are straight and your body is perfectly parallel to the ground. Pull your arms back to roll the wheel and return to the plank position. Repeat. (Instead of the wheel, you can use a stability ball or suspension system.)	Week 1	2 × 5
			Week 2	3 × 8
			Week 3	4 × 10
			Week 4	5 × 12
3. Suspension single-arm row		Hold a suspension handle in your left hand in a reclined position. Keeping your chest facing forward and body completely straight, flex your left elbow, pulling yourself up until your left arm is by your left side. Extend your arm to the starting position. Repeat for the desired number of repetitions, then switch to the other side. Use clamps or lockdown handles for additional grip strength.	Week 1	2 × 5 per side
			Week 2	3 × 8 per side
			Week 3	4 × 10 per side
			Week 4	5 × 8 per side
4. Cable staggered stance single-arm CLA compound row		Stand in a staggered stance, your left leg forward. Hold the handle of a low cable in your right hand in a neutral grip. (Use a band if you don't have access to a cable machine.) Hinge at the hips and lean your shoulders forward until your torso is parallel to the ground and you feel a good stretch in your left hamstrings. Simultaneously extend the hips and row with your right arm until your right hand is next to the right side of your ribs. Repeat for the desired number of repetitions, then switch to the other side.	Week 1	2 × 8 per side
			Week 2	3 × 10 per side
			Week 3	4 × 12 per side
			Week 4	5 × 10 per side
5. DB 45-degree row		Stand with your feet shoulder-width apart. Keep a slight bend in the knees. Lean forward, hinging at the hips to a 45-degree angle. Hold a dumbbell in each hand and allow your arms to extend down. Keep your palms facing the front. Row the dumbbells up, pulling them toward the sides of your ribs. Lower the dumbbells to the starting position. Repeat.	Week 1	2 × 10
			Week 2	3 × 12
			Week 3	4 × 15
			Week 4	5 × 12

HIS BACK 4: HIGH VOLUME

This 4-week program is a monster high-volume workout designed for maximum growth. Pack a lunch; you are going to be here for a while. I caution everyone against tackling this workout with maximum weight; it will destroy you if you do. Pace yourself and let the volume, not the load, do the work. Use lighter loads and slow down so you can feel each contraction. If you take the steady approach, you will feel your muscle pump over the workout; if you go too fast, you will gas out and lose your pump. For a faster and more efficient workout, this routine can also be done in sets of pairs (1 and 2, 3 and 4) with 5 as a finisher. Weeks 1 and 2 will be enough for most people. Weeks 3 and 4 should be attempted only by professionals and those who have a considerable training base.

Equipment

Lat pull-down machine with wide bar attachment, rowing machine with V-bar attachment, barbell, weight bench, dumbbells, cable machine with straight bar attachment or bands

Notes

Weeks 1 and 2: Perform 2 times per week.

Weeks 3 and 4: Perform 1 time per week (for very advanced trainees only).

Table 9.4   His Back 4: High Volume

Exercise	Photo	Instructions	Weeks	Sets × reps
1. Wide-grip pull-down (may use normal or neutral bar)		Attach a wide bar to the lat pull-down machine. Hold on to the bar with your palms facing away and wider than shoulder-width. Flexing your elbows, pull the bar down until it touches your upper chest. Extend your elbows, returning to the starting position. Repeat.	Week 1	2 × 8
			Week 2	3 × 10
			Week 3	4 × 10
			Week 4	5 × 8
2. Cable V-bar row		Attach a V-bar to the row pulley. Sit on a flat bench with your feet on the platform in front. Flex your elbows and row (pull) the V-bar toward your ribs until it touches your body. Extend your elbows and push the V-bar forward until full extension. Repeat.	Week 1	2 × 10
			Week 2	3 × 12
			Week 3	4 × 12
			Week 4	5 × 10
3. Barbell bent-over row		Hold a barbell in a pronated grip with your hands shoulder-width apart. Bend your knees slightly and lean your torso forward until it is parallel to the ground. With your arms extending down, palms facing the body, row the barbell up, pulling it toward your ribs. Lower the barbell to the starting position. Repeat.	Week 1	2 × 8
			Week 2	3 × 10
			Week 3	4 × 10
			Week 4	5 × 8

(continued)

Table 9.4 His Back 4: High Volume *(continued)*

Exercise	Photo	Instructions	Weeks	Sets × reps
4. DB pullover		Lie perpendicularly on a flat bench with only your shoulders on the bench. Bend your legs, and keep your feet shoulder-width apart. Hold the dumbbell in both hands over your chest with your arms fully extended. Lower the dumbbell behind your head, keeping your arms fully extended. Once you feel a stretch in the chest, return the dumbbell to the starting position. Repeat.	Week 1	2 × 10
			Week 2	3 × 12
			Week 3	4 × 10
			Week 4	5 × 12
5. Cable straight-arm pull-down breakdown		Stand in front of a cable machine with feet parallel and shoulder-width apart, knees slightly bent, torso flexed about 20 degrees. Using a pronated grip, hold a bar attached to a high pulley. Keeping your arms fully extended, pull the bar down to your thighs. Return to the starting position. Repeat.	Weeks 1-2	2 supersets
			Weeks 3-4	3 supersets

HIS BACK 5: PRO SHOW BACK WORKOUT

This 4-week professional bodybuilding program dissects the back and develops it from the base, near the hips, all the way past the shoulder blades. It also pays attention to the depth of the back with exercises like the quarter deadlifts. Like the previous workout, I recommend you complete each exercise with plenty of rest in between. However, this routine can also be done in sets of pairs (1 and 2, 3 and 4) with 5 as a finisher if you want to work in a time-efficient circuit fashion. I can't emphasize enough that this is a professional workout. Even the equipment used is available only at professional gyms. However, you can substitute exercises and equipment to make it happen in your gym. If you don't have a few years of training under your belt, stick to weeks 1 and 2. If you are a seasoned veteran with time to train, give weeks 3 and 4 a shot.

Equipment

Barbell, cable machine with V-bar and handle attachment, weight bench, dumbbells, back extension bench, resistance bands (such as the JC Predator), T-bar and pad, pull-down machine

Notes

Weeks 1 and 2: Perform 2 times per week.

Weeks 3 and 4: Perform 1 time per week (for very advanced trainees only).

Table 9.5 His Back 5: Pro Show Back Workout

Exercise	Photo	Instructions	Weeks	Sets × reps
DAY 1				
1. Barbell quarter flexed (bent-over) low row		Hold a barbell in a supinated grip with your hands shoulder-width apart, knees slightly bent, and feet shoulder-width apart. Lean your torso forward to a 45-degree angle. With your arms hanging down, row the barbell up, pulling it toward your belly. Lower the barbell a quarter of the way down and repeat.	Week 1	2 × 8
			Week 2	3 × 10
			Week 3	4 × 10
			Week 4	5 × 8
2. V-bar pull-down to chest		Hold a V-bar attached to a high pulley. Sit down with your knees bent, your feet shoulder-width apart, and your arms extended overhead. Flex your elbows and pull the V-bar to the chest. Extend your arms to the starting position. Repeat.	Week 1	2 × 10
			Week 2	3 × 12
			Week 3	4 × 10
			Week 4	5 × 12
3. DB pullover		Lie perpendicularly on a flat bench with only your shoulders on the bench. Bend your legs and keep your feet shoulder-width apart on the ground. Hold a dumbbell in both hands over your chest with your arms fully extended. Lower the dumbbell behind your head, keeping your arms fully extended. Once you feel a stretch in the chest, return the dumbbell to starting position. Repeat.	Week 1	2 × 10
			Week 2	3 × 12
			Week 3	4 × 10
			Week 4	5 × 12
4. DB back extension compound row (45-degree bench)		Tucking your ankles under the pads, place your thighs on the pads of the back extension bench, with the pads at hip level. Flex the hips and grab dumbbells in each hand. Simultaneously extend your hips and row the dumbbells to your sides. Flex your hips and lower the dumbbells to the starting position. Repeat.	Week 1	2 × 8
			Week 2	3 × 10
			Week 3	4 × 12
			Week 4	5 × 1
5. Band finisher: BP row + BP bent-over alternating row + BP swim (meta back)		BP row: Hold the handle of a band in each hand with a pronated grip. Stand upright with your feet shoulder-width apart and your elbows extended. Flex your elbows, pulling the handles to your sides. Extend your elbows out in front. Repeat. BP bent-over alternating row: Hinge at the hips until the torso is parallel to the ground. Row in an alternating fashion (20 reps per side). BP swim: Stand. Keeping the arms extended through the entire motion, pull the bands down while flexing your torso until your hands are near your back pockets and the bands are touching the shoulders. Return to the starting position. Repeat.	Weeks 1-2	2 (20 + 20 per side + 20)
			Weeks 3-4	3 (20 + 20 per side + 20)

(continued)

Table 9.5 His Back 5: Pro Show Back Workout *(continued)*

Exercise	Photo	Instructions	Weeks	Sets × reps
DAY 2				
1. Barbell partial deadlift (off racks)		Stand behind the barbell, your feet shoulder-width apart. Hold the barbell with both hands, your hands shoulder-width apart. Lower your hips and bend your knees. Push through your heels and lift the weight, driving your hips into the bar. Lower the barbell a quarter of the way down, then pull back up until your hips hit the bar again. Repeat this quarter movement for the desired number of reps, then lower the barbell to the rack.	Week 1	2 × 8
			Week 2	3 × 10
			Week 3	4 × 10
			Week 4	5 × 8
2. Cable staggered stance quarter flexed single-arm high-to-low wide cable pull-down		Stand in a staggered stance with your left leg forward. Hold the handle of a high cable secured above head level in your right hand. Keep your arm extended and torso flexed at 45 degrees. Pull down in a wide fashion, as if you were doing a single-arm pull-down. When your elbow is fully flexed, raise and extend the arm to the original position. Switch arms and repeat.	Week 1	2 × 10 per side
			Week 2	3 × 12 per side
			Week 3	4 × 10 per side
			Week 4	5 × 12 per side
3. Chest-supported Barbell row		Lie prone on the T-bar row pad, making sure your upper chest is at the top of the pad. (Perform unsupported if you don't have a supported T-bar set up.) Once in position, hold the T-bar handles with your arms extended. Flexing at your elbows, pull the weight up until your elbows are fully flexed. Extend your elbows to the starting position. Repeat.	Week 1	2 × 8
			Week 2	3 × 10
			Week 3	4 × 10
			Week 4	5 × 8
4. Single-arm cable pull-down		Sit at a cable machine with a single handle attached to a high pulley. Reach above you and hold the handle in your right hand with the elbow fully extended. Flexing your elbow, pull the handle down until it is close to your shoulder. Extend your arm back up to the starting position. Repeat. Switch sides.	Week 1	2 × 10 per side
			Week 2	3 × 12 per side
			Week 3	4 × 10 per side
			Week 4	5 × 12 per side
5. DB finisher: DB bent-over row breakdown superset		Hold a dumbbell in a pronated grip in each hand. Bend your knees slightly, keep your feet shoulder-width apart, and lean forward at a 45-degree angle at the hips. Flex your elbows to pull the dumbbells toward you, keeping them close to your body. Once the dumbbells are right beneath your ribs, extend your arms and return to the starting position. Repeat. Start with a weight that allows you to perform 15 reps. Drop the weight 20%-25% for 3 drop sets to failure in each superset; do the first set and 2 drop sets.	Weeks 1-2	2 supersets
			Weeks 3-4	3 supersets

HER BACK 1: HOME OR PARK BACK WORKOUT

This 4-week program can be done in a park or at home using a portable pull-up bar on a door. Most women think they can't do pull-ups, but I routinely get fit females to do 5-10 pull-ups with no problems. If you need help, use a large band to assist you or ask a partner. This is a fantastic workout for the woman who thought she could never do a pull-up and wants to get strong without getting big. With just a portable pull-up bar on a door in your house, this low-volume, high-intensity workout can develop a very strong back without creating a wide back. Weeks 1 and 2 will be enough for most people, while weeks 3 and 4 should be attempted only by more advanced individuals who have a considerable training base.

Equipment

Pull-up bar, beach towel, box, suspension system (optional), wheel (optional), large band (optional)

Notes

For all pull-up and chin-up variations, you can use a band to assist you.

Weeks 1 and 2: Perform 2 times per week.

Weeks 3 and 4: Perform 1 time per week (for very advanced trainees only).

Table 9.6 Her Back 1: Home or Park Back Workout

Exercise	Photo	Instructions	Weeks	Sets × reps
1. Pull-up		Grab the pull-up bar with your palms facing away from you and your hands shoulder-width apart, both elbows extended. Flex at your elbows, bringing your chest toward the bar until your chin is above the bar. Lower until your elbows reach full extension. (If you're unable to pull your body weight, use a band for assistance.) Repeat.	Week 1	2 × 2-4
			Week 2	3 × 3-5
			Week 3	4 × 4-6
			Week 4	5 × 5-8
2. Chin-up		Grab the pull-up bar with your palms facing you and both elbows extended. Flex at your elbows, bringing your chest toward the bar until your chin is above the bar. Lower your chest until your elbows reach full extension. (If you're unable to pull your body weight, use a band for assistance.) Repeat.	Week 1	2 × 2-3
			Week 2	3 × 3-4
			Week 3	4 × 4-5
			Week 4	5 × 5
3. Partial pump at midway (chin-up grip)		Grab the pull-up bar with your palms facing you, both elbows extended. Flex at your elbows, bringing your chest toward the bar until your elbows flex at 90 degrees. You may use a box to get you to that position. Hold this suspended position and perform small pumps at about 90-110 degrees of elbow flexion.	Week 1	2 × 2-3
			Week 2	3 × 3-4
			Week 3	4 × 4-5
			Week 4	5 × 5

(continued)

Table 9.6 Her Back 1: Home or Park Back Workout *(continued)*

Exercise	Photo	Instructions	Weeks	Sets × reps
4. Rope or towel recline row		Wrap a rope or a big beach towel over the pull-up bar. Hold the ends in each hand, palms facing each other, and assume a reclined position. Flex your elbows and pull yourself up until your elbows reach full flexion and your hands are at the sides of your chest. Lower your body until your elbows are at full extension. Repeat. (You may use a suspension system instead, if available.)	Week 1	2 × 8
			Week 2	3 × 10
			Week 3	4 × 12
			Week 4	5 × 10
5. Rope or towel roll-out		Wrap a rope or a big beach towel over the pull-up bar. Hold the ends in each hand, palms facing each other, and assume a comfortable inclined position (about 70 degrees facing down) as if you were going to do a push-up. Keeping your arms extended, allow your shoulders to flex and your arms to move out and up until your entire body is in a straight line. Pull your arms back to the push-up position. Repeat. As you get stronger, reduce your incline angle. (You may use a wheel instead, if available.)	Week 1	2 × 2-3
			Week 2	3 × 3-4
			Week 3	4 × 4-5
			Week 4	5 × 5

HER BACK 2: CABLE OR BAND BACK TONING WORKOUT

This 4-week band/pulley program is easy to execute but very effective. Since it uses a band or a cable system, the workout can be done at home, while traveling, or at a gym. The workout uses the staggered stance for half of the exercises, making it a great workout to help supplement your glute work. If you are tight for time, you can hit the back and glutes at the same time. Because of the good glute activation in this workout, I recommend you complete this workout a couple days after your main glute/hip training or perform it the day before. Although it's a back routine, the glutes stabilize some exercises. You don't want your glutes to fail due to fatigue. Weeks 1 and 2 will be enough for most people, while weeks 3 and 4 should be attempted only by more advanced individuals who have a considerable training base.

Equipment

Cable machine with handle attachment or bands with handles

Notes

Weeks 1 and 2: Perform 2 times per week.

Weeks 3 and 4: Perform 1 time per week (for very advanced trainees only).

Table 9.7 Her Back 2: Cable or Band Back Toning Workout

Exercise	Photo	Instructions	Weeks	Sets × reps
1. BP parallel stance compound low row		Set a band or cable at a low position. Stand with your feet shoulder-width apart, a slight bend in your knees. Hold the handles in a pronated grip. Keep your back straight through the entire movement. With your arms fully extended, flex your hips until you feel a good stretch in your hamstrings. Simultaneously extend your hips and elbows to row the handles to the side of your ribs. Extend your arms and flex your hips back to the original position. Repeat.	Week 1 Week 2 Week 3 Week 4	2 × 8 3 × 10 4 × 12 5 × 10
2. BP staggered stance bent-over alternating row		Set a band or cable at waist to chest height. Stand in a staggered stance (left leg forward) and hold a band or cable handle in each hand in a pronated grip. Flex at the hips until you feel a good stretch in your left hamstrings. Start with your left arm extended and your right elbow flexed to 90 degrees and away from your body. Perform alternating one-arm pulls from the bent-over position. Switch leg position and repeat.	Week 1 Week 2 Week 3 Week 4	2 × 10 per side 3 × 12 per side 4 × 15 per side 5 × 12 per side
3. BP staggered stance single-arm CLA mid row		Set a band or cable at waist to chest height. Stand in a staggered stance, your left foot forward. Hold a handle in your right hand in a neutral position, your palm facing in. Flex your elbow by pulling the handle to the right side of your ribcage. Extend your arm to the original position. Repeat for the desired number of repetitions, then switch arms and leg positions and repeat to the other side.	Week 1 Week 2 Week 3 Week 4	2 × 8 per side 3 × 10 per side 4 × 12 per side 5 × 10 per side
4. BP single-arm swim (straight-arm pull-down)		Set a band or cable at a high point above your head. Stand with your feet shoulder-width apart, a slight bend in the knees. Hold the handle with your right hand and hinge at the hips to lean forward about 45 degrees. Keeping your arm fully extended, hinge at the shoulder to pull your arm down until your right hand is next to your right hip. Return to the starting position. Repeat for the desired number of repetitions, then switch to the other arm.	Week 1 Week 2 Week 3 Week 4	2 × 10 per side 3 × 12 per side 4 × 15 per side 5 × 12 per side

HER BACK 3: FUNCTIONAL BACK SHAPING WORKOUT

This 4-week program is a fun functional workout with some unique exercises. Although this workout is a back workout, the core is really activated by the plank position, lateral flexion, and long-lever bent-over positions used in some of these exercises. Most homes can be equipped with the functional equipment needed for this workout, so this is a great home routine that really delivers on the performance side of things. Weeks 1 and 2 will be enough for most people, while weeks 3 and 4 should be attempted only by more advanced individuals who have a considerable training base.

Equipment

Suspension system with handles, resistance bands with handles (such as JC Traveler or Predator Jr.), stable object such as a door, stability ball, barbell, dumbbells (optional)

Notes

Weeks 1 and 2: Perform 2 times per week.

Weeks 3 and 4: Perform 1 time per week (for very advanced trainees only).

Table 9.8 Her Back 3: Functional Back Shaping Workout

Exercise	Photo	Instructions	Weeks	Sets × reps
1. Suspension L-pull (seated from feet)		Sit on the ground, your legs straight out in front. Hold the suspension system handles with arms fully extended. Flex at your elbows, pulling yourself up from the ground. Make sure to keep your L position with your legs straight and feet on the floor. Once in full flexion, extend your elbows, and lower yourself back to the ground. Repeat.	Week 1	2 × 8
			Week 2	3 × 10
			Week 3	4 × 12
			Week 4	5 × 10
2. BP single-arm lateral pull-down (with lat flexion)		Stand with a band secured at the top of a door on your right-hand side. Hold the handle with your right hand, your arm straight and palm facing the front. Simultaneously flex your torso to the right, while flexing your right elbow to pull the band until your right elbow is fully flexed and touches your right hip. Slowly return your body and right arm to the starting position. Repeat for the desired number of repetitions, then switch to the other side.	Week 1	2 × 8 per side
			Week 2	3 × 10 per side
			Week 3	4 × 12 per side
			Week 4	5 × 10 per side
3. SB elbow roll-out		Assume a plank position on a stability ball, your elbows on the stability ball and your knees or feet on the ground. Keeping this plank position, roll the ball forward, extending your arms as far as your core can tolerate and stay pain-free. Roll the ball back to the plank position. Repeat.	Week 1	2 × 8
			Week 2	3 × 10
			Week 3	4 × 12
			Week 4	5 × 10

Exercise	Photo	Instructions	Weeks	Sets × reps
4. DB quarter flexed (bent-over) low row		Hold the dumbbells in a pronated grip. Bend your knees slightly. Keep your feet shoulder-width apart and lean forward at a 45-degree angle at the hips. Starting with your arms straight and vertical, flex your elbows to pull the dumbbells to the sides of your lower ribs. Lower the dumbbells to the starting position. Repeat.	Week 1	2 × 10
			Week 2	3 × 12
			Week 3	4 × 10
			Week 4	5 × 12

HER BACK 4: MS. FITNESS PRO BACK WORKOUT

This 4-week program is the first of two pro-grade workouts. This is a full-fledged, high-volume bodybuilding workout with a ton of work in it. The exercises are nothing fancy, just good old-fashioned work. If you are using heavy weights, this workout will take 90 to 120 min, but you can always use lighter loads and cut the volume of sets and reps. Weeks 1 and 2 will be enough for most people. Only professionals should attempt weeks 3 and 4.

Equipment

Cable machine with wide bar attachment and straight bar attachment, incline bench, weight bench, dumbbells

Notes

Weeks 1 and 2: Perform 2 times per week.

Weeks 3 and 4: Perform 1 time per week (for very advanced trainees only).

Table 9.9 Her Back 4: Ms. Fitness Pro Back Workout

Exercise	Photo	Instructions	Weeks	Sets × reps
1. Neutral grip sternum pull-down		Attach a wide bar to a high pulley and hold it in a neutral grip at each end, your palms facing in. Extend your elbows, keeping your arms overhead. Sit with your feet shoulder-width apart. Flex your elbows and pull the bar down to your sternum. Return to the starting position. Repeat.	Week 1	2 × 8
			Week 2	3 × 10
			Week 3	4 × 12
			Week 4	5 × 10
2. DB prone incline bench row		Lie prone on an incline bench, your chest and belly on the inclined portion of the bench. Hold a dumbbell in each hand with your arms fully extended. Flex your elbows, pulling the dumbbells up to the sides of your rib cage. Lower the dumbbells to the starting position. Repeat.	Week 1	2 × 8
			Week 2	3 × 10
			Week 3	4 × 12
			Week 4	5 × 10

(continued)

Table 9.9 Her Back 4: Ms. Fitness Pro Back Workout *(continued)*

Exercise	Photo	Instructions	Weeks	Sets × reps
3. DB bent-over row (supported)		Hold a dumbbell in your right hand using a neutral grip. Bend your knees slightly, your feet shoulder-width apart. Lean forward at a 45-degree angle at the hips. Rest your left hand on a bench or other stable structure. Flex your right elbow and row the dumbbell to the right side of your rib cage. Extend your elbow back to the starting position. Repeat for the desired number of repetitions, then switch to the other side.	Week 1	2 × 10 per side
			Week 2	3 × 12 per side
			Week 3	4 × 15 per side
			Week 4	5 × 12 per side
4. Cable straight-arm pull-down		Attach a straight bar to a high cable pulley. Hold the bar in a pronated grip, your arms extended and the bar at shoulder height. Lean forward at a 45-degree angle at the hips so that the bar is above head height and your arms are in line with the torso. Pull the bar down until it touches your thighs. Raise the bar back to the starting position. Repeat.	Week 1	2 × 10
			Week 2	3 × 12
			Week 3	4 × 15
			Week 4	5 × 15
5. DB pullover breakdown set		Lie perpendicularly on a flat bench with only your shoulders on the bench. Your legs are bent, and your feet are shoulder-width apart. Hold the dumbbell in both hands over your chest, your arms fully extended. Lower the dumbbell behind your head, keeping your arms extended. Once you feel a stretch in the chest, bring the dumbbell back over your chest. Repeat. Start with a weight that allows you to perform 15 reps. Drop the weight 20%-25% for each set and perform the reps to failure. Perform 3 sets total in each superset: first set and 2 drop sets.	Weeks 1-2	2 supersets
			Weeks 3-4	3 supersets

HER BACK 5:
PROFESSIONAL-GRADE BODYBUILDING BACK WORKOUT

The last body transformation workout is this 4-week, 2-day professional-grade split routine for the back. This workout pays particular attention to the tie-in of the lower back and lats, something neglected in many workouts. This is another back workout that serves as a great supplementary workout for the glutes. You can superset exercises 1, 2, 3, and 4 (about 70 min) or take your time and run the workout in succession (about 90 min). Weeks 1 and 2 will be enough for most people, while weeks 3 and 4 should be attempted only by more advanced individuals who have a considerable training base.

Equipment

Dumbbells; medicine balls; cable machine with handle, rope, wide-grip straight bar, and regular bar attachments; bench; stability ball; pull-down machine; T-bar machine; rowing machine with wide-grip bar; bands (such as JC Sports or Predator)

Notes

Weeks 1 and 2: Perform 2 times per week.

Weeks 3 and 4: Perform 1 time per week (for very advanced trainees only).

Table 9.10   Her Back 5: Professional-Grade Bodybuilding Back Workout

Exercise	Photo	Instructions	Weeks	Sets × reps
DAY 1				
1. DB quarter flexed (bent-over) low row		Hold the dumbbells in a pronated grip. Bend your knees slightly. Keep your feet shoulder-width apart and lean forward at a 45-degree angle at the hips. Starting with your arms straight and vertical, flex your elbows to pull the dumbbells to the sides of your lower ribs. Lower the dumbbells to the starting position. Repeat.	Week 1	2 × 8
			Week 2	3 × 10
			Week 3	4 × 8
			Week 4	5 × 6
2. Cable kneeling single-arm row (Moto row variation)		Kneel facing a low cable or band. Hold the handle in your right hand with your elbow extended and palm facing down (or in). Place your left hand in front of you for stability. Flex your right elbow and pull the handle to the side of the right chest. Extend your elbow back to the starting position. Repeat for the desired number of repetitions, then switch arms and repeat.	Week 1	2 × 8 per side
			Week 2	3 × 10 per side
			Week 3	4 × 12 per side
			Week 4	5 × 10 per side
3. Cable incline bench pullover		Place an incline bench in front of a cable set at about hip height with a rope attachment at the end of the cable. Lie on the incline bench, with your feet shoulder-width apart. Hold the rope ends with your arms straight and your hands behind your head, feeling a good stretch on your back. Keeping your arms straight, pull the rope until your arms are at 90 degrees to your body. Return your hands to the starting position behind your head. Repeat.	Week 1	2 × 10
			Week 2	3 × 10
			Week 3	4 × 12
			Week 4	5 × 12

(continued)

Table 9.10 Her Back 5: Professional-Grade Bodybuilding Back Workout *(continued)*

Exercise	Photo	Instructions	Weeks	Sets × reps
4. SB reverse extension with weight between feet		Lie on a small stability ball (55 cm) so your pelvis is on the top and your elbows are on the ground. Have someone put a dumbbell or medicine ball between your feet. Squeeze the legs to make sure you don't drop the weight. Keep your knees slightly flexed while squeezing the dumbbell or medicine ball. Extend the hips to raise your legs and the weight. Slowly lower your legs to the starting position. Repeat.	Week 1	2 × 10
			Week 2	3 × 12
			Week 3	4 × 15
			Week 4	5 × 12
5. Finisher: cable standing wide-grip high row to chin + cable row to hip + cable bent-over straight-arm pull-down		Attach a wide-grip straight bar to a cable pulley at shoulder height. Stand facing the cable machine, your elbows fully extended and your knees slightly bent. Cable standing wide-grip high row to chin: Holding the bar in a pronated grip, flex your elbows to pull the bar toward your chin. Extend your elbows back to the starting position. Repeat for 20 reps. Cable row to hips: Flex your elbows again, this time rowing the bar down to your hips. Extend your elbows back to the starting position. Repeat to failure. Cable bent-over straight-arm pull-down: Lean forward at a 45-degree angle at the hips. Keeping your arms extended, pull the bar to your hips. Allow the bar to go back to the starting position. Repeat to failure. This is one superset. Do not rest between exercises.	Weeks 1-2	2 (20 + failure + failure) supersets
			Week 3-4	3 (20 + failure + failure) supersets
DAY 2				
1. Cable standing row to belly		Stand facing the cable machine, your elbows fully extended and your knees slightly bent. Holding the bar in a pronated grip, flex your elbows to pull the bar toward your belly. Extend your elbows, returning to the starting position. Repeat.	Week 1	2 × 8
			Week 2	3 × 10
			Week 3	4 × 10
			Week 4	5 × 8
2. Machine seated single-arm pull-down		Sit at a pull-down machine. Reach above you and hold one handle with your right hand, your elbow fully extended. Flex your elbow, pulling the handle down to the right side of your ribcage. Extend your elbow back to the starting position. Repeat for the desired number of repetitions, then switch to the other side.	Week 1	2 × 8 per side
			Week 2	3 × 10 per side
			Week 3	4 × 12 per side
			Week 4	5 × 10 per side

Exercise	Photo	Instructions	Weeks	Sets × reps
3. T-bar quarter deadlift + T-bar row		Stand over the T-bar so it is underneath you. Once in position, hold on to the T-bar handles with your arms extended. Perform a quarter deadlift (lean your body 45 degrees forward) and hold the position, lowering the bar and keeping your elbows at full extension. Flex your elbows to pull the weight below your chest. Extend your elbows to lower the T-bar to the starting position. Repeat.	Week 1	2 × 8
			Week 2	3 × 10
			Week 3	4 × 8
			Week 4	5 × 6
4. Cable seated wide-grip high row		Attach a wide-grip bar to the row pulley. Sit on a flat bench with your feet flat, keeping your arms extended. Flex your elbows and pull the bar toward you until it touches your collarbone. Extend your elbows to return to the starting position. Repeat.	Week 1	2 × 8
			Week 2	3 × 10
			Week 3	4 × 12
			Week 4	5 × 10
5. Band finisher: BP row + BP bent-over alternating band row + BP swim (meta back)		BP row: Hold the handle of a band in each hand with a pronated grip. Stand upright with your feet shoulder-width apart and elbows extended. Flex your elbows, pulling the handles to your sides. Extend your elbows out in front. Repeat. BP bent-over alternating row: Hold a handle in each hand in a pronated grip. Hinge at the hips until the torso is parallel to the ground. Row in an alternating fashion (20 reps per side). BP swim: Stand. Hold a handle in each hand in a pronated grip. Keeping your arms extended through the entire motion, pull the bands down while flexing your torso until your hands are near your back pockets and the bands are touching the shoulders. Return to the starting position. Repeat.	Weeks 1-2	2 (20 + 20 per arm + 20) supersets
			Weeks 3-4	3 (20 + 20 per arm + 20) supersets

Summary

I hope this chapter inspired a new appreciation for how important and complex back training really is yet simplified your training approach. At the end of day, it's not about an exercise or how much weight you use. Yes, those factors play a role in your training, but they play a role because of what they do, not because of what they are! They stimulate the muscle. However, no one exercise reigns supreme over another because how much a muscle is stimulated is in the mind of the person doing the exercise. In essence, whatever exercise allows an individual to connect with a muscle and contract it (stimulate it) is the best exercise. I have seen exercises I consider useless pump up my training partner to no end! So, if you feel the exercise and can connect with the muscle you are working, keep doing it. This chapter provides a variety sure to give you four to eight exercises that will connect you with your body and give you that pump that indicates the training is on target. Mix and match until you create that perfect workout and then run with it for four weeks.

PART III

Athletic Movement

Part III concentrates on athletic movements and abilities, such as jumping power, speed, and agility. The chapter on jumping considers the various ways athletes jump and does not lump all of jumping into one category. You also will see that we do not use Olympic lifts, depth jumps, or other training that is overrated, sometimes inefficient, and is not specific to much of the jumping that occurs in sports. Although IHP has about $400,000 worth of equipment, we train jumping simply, and this simple approach to jump training improves jump height as well as anything else. This simple programming is shared with you in that chapter.

The chapter on speed addresses different aspects of sport locomotion that often are thrown together into the speed bucket. Although speed is certainly important in sports, I would argue a more important ability is acceleration. Therefore I include workouts for both speed and acceleration. Likewise, although linear speed gets a ton of attention, often changes of direction are far more important in athletics. Both are covered in this chapter.

Finally, agility is another important athletic ability that does not get the attention it deserves. In the agility chapter, I cover everything from cone drills to situational position changes. Some of the cone agility drills have an enormous conditioning component and so serve as both conditioning and agility training. This chapter is one of the shortest in the book, but packs a big punch. I am certain you will be a much more explosive and agile athlete after completing some of the workouts that await you in part III.

CHAPTER 10

Jumping

Of all valuable athletic skills, jumping is at the top of the list. Whether it's jumping to block a spike in volleyball, dunk a ball in basketball, or make a catch in football, jumping is at the forefront of many sports. All jumping is similar but not the same. Although I could get into the physics of jumps, I want to keep things simple and practical. Therefore, let's separate jumps into two basic categories: standing and running vertical jumps. This way, we can better understand how to train them specifically.

First, we have the parallel stance standing vertical jump. Of all jumps, I consider this the most popular, the most trained, and the one most dependent on strength, yet it's possibly the least functional for life (i.e., sports). I know that seems odd, but let's look at it from a practical standpoint. Few jumps in life occur from a stationary position, use both legs symmetrically, and launch a person vertically upward. Other than a jump ball in basketball or some blocks in volleyball, most jumps use a running start to convert horizontal energy into vertical energy, just like skimming a rock on water.

Standing vertical jumps use the largest amount of leg strength. This is why squatting has traditionally been the most common strength exercise used to improve vertical jump. Squatting improves the amount and magnitude of contraction. Various speed and power exercises are added to squats to help develop the speed of contraction. These include some partial lifts from the Olympic weightlifting world, such as cleans and high pulls, as well as various jumping-related exercises, such as box jumps, vertical jumps, and medicine ball scoop tosses. There is no doubt these exercises improve lower-body power and have a place in just about any jump enhancement program.

Second, we have running vertical jumps. Running jumps are separated into two categories: double-leg and single-leg takeoffs, regardless of landing position. Therefore, one needs to understand that double-leg vertical jumps use the A-frame for takeoff, while the single-leg jumps utilize the 7-frame. This distinction must be made if the principle of specificity of training is to be adhered to. Training on two legs is very different than training on one leg, and we need to look at things from a functional standpoint, even if we have to question traditional dogma.

Whether it's a jump serve in volleyball, a single-leg takeoff for a dunk in basketball, or any jump in track and field, all these jumps use muscular contraction. A significant amount of vertical lift is generated by the horizontal energy provided by running and the elastic components of the body (e.g., bone, ligaments, tendons, and other noncontractile tissue). Running vertical jumps require the least amount of range of motion and the least amount of leg and hip strength (as we usually understand strength), but they utilize the most elastic recoil. These jumps don't require a lot of leg movement through large ranges of motion; rather, they require leg and hip stiffness through very short ranges of motion. If you look at these jumps in slow motion, you will see small ranges of motion of the ankles, knees, and hips at the moment of takeoff (i.e., where horizontal momentum is converted to vertical lift). Therefore, this chapter has many partial-range-of-motion exercises that develop the lower-body stiffness characteristic of elastic power movements.

This chapter includes easy-to-follow workouts that will improve all versions of vertical jumps, from standing to running, and from double-leg to single-leg. Many workouts follow the succession format in which all the sets of a particular exercise are completed before going on to the next exercise. I also use the sequence method, pairing a strength exercise and an explosive exercise that looks like the strength exercise (i.e., uses the same muscles). This pairing of a strength exercise and an explosive exercise has been referred to as *complex* or *contrast training*. In complex training, the CNS is excited but not fatigued by a few reps of the strength exercise. A short rest (about a minute) allows the muscles to recover, while the CNS is still excited (i.e., potentiated). Then the light explosive exercise is performed to a much higher power output than if it were done without the prior heavy work. This process works just like a batter who warms up by swinging a bat weighted with a doughnut, then removes the doughnut and swings the bat by itself.

I also vary the equipment so you can train in any field or gym. This chapter contains medicine ball and dumbbell workouts that can be performed on any field, as well as workouts that require standard equipment such as barbells, dumbbells, and medicine balls. A few workouts require specialized equipment, such as sleds, in case you have them available. If you like a workout, but it uses equipment you don't have, substitute a similar exercise that uses available equipment. For example, if you don't have a leg press machine for a double-leg or single-leg leg press, substitute a barbell squat or weighted step-up, respectively. If you don't have a sled to drag, push, or pull, use a tire to provide resistance. Equipment shouldn't determine the effectiveness of your training. Options are available, so no excuses. Make it happen.

Power training should not be done without a training base. In order to learn to be explosive, you must practice being explosive; it is a learned behavior. This means each explosive repetition has to be an attempt at a personal record, and ample rest (5-10 sec) between each rep must be taken in order to repeatedly provide your best effort. This is not conditioning; this is power development. Take your time and learn to be explosive by constantly performing quality power repetitions.

Fast, explosive movements put a lot of strain on the entire jumping mechanism (e.g., bone, ligaments, tendons, and muscles). If the specific structure involved in generating the force required for the jump is not ready, some form of injury is almost certain. Therefore, I recommend everyone complete a leg and hip program from chapter 4 to develop a proper training base for jump training. Ideally you want a week of active recovery between the month of strength work and the jump training in this chapter, but since the workouts are progressive (i.e., they start light and progressively get heavier) you may proceed with caution into these workouts after completing your base training. If at any time your ankles, knees, or hips become achy, stop training or, at the very least, reduce your volume and intensity. Pain is a sign the work you are doing is too much for your joints and more strength may be needed, or it means that the training just does not agree with you. Pain can come from many things, such as being too heavy for your structure, lack of strength, insufficient training base, incorrect execution of an exercise, too much weight for an exercise, or an incorrect warm-up. Don't worry; we can always train around pain and improve performance to some degree without doing more damage. Above all, be smart about your training! If an exercise doesn't feel good, stop and substitute an exercise that does feel good. Train pain free.

Warming up for jump training is more important than for hypertrophy training, perhaps because hypertrophy training does not start as an all-out effort and jump training does. In hypertrophy training, the muscle has time to adjust to the load over 8 to 15 repetitions. In jump training, it has to be ready on the first jump. Therefore, here is a basic warm-up protocol to get you ready for your jump workouts.

WARM-UP FOR DOUBLE-LEG JUMPING

MB chopper (MB chop, rotation with pivot, diagonal wood chop) 3 × 10 + 10 + 10 (to each side)

Vertical jump 3 × 3 (1 × 3 at 50% effort, 1 × 3 at 75% effort, and 1 × 3 at 100% effort)

WARM-UP FOR SINGLE-LEG JUMPING

Single-leg CLA anterior reach 2 × 10 per leg

Single-leg short squat 2 × 5 per leg

Single-leg hop 2 × 2-3 per leg

JUMP 1: STATIONARY DOUBLE-LEG JUMP FIELD WORKOUT

This is a basic 4-week program to develop stationary double-leg jumping. It requires simple equipment, including a weight plate or heavy and light medicine balls (heavy for chopping and light for throwing). This workout is perfect for young athletes or those wanting to improve their jumping ability for a weekend game of beach volleyball or basketball. The workout is set up as a sequence: Perform the A exercise, rest for 1 min, perform the B exercise, and rest 2-3 min before going back to the A exercise. Perform each B exercise with maximum effort, and rest for 5-10 sec between each rep to ensure maximal training intensity. You can also perform this workout in succession and complete the prescribed sets and reps of each exercise before going on to the next exercise, resting 1 min between each exercise.

Equipment

Heavy weight plate, medicine ball, dumbbells

Notes

Rest for 1 min between the A and B exercises in each complex. Rest 2-3 min between each complex.

JUMP WORKOUTS

Table 10.1 Jump 1: Stationary Double-Leg Jump Field Workout

Exercise	Photo	Instructions	Weeks	Sets × reps
1a. Weight plate speed chop		Stand upright, your feet shoulder-width apart. Hold a heavy weight plate in both hands over your head. Squat and lower the plate between your legs while leaning your shoulders forward and keeping your back straight. Stand up to return to the starting position. Repeat. Use a heavy weight that allows you to perform 8-10 repetitions.	Weeks 1-2	2 × 5
			Weeks 3-4	3 × 5

(continued)

Table 10.1   Jump 1: Stationary Double-Leg Jump Field Workout *(continued)*

Exercise	Photo	Instructions	Weeks	Sets × reps
1b. MB reverse scoop throw		Hold the medicine ball in your hands, your arms extended and feet shoulder-width apart. Squat, lowering the medicine ball between your legs. Thrust the hips forward, throwing the ball backward over your head. Repeat. Use a light weight you can throw fast.	Weeks 1-2	2 × 5
			Weeks 3-4	3 × 5
2a. DB squat jump		Stand upright, your feet shoulder-width apart. Hold a dumbbell in each hand by your sides. Sit your hips back into a squat until your thighs are parallel to the floor. Jump straight up, pushing through your toes, and land softly. Repeat. Use a heavy weight that allows you to perform 8-10 repetitions.	Weeks 1-2	2 × 5
			Weeks 3-4	3 × 5
2b. Vertical jump		Stand upright with your feet shoulder-width apart. Squat, swinging the arms back. Explode up and swing the arms forward, reaching as high as you can. Land softly on both feet. Repeat.	Weeks 1-2	2 × 5
			Weeks 3-4	3 × 5
3a. MB burpee		With a medicine ball in front of you, squat down and place your hands on the medicine ball while jumping your feet out into a plank position. Quickly bring your feet back toward the medicine ball, then stand upright with the medicine ball. Lower the medicine ball back to the starting position. Repeat. Use a heavy weight that allows you to perform 8-10 repetitions.	Weeks 1-2	2 × 5
			Weeks 3-4	3 × 5
3b. MB jump and reach		Hold a medicine ball in front of you at chest level with your feet shoulder-width apart. Squat down and jump up while reaching up with the medicine ball. Return to the starting position. Repeat. Use a light weight that you can lift as high as possible.	Weeks 1-2	2 × 5
			Weeks 3-4	3 × 5

JUMP 2: STATIONARY DOUBLE-LEG JUMP GYM WORKOUT

This basic 4-week program develops stationary double-leg jumping and is perfect for a gym since it requires barbells, racks, and boxes. This workout is appropriate for intermediate athletes or those who have a training base and want to improve their stationary vertical jumps. The sequence format is used: Perform the A exercise, rest 1 min, perform the B exercise, and rest 2-3 min before going back to the A exercise. Perform each B exercise with a maximum effort, and rest 3-5 sec between each rep to ensure maximal training intensity. Although the sequence format is my preference for power training, you can also perform this workout in succession fashion and complete the prescribed sets and reps of each exercise before going on to the next exercise.

Equipment

Barbell, plyometric box, medicine ball

Notes

Rest for 1 min between the A and B exercises in each complex. Rest 2-3 min between each complex.

Table 10.2 Jump 2: Stationary Double-Leg Jump Gym Workout

Exercise	Photo	Instructions	Weeks	Sets × reps
1a. Barbell high pull		Hold the barbell in a pronated grip with hands just outside hip-width, your feet shoulder-width apart. Keeping your back straight, move your hips back as you bend your knees. Keeping your arms straight, simultaneously extend your ankles, knees, and hips while shrugging, lifting the bar to your abdomen. Lower the barbell to the starting position. Repeat. Use a heavy weight that allows you to perform 7-8 reps.	Weeks 1-2	2 × 5
			Weeks 3-4	3 × 5
1b. Vertical jump		Stand upright with your feet shoulder-width apart. Squat, swinging your arms back. As you explode up, swing your arms forward, reaching as high as you can. Land softly. Repeat.	Weeks 1-2	2 × 5
			Weeks 3-4	3 × 5
2a. Barbell squat		Stand upright, your feet shoulder-width apart. Hold the barbell on your traps below your neck. Sit the hips back as you squat until your thighs are parallel to the ground. Push through your heels to return to the starting position. Repeat. Use a heavy weight that allows you to perform 7-8 reps.	Weeks 1-2	2 × 5
			Weeks 3-4	3 × 5

(continued)

Table 10.2 Jump 2: Stationary Double-Leg Jump Gym Workout *(continued)*

Exercise	Photo	Instructions	Weeks	Sets × reps
2b. Box jump		Stand upright, facing a plyometric box. Lower your hips into a quarter squat, swinging your arms back. Jump onto the box as you swing your arms up. Step down from the box. Repeat.	Weeks 1-2	2 × 5
			Weeks 3-4	3 × 5
3a. Barbell deadlift		Hold the barbell in a pronated grip, your hands just outside hip-width and your feet shoulder-width apart. Keeping your back straight, move your hips back as you bend your knees. Squat so your shins are right behind the bar. Protract the shoulder blades and begin to push through the heels while driving your hips forward into an upright position. Lower the barbell by squatting down. Repeat. Use a heavy weight that allows you to perform 7-8 reps.	Weeks 1-2	2 × 5
			Weeks 3-4	3 × 5
3b. MB burpee to jump		With a medicine ball in front of you, squat and place your hands on the medicine ball while jumping your feet out into a plank position. Quickly bring your feet back toward the medicine ball. Stand upright with the medicine ball and jump. Lower the medicine ball to the starting position. Repeat.	Weeks 1-2	2 × 5
			Weeks 3-4	3 × 5

JUMP 3: DOUBLE-LEG JUMPING WITH RUNNING START HOME WORKOUT

This basic 4-week program develops all double-leg jumping that uses a running start. I use this workout with clients who need something easy to do at home using dumbbells, medicine balls, and body weight. Although this workout is simple enough to be used by beginners, it also can be used by advanced athletes if you increase the loads of the resistance exercises and the amplitude of the jumps. The sequence format is used: Perform the A exercise, rest 1 min, perform the B exercise, and rest 2-3 min before going back to the A exercise. Perform each B exercise with a maximum effort, and rest 3-5 sec between each rep to ensure maximal training intensity. Although the sequence method is preferred, you can also perform this workout in succession fashion and complete the prescribed sets and reps of each exercise before going on to the next exercise.

Equipment

Dumbbells, medicine ball, basketball hoop (or wall), barbell, standing calf machine, Smith machine, board or platform

Notes

Rest for 1 min between the A and B exercises in each complex. Rest 2-3 min between each complex.

Table 10.3 Jump 3: Double-Leg Jumping With Running Start Home Workout

Exercise	Photo	Instructions	Weeks	Sets × reps
1a. DB lateral reaching lunge		Stand upright, your feet shoulder-width apart. Hold a dumbbell in both hands at at your sides. Step to your right with your right leg, bending at the hips, and reach with the dumbbell to your right foot. Push off with your right leg back to the starting position and repeat to the left side. Use a heavy weight that allows you to perform 7-8 reps.	Weeks 1-2	2 × 5 per side
			Weeks 3-4	3 × 5 per side
1b. MB lateral step and rim touch		Stand underneath a basketball hoop and hold a medicine ball at chest level. Take a lateral step to your right. Immediately jump explosively into the air and touch the rim with the medicine ball. Repeat to the left side. You may use a wall if you cannot jump high enough to touch a rim. Use a light ball (1-2 lb [1 kg]) that allows you to jump high.	Weeks 1-2	2 × 5 per side
			Weeks 3-4	3 × 5 per side
2a. DB rotating reaching lunge		Stand upright, your feet shoulder-width apart. Hold a dumbbell in both hands at chest level. Step to your right and back (135 degrees) with your right leg, bending at the hips, and reach with the dumbbell to your right foot. Push off with your right leg back to the starting position and repeat to the left. Use a heavy weight that allows you to perform 7-8 reps.	Weeks 1-2	2 × 5 per side
			Weeks 3-4	3 × 5 per side
2b. MB rotational step and rim touch		Stand with your back to a basketball hoop or wall. Hold a medicine ball at chest level. Take a rotational step back to your right so your end position is facing the hoop. Immediately jump explosively into the air and touch the rim with the medicine ball. Repeat to the left side. Note: You may use a wall if you cannot jump high enough to touch a rim. Use a light ball (1-2 lb [1 kg]) that allows you to jump high.	Weeks 1-2	2 × 5 per side
			Weeks 3-4	3 × 5 per side
3a. Weighted ankle pump		Use a standing calf machine, Smith machine, dumbbells, or a barbell to load this exercise. Stand upright, your feet shoulder-width apart, with the barbell (or shoulder pads) on your traps below your neck. Stand on the ground or place the balls of your feet on a board, low box, or platform. Perform quick and pulsating heel raises, barely flexing your knees and ankles. Use your legs like a strong spring. Use a heavy weight that allows you to perform 10-15 reps with no rest between reps.	Weeks 1-2	2 × 5-10
			Weeks 3-4	3 × 5-10

(continued)

Exercise	Photo	Instructions	Weeks	Sets × reps
3b. Ankle jump		This exercise is like skipping rope. Stand with your feet shoulder-width apart. Using only your ankles, push off the ground into the air as if skipping a rope. Get as high as you can on each jump without your heels touching the ground. No rest between reps.	Weeks 1-2	2 × 5-10
			Weeks 3-4	3 × 5-10

JUMP 4: DOUBLE-LEG JUMP FROM RUNNING START WORKOUT

This basic 4-week program develops power for all double-leg jumping from a running start. This is one of our favorite workouts at IHP because we have really cool leg presses and various other pieces of power equipment. Like the previous workout, this workout can be used with low intensity for a beginner or ramped up in loads and amplitude for pro athletes. The sequence format is used: Perform the A exercise, rest 1 min, perform the B exercise, and rest 2-3 min before going back to the A exercise. Perform each B exercise with a maximum effort, and rest 3-5 sec between each rep to ensure maximal training intensity. At IHP we prefer the sequence method, but you can also perform this workout in succession and complete the prescribed sets and reps of each exercise before going on to the next exercise.

Equipment

Barbell, Smith machine, standing calf machine, leg press machine, plyometric box, dumbbells

Notes

Rest for 1 min between the A and B exercises in each complex. Rest 2-3 min between each complex.

Table 10.4 Jump 4: Double-Leg Jump From Running Start Workout

Exercise	Photo	Instructions	Weeks	Sets × reps
1a. Quarter barbell squat		You can use a regular barbell, a Smith machine, or some standing calf machines. Stand upright, your feet shoulder-width apart, with the barbell on your traps below your neck. Squat a quarter of the way down, controlled. Make sure your knees do not extend past your toes. Push through your heels until you are back in the starting position. Repeat. Use a heavy weight that allows you to perform 7-8 reps.	Weeks 1-2	2 × 5
			Weeks 3-4	3 × 5
1b. Double-leg lead-up vertical jump		With your feet shoulder-width apart, take 2 or 3 quick lead-up steps and jump as high as you can, as if you were going to dunk a basketball. Land softly and repeat.	Weeks 1-2	2 × 5
			Weeks 3-4	3 × 5

Exercise	Photo	Instructions	Weeks	Sets × reps
2a. Leg half-press		Sit in a leg press machine with your feet shoulder-width apart on the platform. Hold on to the handles at your sides and push through your heels until your knees have slight flexion. Lower the platform until your knees are about 90-110 degrees flexed. Quickly push the sled back to the starting position. Repeat. Use a heavy weight that allows you to perform 7-8 reps. Since some jumps require taking off from the balls of the feet, you may drive the leg press from the balls of the feet.	Weeks 1-2	2 × 5
			Weeks 3-4	3 × 5
2b. Double-leg lead-up box jump		With your feet shoulder-width apart, take 2 or 3 quick steps toward a plyometric box. Jump onto the box, landing softly. Step down and repeat. Use a box that allows you to land with your knees slightly bent. Also try approaching the box from different angles.	Weeks 1-2	2 × 5
			Weeks 3-4	3 × 5
3a. DB lateral reaching lunge		Stand upright, your feet shoulder-width apart. Hold one dumbbell in each hand at chest level. Step to your right with your right leg, bending at the hips, and reach with the dumbbell to your right foot. Push off with your right leg back to the starting position and repeat to the left. Use a heavy weight that allows you to perform 7-10 reps.	Weeks 1-2	2 × 5 per side
			Weeks 3-4	3 × 5 per side
3b. MB lateral step and rim touch		Stand underneath a basketball hoop and hold a medicine ball at chest level. Take a lateral step to your right. Immediately jump explosively into the air and touch the rim with the medicine ball. Repeat to the left side. You may use a wall if you cannot jump high enough to touch a rim. Use a light ball (1-2 lb [1 kg]) that allows you to jump high.	Weeks 1-2	2 × 5 per side
			Weeks 3-4	3 × 5 per side

JUMP 5: SINGLE-LEG JUMP FROM RUNNING START WORKOUT

This basic 4-week program develops power in single-leg jumps from a running start. This simple but very effective workout uses body weight, medicine balls, and dumbbells. However, do not let the simplicity of the workout fool you. I use this workout with elite high school and college athletes, and it works like a charm! The sequence format is used: Perform the A exercise, rest 1 min, perform the B exercise, and rest 2-3 min before going back to the A exercise. Perform each B exercise with a maximum effort, and rest 5-10 sec between each rep to ensure maximal training intensity. At IHP we prefer the sequence method for complex training, but you can also perform this workout in succession fashion and complete the prescribed sets and reps of each exercise before going on to the next exercise.

Equipment

Dumbbells, plyometric box, medicine ball, low hurdles

Notes

Rest for 1 min between the A and B exercises in each complex. Rest 2-3 min between each complex.

Table 10.5 Jump 5: Single-Leg Jump From Running Start Workout

Exercise	Photo	Instructions	Weeks	Sets × reps
1a. Single-leg DB step-up		Stand upright, holding a dumbbell in each hand and facing a plyometric box. Place your left foot on the plyometric box. Push through your left heel, raising your body and right leg onto the plyometric box. Step off the plyometric box with your right foot first back to the starting position. Perform all repetitions leading with your left foot, then switch to leading with your right foot. Use a heavy weight that allows you to perform 7-8 reps.	Weeks 1-2	2 × 5 per side
			Weeks 3-4	3 × 5 per side
1b. Single-leg hop		Balance on your right leg. Using only your right leg, push off in a heel-to-toes fashion and hop in a straight line. Perform for desired reps, then repeat with your left leg. Hop for distance each time with minimum ground contact time.	Weeks 1-2	2 × 5 per side
			Weeks 3-4	3 × 5 per side
2a. Single-leg MB wood chop		Stand on your right leg and hold a medicine ball in both hands overhead. Slightly squat and lower the medicine ball toward your right foot. Return to the starting position, raising the medicine ball above your head. Perform all repetitions while balancing on your right leg, then switch to your left leg. Use a heavy weight that allows you to perform 7-8 reps.	Weeks 1-2	2 × 5 per side
			Weeks 3-4	3 × 5 per side

Exercise	Photo	Instructions	Weeks	Sets × reps
2b. Power skip		Stand with your feet shoulder-width apart and your elbows at 90 degrees. Keeping your elbows at 90 degrees, simultaneously raise your right knee and swing your left arm forward, launching your body up and forward. Land on your left foot and immediately step onto your right foot. Perform the skipping sequence to the other side of the body. Continue alternating legs in a skipping motion, always moving the lower and upper body in opposition. Skip for distance each time with minimum ground contact time.	Weeks 1-2	2 × 5 per side
			Weeks 3-4	3 × 5 per side
3a. DB rear lunge		Stand with your feet shoulder-width apart and hold a dumbbell in each hand at your sides. Step backward into a lunge with your right leg. Return to the starting position and repeat, lunging backward with your left leg. Use a heavy weight that allows you to perform 7-8 reps.	Weeks 1-2	2 × 5 per side
			Weeks 3-4	3 × 5 per side
3b. Single-leg low-hurdle jump		Set up 5 hurdles (6-8 in. [15-20 cm]) 2-3 ft (1 m) apart. Balance on your right leg in front of the first hurdle. Using only your right leg, push through your heel and toes and jump over each hurdle until you jump all 5 hurdles. Turn around and repeat, jumping off your left leg. Jump with minimum ground contact time.	Weeks 1-2	2 × 5 per side
			Weeks 3-4	3 × 5 per side

Summary

This chapter includes some of the most effective jumping workouts I have used at IHP over the last 20 years. Although many seem simple, our coaching and insistence on perfect execution make these workouts extremely powerful. Whether it's a double-leg jump or a single-leg jump, these workouts deliver quick results in a safe and effective manner. No high-level plyometric training is needed in order to participate in effective and advanced power training, and these workouts are proof of that. The complex methods introduced in this book increase not only the effectiveness of power training, but they do so with an inclusion of strength training, an added bonus and why I prefer this method of power development. Take any of these workouts for a test drive, and you will be amazed at the gains in your vertical jumping capacity.

CHAPTER 11

Speed

I f any athletic attribute can topple jumping in terms of popularity, running speed has to be it. Speed is, without a doubt, the most sought-after physical attribute that athletes ask for at IHP. It does not matter if the athletes play football, soccer, basketball, rugby, or lacrosse or run track and field or even a triathlon, they all ask for more speed. Traditionally, the enhancement of locomotive speed was approached by improving leg power through traditional lifts (e.g., squat, clean, deadlift, leg press) and various running drills (e.g., skips, hops, jumps, and bounds). The speed, agility, and quickness training popularized by Randy Smyth in the late 1980s and early 1990s brought attention to the training of speed. Speed training provided by sprint coaches and U.S.A. Track and Field contributed to the body of knowledge about making athletes faster. Most recently functional training added to the training options available and forced us to look at training more realistically and practically, question tradition, and dare to try new training methods. This chapter provides the new flavor of functional training for speed mixed into the traditional training for speed.

The most common characteristic of human locomotion is that it occurs a single leg at a time. If the main training principle is the specificity principle of training, we must ask why practically all strength training intended to improve leg strength for the enhancement of running speed has been done on two legs. I don't know the reason, and it does not matter. At IHP, we broke the tradition a long time ago, and I outlined our approach to single-leg training in my 2001 NSCA *Strength and Conditioning Journal* article, "Single-Leg Training for 2-Legged Sports: Efficacy of Strength Development in Athletic Performance." In that article, as well as in *Functional Training*, I show how running is all about single-leg (e.g., the 7-frame) strength and power. As a matter of fact, changes of direction and all rotating sport skills depend on single-leg strength and power and lots of rotation.

The functional training movement paid specific attention to this single-leg phenomenon. However, at times, it's been lost in flexibility, balance, and all the "proprioceptively enriched" verbiage. At IHP, we improve running by developing single-leg stiffness at very conservative flexion angles at the ankles, knees, and hips. When you look at running, you will never see deep positions or extreme ranges of motion at any of these joints. You see them generating enormous forces like springs: tight ranges with a lot of power are being driven through these joints. Therefore, in this chapter, you will see many partial-range-of-motion strength training and a lot of single-leg training.

Equipment varies from body weight to the standard functional favorites, such as medicine balls, stability balls, bands, and dumbbells. However, I also include more specialized equipment, such as leg press machines, shuttles, sleds, and even trucks and cars so you can experience the breadth of IHP training. Yes, I said trucks and cars! If you want a peek at what we have been doing at IHP since 2001 for running speed, search YouTube for "truck push at IHP" (https://www.youtube.com/watch?v=fhS3E_NGQME), and you will see how everyone uses a Lincoln Navigator to specifically improve leg strength for running speed and pushing power. Don't worry; I always offer alternatives in case you don't have some of this specialized equipment.

The format of the workouts in this chapter range from the complex model used for jumping workouts to the more standard succession format using strength and functional exercises. However, I am adding a twist to this chapter, since running speed is such a coveted athletic ability. I'm adding a supplemental protocol for everyone

Triple Threat

The triple threat is a combination of three stability ball exercises in succession, consisting of the SB bridge (figure 11.1), the SB leg curl (figure 11.2), and the SB hip lift (figure 11.3). This protocol keeps constant tension on the hamstrings by requiring the hips to come up and remain off the floor during the entire protocol.

Begin the progression by using both legs simultaneously. On week 1, perform 3 sets of 5 repetitions for each exercise in sequence without rest. Perform 15 nonstop repetitions per set—5 bridges, 5 leg curls, walk the ball out, and perform 5 hip lifts (this is a triple threat set). Rest 1 to 2 minutes between each triple threat set. Each week, add 2 repetitions to each exercise. By week 10, you will be doing 15 repetitions of each exercise, 45 continuous repetitions per triple threat set, for 3 sets. On week 11, the progression gets much more interesting; it goes to single-leg work. The repetition and set scheme starts at week 1 again. Perform 15 nonstop repetitions per set per leg—5 bridges, 5 leg curls, walk the ball out, and perform 5 hip lifts (this is a triple threat set). Perform the same sequence with the other leg. Each week, add 2 repetitions to each exercise. Since one leg is resting while the other is exercising, there is no need to rest between sets. By week 20, you are doing 15 repetitions of each exercise, 45 continuous repetitions per set, for 3 sets, on each leg. This workout can be performed 2 or 3 times per week for an eternity and will give you hamstrings of steel! We have not had hamstring pulls at IHP since we started to use the triple threat with our other single-leg protocols.

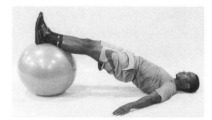

Figure 11.1 SB bridge.

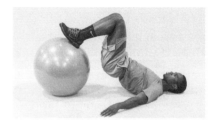

Figure 11.2 SB leg curl.

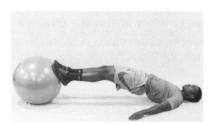

Figure 11.3 SB hip lift.

performing any one of these workouts: the famous triple threat. The triple threat was also featured in the 2001 NSCA *Strength and Conditioning Journal* article "Hamstrings of Steel: Preventing the Pull, Part II—Training the 'Triple Threat'" (volume 23, issue 1, page 18) and *Functional Training*.

I have added a couple killer warm-up workouts that will add speed. These warm-ups excite the CNS and add a little spring to your ankles and knees. All athletes can use these simple warm-ups to prepare for speed workouts and improve running speed. These protocols are much more effective than jogging on a treadmill or even stretching for 5 to 10 minutes.

WARM-UP FOR LINEAR SPEED

Double-leg weighted rope jump (ropes of 1-2 lb [1 kg]) 2 × 20-30

Single-leg weighted rope jump (ropes of 0.5-1 lb [0.2-1 kg)) 2 × 10-20 per leg

Single-leg anterior reach 2 × 10 per leg

Single-leg band-resisted knee-up 2 × 10 per leg

V-up 2 × 10

WARM-UP FOR LATERAL SPEED AND CHANGES OF DIRECTION

Double-leg weighted rope jump (ropes of 1-2 lb [1 kg]) 2 × 20-30

Single-leg weighted rope jump (ropes of 0.5-1 lb [0.2-1 kg]) 2 × 10-20 per leg

MB 3D reaching lunge 2 × 6 (3 per side): 6 anterior, 6 lateral, and 6 rotational

Skater 2 × 10 (5 per side)

Single-leg lateral band-resisted knee-up 2 × 10

X-up 2 × 10

Just these warm-ups and the triple threat alone are enough to improve anyone's speed. However, when you combine them with the workouts in this chapter, there is no telling the improvements you will experience in your running speed. Many of our high school athletes attribute these workouts to allowing them to be recruited by some of the top universities in the country, with full-ride scholarships. Now, if that's not exciting, I don't know what is. Try some of these workouts and see where they take your speed.

SPEED 1: BIOMOTOR SKILL SPEED WORKOUT

This 4-week program focuses on developing biomotor skills through light plyometrics. Once you establish a good base of training (complete 4 weeks), you can even use a reduced volume version of this workout as a warm-up to running drills and skills training. This is a perfect workout for any person wanting to improve running mechanics and speed, such as recreational runners and field and court athletes. Weeks 1 and 2 will be enough for most people, while weeks 3 and 4 should be attempted only by more advanced individuals who have a considerable training base.

Equipment

Wall

Notes

Perform 2-4 times per week.

Table 11.1 Speed 1: Biomotor Skill Speed Workout

Exercise	Photo	Instructions	Weeks	Sets × reps
1. Ankling		This exercise is a fast, low-amplitude run using only the balls of your feet. Stand with your feet shoulder-width apart. Using only dorsiflexion and plantar flexion of your ankles, pull one heel off the ground. Continue alternating ankles in a running motion.	Week 1	2 × 15 yd (14 m)
			Week 2	3 × 20 yd (18 m)
			Week 3	4 × 20 yd (18 m)
			Week 4	4 × 25 yd (23 m)
2. Frankenstein run		Stand upright with your feet shoulder-width apart and your arms extended out in front. Keeping your legs straight, bring your leg up to your hand with each step. Lower your leg back to the ground and repeat with the other leg.	Week 1	2 × 15 yd (14 m)
			Week 2	3 × 20 yd (18 m)
			Week 3	4 × 20 yd (18 m)
			Week 4	4 × 25 yd (23 m)
3. Wall run		Place your hands on a wall and lean into it at a 45-70-degree angle. As you quickly run in place, drive your knees up toward the wall. Repeat for desired reps.	Week 1	2 × 3 per side
			Week 2	3 × 5 per side
			Week 3	4 × 7 per side
			Week 4	4 × 9 per side
4. Power skip		Stand upright with your feet shoulder-width apart. Begin skipping, making sure to push through your toes, driving your knee up each time and gaining distance. Repeat for the desired reps or distance.	Week 1	2 × 15 per side
			Week 2	3 × 20 yd (18 m)
			Week 3	4 × 20 yd (18 m)
			Week 4	4 × 25 yd (23 m)
5. Single-leg hop		Stand upright, balancing on one leg. Using just this leg, hop for the desired distance. Repeat using the other leg.	Week 1	2 × 10 yd (9 m)
			Week 2	3 × 15 yd (14 m)
			Week 3	4 × 20 yd (18 m)
			Week 4	4 × 20 yd (18 m)

Exercise	Photo	Instructions	Weeks	Sets × reps
6. 45-degree calf pump		Place your hands on a wall and lean into it at a 45-70-degree angle. Balance on the ball of your left foot, and bring your right leg up in a knee-up, toe-up fashion. Perform mini ankle extensions (pumps). Repeat using the other leg.	Week 1	2 × 10 per leg
			Week 2	3 × 20 per leg
			Week 3	4 × 30 per leg
			Week 4	4 × 40 per leg

SPEED 2: RUNNING POWER GYM WORKOUT

This 4-week program develops running power. As written, you will need lifting equipment close to a running area. Perform the A exercise, rest 1-2 min, then perform the B exercise. If your facility doesn't allow this set-up, perform 1a, 2a, 3a, and 3b in the weight area, then go to the running area and perform 1b and 2b. This workout is very effective in developing top-end speed and is also a great workout for endurance runners, especially those who run hills. Weeks 1 and 2 will be enough for most people. Weeks 3 and 4 should be attempted only by college-level and professional athletes who have several years of training experience.

Equipment

Sled, weights, treadmill (optional), leg press machine, start blocks, band (such as JC Sport or Predator), power slings, dumbbells

Notes

For the single-leg ball-of-foot leg press, band-resisted stationary A run, and running curl, the repetition range or time drops from week to week. For these exercises, the weights used must go up in order to keep the exercise challenging and strength gains continuous.

Weeks 1 and 2: Perform 2 times per week.

Weeks 3 and 4: Perform 1 time per week (very advanced trainees only).

Table 11.2 Speed 2: Running Power Gym Workout

Exercise	Photo	Instructions	Weeks	Sets × reps
1a. Sled run		Load the sled with a weight that allows you to run. Attach the sled to your waist via a power sling and face away from the sled. Run as fast as possible, pulling the sled behind you for the prescribed distance. Pull a small tire if you don't have a sled.	Week 1	2 × 15 yd (14 m)
			Week 2	3 × 20 yd (18 m)
			Week 3	4 × 20 yd (18 m)
			Week 4	4 × 25 yd (23 m)
1b. 30-yard run		A treadmill can be used, if you prefer. Run slowly for the first 10 yd (9 m). Increase your speed for the second 10 yd (9 m) and sprint the last 10 yd (9 m) at 100% speed. Build to your top speed. Repeat.	Week 1	2 × 30 yd
			Week 2	3 × 30 yd
			Week 3	4 × 30 yd
			Week 4	4 × 30 yd

(continued)

Table 11.2 Speed 2: Running Power Gym Workout *(continued)*

Exercise	Photo	Instructions	Weeks	Sets × reps
2a. Single-leg ball-of-foot leg press		Sit on the leg press machine, planting one foot on the platform. Using just the ball of your foot, extend your knee, pushing on the platform. Do not lock out your knee. After the leg is extended, flex the knee and lower the weight until the knee is flexed to 90 degrees. Repeat for the desired number of reps, then switch to the other leg.	Week 1	2 × 10 per side
			Week 2	3 × 8 per side
			Week 3	4 × 6 per side
			Week 4	4 × 4 per side
2b. 10-yard start		Position yourself in the start blocks. Explode out of the blocks by staying low and driving your leading knee. Make sure to stay low for the entire 10 yd (9 m) as you sprint.	Week 1	2
			Week 2	3
			Week 3	4
			Week 4	4
3a. Band-resisted stationary A run		Put a band around your waist with the anchor point behind you. Make sure there is tension in the band to start. Run in place while resisting the band, driving your knees up with each step. Stay on the balls of your feet the whole time.	Week 1	2 × 15 sec
			Week 2	3 × 15 sec
			Week 3	4 × 10 sec
			Week 4	4 × 10 sec
3b. Running curl		Hold a dumbbell in each hand while standing in place with your feet shoulder-width apart. Pump your arms as if running, keeping your lower body still. Focus on controlling the pushing and pulling with speed.	Week 1	2 × 15 sec
			Week 2	3 × 15 sec
			Week 3	4 × 10 sec
			Week 4	4 × 10 sec

SPEED 3: LATERAL SPEED AND LATERAL CHANGES OF DIRECTION WORKOUT

This 4-week program improves lateral speed and lateral changes of directions. Similar to speed workout 1, you can use a reduced-volume version of this workout as a warm-up to running drills on your lateral speed days. This is a perfect workout to improve the quickness needed in short lateral changes of direction in court sports such as tennis and basketball. Weeks 1 and 2 will be enough for most people. Weeks 3 and 4 should be attempted only by college-level and professional athletes who have several years of training experience.

Equipment

None

Notes

Weeks 1 and 2: Perform 2 times per week.

Weeks 3 and 4: Perform 1 time per week (very advanced trainees only).

Table 11.3 Speed 3: Lateral Speed and Lateral Changes of Direction Workout

Exercise	Photo	Instructions	Weeks	Sets × reps
1. Carioca		Stand upright with your feet shoulder-width apart, a slight bend in your knees. Put the right foot on the starting line and left foot downfield. Cross your right foot in front of your left foot with your arms at your sides. Then take your left foot and step out to the side, while taking your right foot and crossing it behind you. Continue moving laterally for the desired distance. Repeat for the desired distance, switching direction each time.	Week 1	1 × 15 yd (14 m) per side
			Week 2	1 × 20 yd (18 m) per side
			Week 3	2 × 20 yd (18 m) per side
			Week 4	3 × 25 yd (23 m) per side
2. Lateral shuffle		Stand upright with your feet shoulder-width apart, the right foot on the starting line and the left foot downfield. Bend your knees slightly. Take a long lateral step with your left foot. While staying in a low position, take a step with your right foot to the original athletic position. Repeat taking lateral shuffles as fast as you can control.	Week 1	1 × 15 yd (14 m) per side
			Week 2	1 × 20 yd (18 m) per side
			Week 3	2 × 20 yd (18 m) per side
			Week 4	3 × 25 yd (23 m) per side
3. Side push-off skip (no crossover)		Stand upright with your feet shoulder-width apart, a slight bend in the knees. Put your right foot on the starting line and the left foot downfield. Start skipping in place to get your rhythm. Once you establish your rhythm, push off with your right leg laterally to your left so that each skip with your right leg launches you further downfield to your left. Complete the desired distance, then switch directions and skip to the other side.	Week 1	1 × 15 yd (14 m) per side
			Week 2	1 × 20 yd (18 m) per side
			Week 3	2 × 20 yd (18 m) per side
			Week 4	3 × 25 yd (23 m) per side
4. Crossover skip		Stand upright with your feet shoulder-width apart, a slight bend in the knees. Put your right foot on the starting line and the left foot downfield. Start skipping in place to get your rhythm. Once you establish your rhythm, skip your right foot across and in front of your left foot, and skip your left leg downfield. Continue to skip laterally downfield to your left, with your right foot always going over your left foot. Move your arms as if running. Complete the desired distance, then switch directions, skipping to the other side.	Week 1	1 × 15 yd (14 m) per side
			Week 2	1 × 20 yd (18 m) per side
			Week 3	2 × 20 yd (18 m) per side
			Week 4	3 × 25 yd (23 m) per side
5. Skater		Start in a half squat with your feet shoulder-width apart. Jump to your left, landing on your left foot, while bringing your right leg across and behind your left leg, without touching the floor. Once stable, jump back to your right, landing on your right foot as your left leg goes behind your right leg. Repeat the skating motion.	Week 1	1 × 5 per side
			Week 2	1 × 7 per side
			Week 3	2 × 10 per side
			Week 4	3 × 12 per side

SPEED 4: LATERAL SPEED AND CHANGES OF DIRECTION

This 4-week program develops lateral speed and lateral changes of direction. As written, you will need lifting equipment close to an area for running. Perform the A exercise, rest 1-2 min, and then perform the B exercise. If your facility doesn't allow this set-up, perform 1a, 2a, 3a, and 3b in the weight area, then go to the running area of the facility to perform 1b and 2b. This workout is very effective in developing top-end speed and is a great workout for endurance runners, especially those who run hills. Weeks 1 and 2 will be enough for most people, while weeks 3 and 4 should be attempted only by more advanced individuals who have a considerable training base such as college and professional athletes.

Equipment

Band; slide board; sled; weights; chain, rope, or heavy nylon strap; belt (such as JC Power Sling); small hurdles; wall; stability ball

Notes

Weeks 1 and 2: Perform 2 times per week.

Weeks 3 and 4: Perform 1 time per week (very advanced trainees only).

Table 11.4 Speed 4: Lateral Speed and Changes of Direction

Exercise	Photo	Instructions	Weeks	Sets × reps
1a. Band-resisted unilateral slide		Use a band that does not allow you to get to the other side of the slide. Put a band around your waist and stand on a slide board, with the anchor point of the band to the right side. Get into a quarter squat and and push off your right foot while the band resists. Get as far as you can while staying in a wide athletic position, then slide back to the stopping block. Repeat for the desired number of repetitions, then switch to the other side.	Week 1	2 × 8-10 per side
			Week 2	3 × 10 per side
			Week 3	4 × 5-7 per side
			Week 4	4 × 8-10 per side
1b. Band-resisted shuffle run		Put a band around your waist with the anchor point of the band to the right side. Get into a quarter squat and push off your right foot, shuffling to your left for 3-4 yd (3-4 m). Shuffle back to the starting position and repeat. Perform to other side.	Week 1	2 × 3-4 yd (3-4 m)
			Week 2	3 × 3-4 yd (3-4 m)
			Week 3	4 × 3-4 yd (3-4 m)
			Week 4	5 × 3-4 yd (3-4 m)
2a. Lateral sled pull		You can use a heavy tire or other weighted object. Load your sled with the desired weight and attach a chain, rope, or heavy nylon strap to a belt that wraps around your waist, such as a sling. Stand with the sled to your left. Get into a quarter squat and push off your left foot as you take a wide step to your right. Continue to step to your right for the desired distance. Repeat on the other side.	Week 1	2 × 5 yd (5 m)
			Week 2	3 × 5 yd (5 m)
			Week 3	4 × 7 yd (6 m)
			Week 4	5 × 10 yd (9 m)

Exercise	Photo	Instructions	Weeks	Sets × reps
2b. Single-leg lateral two-hurdle hop to 5-yard sprint		Balance on your right leg, with 2 hurdles to your left. Using your right leg, laterally hop over the 2 hurdles with control. As you land after hopping over the second hurdle, explode into a sprint for 5 yd (5 m). Repeat on the other side.	Week 1	2 × 5 yd (5 m) per side
			Week 2	3 × 5 yd (5 m) per side
			Week 3	4 × 5 yd (5 m) per side
			Week 4	5 × 5 yd (5 m) per side
3a. SB single-leg lateral wall slide (inner and outer leg)		Stand with a wall to your left and place a stability ball under your left armpit between you and the wall. Place your left hand on the wall for balance. Walk your feet to the right to create a comfortable lean. Balancing on your right leg (outer leg), perform 5 short squats (quarter to half squats) with your right leg. Balance on your left leg (inner leg) and perform 5 short squats (quarter to half squats) with your left leg. Repeat with the wall on your right side.	Week 1	2 × 5 per side
			Week 2	3 × 7 per side
			Week 3	4 × 10 per side
			Week 4	5 × 10 per side
3b. Skater to lateral run		Balance on your right leg. Perform a skater jump to the left leg, a skater jump to the right, and a skater jump to the left. As soon as you land the last jump on your left leg, explode into a sprint to your right. Sprint for 5 yards. Repeat.	Week 1	2 × 5 yd (5 m)
			Week 2	3 × 5 yd (5 m)
			Week 3	4 × 5 yd (5 m)
			Week 4	5 × 5 yd (5 m)

SPEED 5: ACCELERATION WORKOUT

This 4-week program develops acceleration. It calls for some special equipment, but you can always substitute as needed. For example, if you don't have a Smith machine for the rear lunge, use dumbbells or even heavy medicine balls. As written, you will need lifting equipment close to an area for running. Perform the A exercise, rest 1-2 min, and then perform the B exercise. If your facility doesn't allow this set-up, perform 1a and 2a, then go to the running area of the facility to perform 1b, 2b, 3a, and 3b. Weeks 1 and 2 will be enough for most people, while weeks 3 and 4 should be attempted only by more advanced individuals who have a considerable training base such as college and professional athletes.

Equipment

Smith machine, treadmill, leg press machine, small hurdles, car or truck, start blocks, step and risers

Notes

Weeks 1 and 2: Perform 2 times per week.

Weeks 3 and 4: Perform 1 time per week (very advanced trainees only).

Table 11.5   Speed 5: Acceleration Workout

Exercise	Photo	Instructions	Weeks	Sets × reps
1a. Smith machine running step		Stand upright with your feet shoulder-width apart and the Smith machine bar on your shoulders. Using your right leg, step back into a lunge while lowering the bar. Return your right leg to the starting position, then step back with your left leg. Repeat.	Week 1	2 × 10 per side
			Week 2	3 × 8 per side
			Week 3	4 × 6 per side
			Week 4	5 × 6 per side
1b. Incline run		Set a treadmill at a 30- to 50-degree incline and a pace you can run. Run for 5 sec at your max speed. Dismount using handles and place feet on side footrails after each set to rest. Repeat for desired reps.	Week 1	2 × 5 sec
			Week 2	3 × 5 sec
			Week 3	4 × 5 sec
			Week 4	5 × 5 sec
2a. Single-leg leg press from toes		Sit in the leg press machine, planting one foot on the platform. Extend your knee, pushing on the platform and extending through your toes. After your leg is extended, flex your knee by lowering yourself back to the starting position. Repeat for the desired number of reps, then switch to the other leg. Do not lock out your knee; make sure to have a soft knee.	Week 1	2 × 10 per side
			Week 2	3 × 8 per side
			Week 3	4 × 6 per side
			Week 4	5 × 6 per side
2b. Single-leg hop to 5-yard sprint		Balance on your right leg. Using your right leg, hop forward with control. As soon as you land, explode into a sprint for 5 yd (5 m). Repeat on the other side.	Week 1	2 × 5 yd (5 m)
			Week 2	3 × 5 yd (5 m)
			Week 3	4 × 5 yd (5 m)
			Week 4	5 × 5 yd (5 m)
3a. Car or truck push start		Start behind a car or truck in neutral. Put your hands on the bumper, your body leaning about 45 degrees. Place your right foot forward, with your right knee bent about 90 degrees and your left leg back and almost straight. Drive hard with your legs to get the car or truck moving as fast as possible for 5 yd.	Week 1	2 × 5 yd (5 m)
			Week 2	3 × 5 yd (5 m)
			Week 3	4 × 5 yd (5 m)
			Week 4	5 × 5 yd (5 m)
3b. Start off the blocks (< 5 yd)		Position yourself in the start blocks. Explode out of the blocks by staying low and driving from the balls of your feet. Make sure to stay low for the entire 5 yd as you sprint.	Week 1	2 × 5 yd (5 m)
			Week 2	3 × 5 yd (5 m)
			Week 3	4 × 5 yd (5 m)
			Week 4	4 × 5 yd (5 m)

Summary

I hope you enjoy this new way of looking at running speed and improving it. I am certain the exercises in this chapter will make anyone faster. More than 3000 athletes have proven them very effective. Whether improving your first-step quickness, acceleration, or top running speed, the workouts in this chapter will help you attain your speed performance goals. These workouts also work wonders for injury prevention, especially hamstring and knee injuries, so you will stay healthy as you get faster. Share these workouts with your friends and teammates and make training for speed a group project. It will be a great experience for everyone.

CHAPTER 12

Agility

Agility is simply the ability to change body direction or position in a fast and fluid manner. Of all abilities that display athleticism, agility has to be it. Agility requires a blend of acceleration, deceleration, kinesthetic awareness, proprioception, quickness, explosiveness, and strength. That all these qualities can be required at any time and from any position makes them an essential part of any athlete's arsenal. In my opinion, agility is often what determines success in sports.

Unlike human locomotion's 7-frame (single-leg dominated), agility does not have a single characteristic, position, or quality that can be trained or focused on. It is a blend of many things, from a sense (e.g., kinesthesia) to a physical ability (e.g., power). Therefore, there is a ton of crossover from quickness drills, accelerations drills, speed drills, and reaction drills. This chapter provides a blend of the various forms of agilities seen in sports and recreation activities. We have combined everything from level changes in a reaction format to tumbling drills for heavy kinesthetic training and total-body power. We have also added popular cone drills for changes of direction and conditioning, as well as agility ladder drills for foot quickness.

Ironically, two of the greatest advantages of agility training are related to its major disadvantage: variety and specificity. Yes, variety and specificity can make agility training fun and very effective. However, because of the infinite variety, poorly planned agility training may lead to training confusion and ridiculous exercises that better resemble circus acts. Therefore, you can tailor any movement you need to make it an effective part of your training. Whether it's a transition within a play—such as a linebacker in American football getting up after being knocked down and running down the field to make a tackle or a tennis player slipping during a volley and regaining control to get to the ball and win the point—you can imitate any similar situation (or as close as possible) and rehearse it over and over again as part of your specific agility training. That's the fun of agility training: You can tailor it to your very specific needs.

The equipment for agility training can certainly get complicated, but we feel controlling the body is the most important and easiest thing to work on, and it requires virtually no equipment. Therefore, most drills and workouts in this chapter use body weight, while a few workouts use inexpensive and simple equipment such as an agility ladder. Some drills can be performed with simple chalk or tape. If you are on a court or cement-type floor, you can use chalk or tape to create five-dot drills, hexagons, and ladders.

Many popular drills did not make it into this chapter, but the drills selected include significant parts or characteristics of some of the popular drills. For example, many of the ladder drills incorporate part of the hexagon drill, and many hurdle and cone drills incorporate the drills performed with dummies on the ground. Another advantage of this comprehensive approach to training is using agility drills as warm-ups.

This approach to program design uses the agility warm-up to not only prepare the body for work but also supplement the workout. Often warm-ups are performed with no rhyme or reason and certainly lack intensity; it's just something you do before a workout. Well, since time is as short and limited as the space in this book, we have to make the warm-up and cool-down count. We have added a few exercises in this section that can be used as an agility warm-up. Start with them slowly and quickly pick up to maximum speed. This process can be extremely fast in warm weather climates, such as at IHP in Florida, where people walk around, sweating under a warm sun. You can select faster exercises for the warm-up, and slower exercises in the cool-down.

During advanced phases of training, we get busy during the cool-down and train quick, precise movements in a fatigued state. This approach teaches focus and perfect execution when fatigued. To use this method, you must have already perfected the exercises performed under fatigue. Also we often leave our short metabolic training for the very end and allow clients to cool down by simply walking around until they are back to normal. Using this approach, athletes get used to pushing while already tired. Intense training at the end of a workout is all part of redefining the human will.

The following two drills can be used individually or together as part of a workout, or as an agility warm-up. This is a great warm-up for biomotor skills training or agility ladder workout.

HEXAGON DRILL

Using chalk or athletic tape (if you don't have a crooked stick), mark a hexagon (six-sided shape) on the floor. The length of each side should be 24 in. (61 cm), and each angle should work out to be 120 degrees (figure 12.1). Start with both feet together in the middle of the hexagon facing the front line. On the command "go," jump forward across the line, then back over the same line into the middle of the hexagon. Then, continuing to face forward with your feet together, jump over the next side and back into the hexagon. Continue this pattern for three full revolutions to complete one set. Perform sets in clockwise and counterclockwise direction. Perform 3-4 sets.

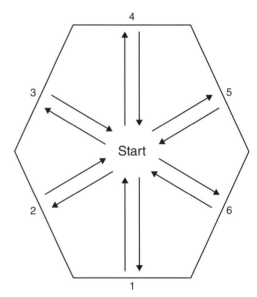

Figure 12.1 Hexagon.

CROSS-ROTATIONAL JUMP DRILL

Using chalk or athletic tape (if you don't have a crooked stick), mark a cross pattern of two perpendicular lines crossing each other (figure 12.2). Stand with a segment between your legs and the intersection and the other three segments in front of you; your left foot in box 1 and your right foot in box 2. Stand with your feet about shoulder-width apart and knees slightly bent. Jump with both feet to the right as you rotate left, landing with your left foot in box 2 and your right foot in box 3. Jump again with both feet to the right as you rotate left; landing with your left foot in box 3 and your right foot in box 4. You are facing opposite where you started. Perform two more rotational jumps until you land in the starting position. Repeat counterclockwise to complete one repetition. Perform 2-4 repetitions per set. Perform 3-4 sets.

The next series of exercises is a sample of a great workout for beginners that can also serve as a warm-up or cool-down for more advanced individuals. These exercises make up one of our favorite warm-ups for our athletes. Many of the moves fit in very nicely to all running-related biomotor skills. You can easily perform higher speed drills after these movements to prepare for more explosive work. When using this workout as a cool-down, you can choose to move slower with perhaps less volume. For example, perform only five minutes of work, but hold positions for a second and increase the flexibility component for the cool-down. What I like most about this application is that it falls in line with our concept of flexibility and strength being one.

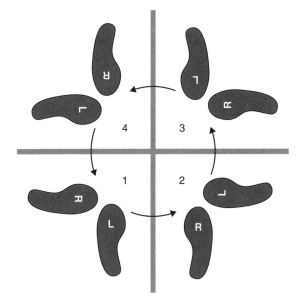

Figure 12.2   Cross-rotational jump drill.

REACHING LUNGE TO OVERHEAD REACH

Perform a long forward step with the right foot and reach with both hands to your right foot (figure 12.3). Step with the left foot to neutral and reach overhead with both arms. Repeat for 10 yards (9 m). Next, perform a long left step and reach with both hands to your left foot, step with right foot to neutral with an overhead reach with both arms. Repeat for 10 yards (9 m).

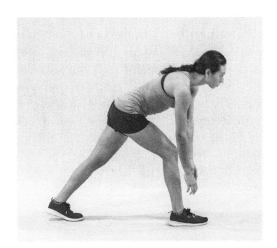

Figure 12.3   Reaching lunge to overhead reach.

LATERAL REACHING LUNGE TO OVERHEAD REACH

Perform a long lateral step to the left and reach with both hands to your left foot (figure 12.4). Step with your right foot to neutral and reach overhead with both arms. Repeat for 10 yards (9 m). Next, perform a long lateral step to the right and reach with both hands to your right foot. Step your left foot to neutral and reach overhead with both arms. Repeat for 10 yards (9 m).

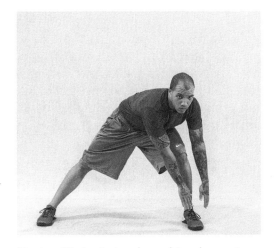

Figure 12.4   Lateral reaching lunge to overhead reach.

LUNGE WITH ROTATION

Perform a right lunge with a right rotation (figure 12.5) and then a left lunge with a left rotation. Continue alternating right and left lunges with rotations for 10 yards (9 m) up and 10 yards (9 m) back.

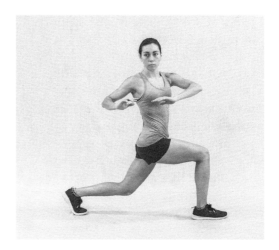

Figure 12.5 Lunge with rotation.

EXAGGERATED LATERAL SHUFFLE WALK

Stand sideways to the starting line in a wide athletic position, your right foot on the starting line (figure 12.6). Take a big step to your left using your left leg, opening up the adductors. Staying in a low position, take a step to your left with your right leg to return to the wide athletic position. Repeat for 10 yards (9 m). Perform 10 yards (9 m) to the other side.

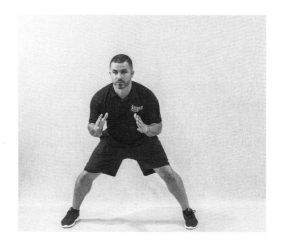

Figure 12.6 Exaggerated lateral shuffle walk.

EXAGGERATED CARIOCA WALK

Stand sideways to the starting line in a wide athletic position, your right foot on the starting line. Take a big crossover step (right leg over left leg) to your left using your right leg (figure 12.7). Keeping a low position, take a big lateral step with your left leg to return to the wide athletic position. Take a big cross step behind to your left using your right leg (right leg behind left leg). Repeat for 10 yards (9 m). Perform 10 yards (9 m) to the other side.

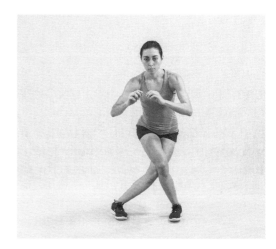

Figure 12.7 Exaggerated carioca walk.

SPIDER-MAN CRAWL

Start in a staggered hand push-up position with your right hand closer to your hips than your left hand. Put your right foot outside of your right hand (figure 12.8). Advance forward with your right hand as you place your left foot outside of your left hand. Advance forward with your left hand as you place your right foot outside of your right hand. Repeat for 10 yards (9 m) up and 10 yards (9 m) back.

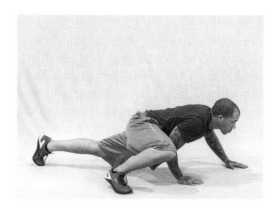

Figure 12.8   Spider-Man crawl.

BEAR CRAWL

Stand with your feet together and knees straight. Place your hands flat in front of you as close to your feet as possible without bending your knees. Keeping your knees straight and feet flat, walk like a bear, keeping your butt up, legs perfectly straight, and feet flat (figure 12.9). Repeat for 10 yards (9 m) up and 10 yards (9 m) back.

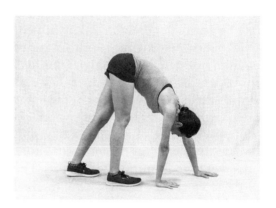

Figure 12.9   Bear crawl.

INCHWORM

Start in a bear crawl position (hands in front of flat feet, knees straight). Walk forward with your hands only, keeping your core tight and rolling to the balls of your feet (figure 12.10). Walk out as far as your core strength will allow without any back pressure or pain. Once you walk your hands out as far as possible, walk your feet toward your hands, keeping your legs straight, until the hamstrings can't stretch anymore. Repeat for 10 yards (9 m) up and 10 yards (9 m) back.

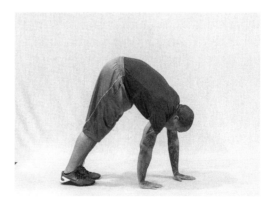

Figure 12.10   Inchworm.

T PUSH-UP

Perform a push-up, then roll to one side as you reach the other arm up in the air so you are in a T position (figure 12.11). You should look like a cross resting on its side. Perform 5-10 repetitions to each side.

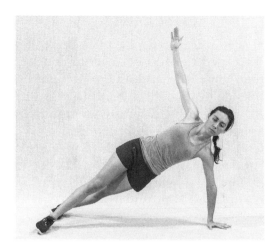

Figure 12.11   T push-up.

I have used some of these exercises as 10-minute warm-ups, 5-minute cool-downs, and as 30-minute workouts with great results. However, when you combine a meaningful warm-up and cool-down with the more intense workouts in this chapter, then you are really cooking with gas. At IHP we do a ton of work with the local high schools, and these workouts pay huge dividends with young athletes. One of the issues we face with young athletes is early specialization in sports and not enough free play when young. Thus, we find incredible athletes who can do incredible things on the field of play, but they can't skip, shuffle, or move their bodies through simple drills. The workouts in this chapter are perfect for those athletes. Even if you are coordinated or just want to add some diversity to your training, these workouts will provide incredible athleticism, prevent injuries, and burn a ton of fun calories.

One final note on the workouts in this chapter. These are 25- to 30-minute workouts, not 5- to 10-minute warm-ups. There is a lot of volume in the advanced versions of these workouts, and they are made that way for a reason. The way I see it, agility training is not supposed to be some hodgepodge of haphazard drills put together. You actually get in shape doing these long workouts. These workouts are effective in not only developing agility but also developing the ability to stay agile when you are tired, which is a big distinction. This intense and high-volume work is our version of what we call body hardening in martial arts, except without crushing your body with repetitive trauma. Most coaches don't see training the way we see it at IHP, and our agility training programs are proof of this. Now, let's get to work.

AGILITY 1: TOTAL-BODY AWARENESS TUMBLING WORKOUT

This 4-week program focuses on total-body tumbling agility. Once you establish a good base of training (complete 3-4 weeks), you can use week 1 or 2 of this program as a warm-up for combat sports and other contact sports in which one falls and has to get up quickly. I have used this workout with all my field sport and combat athletes. I also think it should be mandatory for all children to learn basic tumbling drills. Weeks 1 and 2 will be enough for most people, while weeks 3 and 4 require increased physical endurance that comes from a more advanced training base. These drills can be done for distance, usually about 10 yd (9 m). However, if you have a shorter distance to work with, perform 2 or 3 reps per side of the body per set (4-6 reps total).

Equipment

Small object or partner

Notes

Weeks 1 and 2: Perform 3 or 4 times per week.

Weeks 3 and 4: Perform 2 or 3 times per week (for very advanced trainees only).

Table 12.1 Agility 1: Total-Body Awareness Tumbling Workout

Exercise	Photo	Instructions	Weeks	Sets × reps
1. Forward roll		Initially use a four-point stance to begin until you can begin completely standing upright. Stand in a staggered stance with your right foot forward. Bend over and start to fall forward. As you are about to make contact with the ground, roll over your right shoulder. Come back up to your feet. Repeat and perform to both sides.	Week 1	1 × 2
			Week 2	2 × 2
			Week 3	3 × 2
			Week 4	2 × 4
2. Backward roll		Begin in a seated position until you can begin completely standing upright. From a standing staggered stance, bend your legs and start to sit on the ground behind you. As you are about to make contact with the ground, roll back over your right shoulder. Continue to roll and come up to your feet. Repeat and perform to both sides.	Week 1	1 × 2
			Week 2	2 × 2
			Week 3	3 × 2
			Week 4	2 × 4
3. Backward roll to push-off		From a standing staggered stance, bend your legs and start to sit on the ground behind you. As you are about to make contact with the ground, roll back. Continue to roll as your feet come over your head. Press off using your hands as you roll back up to your feet. Repeat.	Week 1	1 × 2
			Week 2	1 × 3
			Week 3	2 × 2
			Week 4	2 × 3

(continued)

Table 12.1 Agility 1: Total-Body Awareness Tumbling Workout *(continued)*

Exercise	Photo	Instructions	Weeks	Sets × reps
4. Forward roll over object		Set up a barrier that is knee- to hip-height, such as a hurdle or partner on hands and knees. Take a few steps and take off from your right foot, flying over the barrier. Land by rolling over your right shoulder to come back up to your feet. Repeat and perform on both sides.	Week 1	1 × 2 per side
			Week 2	2 × 2 per side
			Week 3	3 × 2 per side
			Week 4	2 × 4 per side
5. Cartwheel		From an open stance, laterally flex to the left and put your left hand on the ground. Continue to turn, putting your right hand on the other side of your left hand as you kick off the ground with your feet, lifting them toward the ceiling. As your feet go over you, your right foot lands and then your left foot lands on the other side. Repeat.	Week 1	1 × 2 per side
			Week 2	2 × 2 per side
			Week 3	3 × 2 per side
			Week 4	2 × 4 per side
6. Roundoff		From a standing staggered stance, laterally flex to the left and put your left hand on the ground. Continue to turn, putting your right hand on the other side of your left hand as you kick off the ground with your feet, lifting them toward the ceiling. As your feet go over you, rotate the body and land with both feet facing the starting position. Repeat.	Week 1	1 × 2 per side
			Week 2	2 × 2 per side
			Week 3	3 × 2 per side
			Week 4	2 × 4 per side

AGILITY 2: RUNNING AGILITY

This 4-week agility program focuses on running agility, and it is a monster conditioning workout. I've included some of the most popular agility tests and drills we have used over the last 15 years. It begins with a low volume of work so you have time to learn and perfect the drills, but eventually this workout becomes a high-volume training session that will condition any athlete. This workout has helped some of our high school athletes prepare to be highly recruited by top universities, and their coaches believe our conditioning is a big part of their athletes' successes. Weeks 1 and 2 will be enough for most people, while weeks 3 and 4 should be attempted only by more advanced individuals who have a considerable training base.

Equipment

Chalk, cones, or tape to mark lines

Notes

Rest 60-120 sec between repetitions. Rest 2-3 min between sets.

Weeks 1 and 2: Perform 3 or 4 times per week.

Weeks 3 and 4: Perform 2 or 3 times per week (for very advanced trainees only).

Table 12.2 Agility 2: Running Agility Workout

Exercise	Instructions	Weeks	Reps
1. 20-yard pro agility drill	Mark 3 lines 5 yd (5 m) apart. Stand in a staggered stance, straddling the starting line (the middle line). Turn to the right, sprint, and touch a line 5 yd (5 m) away with your right hand. Turn back to the left, sprint 10 yd (9 m), and touch the far line with your left hand. Turn back to the right, sprint 5 yd (5 m) though the start line to the finish. Repeat.	Week 1	1
		Week 2	2
		Week 3	2
		Week 4	3
2. T-drill	Set up 3 cones in a line 5 yd (5 m) apart. Set up a fourth cone 10 yd (9 m) from the center cone. Stand in a staggered stance at the fourth cone. Sprint forward 10 yd (9 m) to the center cone, then side shuffle to the right 5 yd (5 m) and touch the far cone with your left hand. Shuffle back to the right for 5 yd (5 m) to the center cone. Touch the center cone, then backpedal 10 yd (9 m) to the starting position at the fourth cone. Repeat alternating the order of turns at the top of the T.	Week 1	1
		Week 2	2
		Week 3	2
		Week 4	3
3. Squirm drill	Stand in a staggered stance. Sprint forward 5 yd (5 m), then rotate 360 degrees and sprint another 5 yd (5 m). Rotate 360 degrees again and sprint another 5 yd (5 m). Sprint right or left for 10 yd (9 m). Return to the starting point and repeat.	Week 1	1
		Week 2	2
		Week 3	2
		Week 4	3
4. 40-yard ladder drill	Mark 3 lines: a starting line, the first line 5 yd (5 m) from the starting line, and the second line 5 yd (5 m) from the first line. Stand in a staggered stance. Sprint 5 yd (5 m) to the first line, touch the line with your right hand, return to the starting line, and touch it with your left hand. Sprint 10 yd (9 m) to the second line, touch with your right hand, return to the starting line, and touch it with your left hand. Sprint 5 yd (5 m) to the first line, touch the line with your right hand, and return to the starting line. Repeat.	Week 1	1
		Week 2	1
		Week 3	2
		Week 4	2

AGILITY 3: AGILITY LADDER WORKOUT

This 4-week program focuses on foot quickness and agility using an agility ladder. If you don't have an agility ladder, draw one with chalk if you are on concrete or mark it with tape if you are on another type of flooring. Just make sure you can clean the surface you are working on and restore it to the original condition. We begin using 10 yd (9 m) (full ladder) to teach the skill, which allows us to get the necessary reps in for learning and conditioning. Once our athletes are comfortable with the correct form, we reduce the length to 5 yd (5 m) (half the ladder) and work on all-out efforts each rep. We even add reactive sprints to a half-ladder drill for more specific reactive work and conditioning. Weeks 1 and 2 will be enough for most people, while weeks 3 and 4 should be attempted only by more advanced individuals who have a considerable training base.

Equipment

Agility ladder

Notes

Rest 15-30 sec between repetitions. Rest 2-3 min between exercises. When performing agility ladders drills, try to look ahead of the ladder and not at the ground.

Weeks 1 and 2: Perform 2 times per week.

Weeks 3 and 4: Perform 1 time per week (very advanced trainees only).

Table 12.3   Agility 3: Agility Ladder Workout

Exercise	Instructions	Weeks	Reps
1. Run through	Run through an agility ladder as fast as possible, touching one foot down between each rung. Emphasize a high knee lift and quick ground reaction. Repeat.	Week 1	2 full ladders
		Week 2	3 full ladders
		Week 3	4 half ladders
		Week 4	6 half ladders
2. Lateral run	Stand lateral to the agility ladder. Laterally run through an agility ladder as fast as possible, touching one foot down between each rung. Emphasize a high knee lift and quick ground reaction. Repeat.	Week 1	2 full ladders
		Week 2	3 full ladders
		Week 3	4 half ladders
		Week 4	6 half ladders
3. Split step	Start in a two-point stance at one end of the agility ladder. Keeping both feet together, jump into the first square. Jump to straddle the next line, with your feet outside the ladder. Jump into the second square with both feet. Repeat, alternating feet together and feet apart down the ladder.	Week 1	2 full ladders
		Week 2	3 full ladders
		Week 3	4 half ladders
		Week 4	6 half ladders
4. Diagonal jump	Start in a two-point stance at one end of the agility ladder with the ladder to your left. Keeping both feet together, jump left into the ladder then left outside the ladder so the ladder is to your right. Jump right into the ladder, one box up, then right outside the ladder so the ladder is to your left. Continue forward in a zigzag pattern. Repeat. This drill may also be performed on one leg as you become more experienced.	Week 1	2 full ladders
		Week 2	3 full ladders
		Week 3	4 half ladders
		Week 4	6 half ladders
5. Icky shuffle	Start on the left side of the ladder. Laterally step with your right foot and place it in the first square. Follow with your left foot into the first square. Laterally step with your right foot to the right side of the ladder, then advance your left foot to the second square in the ladder. Bring your right foot to join your left in the square. Laterally step to the left side of the ladder and advance your right foot to the third square on the ladder. Repeat.	Week 1	2 full ladders
		Week 2	3 full ladders
		Week 3	4 half ladders
		Week 4	6 half ladders
6. Single-leg forward hop	Hop on one leg in every square, emphasizing minimal ground contact. To add difficulty, add a skill to the drill. Repeat with the other leg.	Week 1	1 full ladder per leg
		Week 2	2 full ladders per leg
		Week 3	4 half ladders per leg
		Week 4	6 half ladders per leg
7. Single-leg lateral hop	Laterally hop in every square using only one leg, emphasizing minimal ground contact. To add difficulty, a skill can be added to the drill. Repeat.	Week 1	1 full ladder per leg
		Week 2	2 full ladders per leg
		Week 3	4 half ladders per leg
		Week 4	6 half ladders per leg
8. Single-leg diagonal hop	Stand on one leg at the end of the ladder with the ladder to your left. Keeping both feet together, jump left into the ladder then left outside the ladder so the ladder is to your right. Jump right into the ladder, one box up, then right outside the ladder so the ladder is to your left. Continue forward in a zigzag pattern. Repeat.	Week 1	1 full ladder per leg
		Week 2	2 full ladders per leg
		Week 3	4 half ladders per leg
		Week 4	6 half ladders per leg

AGILITY 4: REACTIVE AGILITY

This 4-week agility program focuses on reactive and positional agility. It uses sound, tactile, or visual cues for athletes to respond to, depending on what they respond to in their sports. You can use these drills as competitions by lining up multiple athletes on a line to see who reacts quickest by getting off the line first and arriving at a destination first (e.g., a line 5 yd [5 m] away). Athletes love to compete, and you can treat it like the Tour de France; give a winner's jersey to the athlete who has the best time or the most wins. This is a perfect drill for all athletes who play contact field sports. Weeks 1 and 2 will be enough for most people, while weeks 3 and 4 should be attempted only by more advanced individuals who have a considerable training base.

Equipment

Partner to cue start

Notes

Rest 60-90 sec between each repetition. Rest 2-3 min between each exercise.

Weeks 1 and 2: Perform 2 times per week.

Weeks 3 and 4: Perform 1 time per week (very advanced trainees only).

Table 12.4 Agility 4: Reactive Agility

Exercise	Instructions	Weeks	Reps
1. Stand from four-point front	Start on the ground on your hands and knees. Explode as fast as possible as you stand up by using the following sequence: hands up, one foot up, then the other foot up. Repeat.	Week 1	1-2
		Week 2	2-3
		Week 3	3
		Week 4	3-4
2. Stand from four-point away	Start on the ground on your hands and knees. Explode as fast as possible as you stand up and turn to face the opposite side using the following sequence: hands up, one foot up, then the other foot up, turn. Repeat.	Week 1	1-2
		Week 2	2-3
		Week 3	3
		Week 4	3-4
3. Stand from sitting facing front	Start in a seated position on the ground. Explode as fast as possible as you stand up. Practice various get-up strategies until you find one that works for you, and rehearse that to each side. Repeat.	Week 1	1-2
		Week 2	2-3
		Week 3	3
		Week 4	3-4
4. Stand from sitting facing away	Start in a seated position on the ground. Explode as fast as possible as you stand up and turn to face the opposite direction. Practice various get-up strategies until you find one that works for you, and rehearse that to each side. Repeat.	Week 1	1-2
		Week 2	1-2
		Week 3	2-3
		Week 4	2-3
5. Sprawl to stand	Start in a two-point stance. Perform a squat thrust, then a roll to either side, and then stand up as fast as possible. Repeat, alternating direction of the roll.	Week 1	1-2
		Week 2	1-2
		Week 3	2-3
		Week 4	2-3
6. Forward fall to sprint	From a standing position, feet together, lean forward until you lose your balance. Accelerate at full speed to keep yourself from falling. Run 20-30 yd (18-27 m). Repeat.	Week 1	1-2
		Week 2	1-2
		Week 3	2-3
		Week 4	2-3

AGILITY 5: CONE DRILL WORKOUT

This 4-week agility program focuses on agility and conditioning. Once you establish a good base of training (complete 4 weeks), you can even use 2 or 3 drills from this workout as a warm-up to skills training. This is a perfect workout for anyone who wants to improve athletic agility and get in game-type conditioning, especially when completing weeks 3 and 4. Weeks 1 and 2 will be enough for most people, but weeks 3 and 4 should be attempted only by more advanced individuals who have a considerable training base.

Equipment

Cones

Notes

Rest 60-90 sec between each repetition. Rest 2-3 min between each exercise.

Weeks 1 and 2: Perform 2 times per week.

Weeks 3 and 4: Perform 1 time per week (very advanced trainees only).

Table 12.5 Agility 5: Cone Drill Workout

Exercise	Instructions	Weeks	Reps
1. 15-yard turn drill	Stand in a ready-to-start position. Sprint forward 5 yd (5 m) to the first cone and make a sharp right turn around it. Sprint to the second cone and make a left turn around the cone. Sprint 5 yd (5 m) through the finish. Repeat.	Week 1	1
		Week 2	2
		Week 3	2-3
		Week 4	3
2. 20-yard square	Stand in a ready-to-start position. Sprint forward 5 yd (5 m) to the first cone and make a sharp right cut. Shuffle right 5 yd (5 m) and make a sharp cut back. Backpedal 5 yd (5 m) to the next cone, and make a sharp left cut. Shuffle to the left and back to the start position. Repeat.	Week 1	1
		Week 2	2
		Week 3	2-3
		Week 4	3
3. X-pattern multi-skill	Stand in a ready-to-start position. Sprint 10 yd (9 m) to the first cone, then sprint diagonally 14 yd (13 m) to the second cone. Backpedal 10 yd (9 m) to the third cone. At the third cone, sprint diagonally 14 yd (13 m) to the fourth cone. Repeat.	Week 1	1
		Week 2	2
		Week 3	2-3
		Week 4	3
4. Zigzag	Stand in a ready-to-start position. Stand facing a row of 5-10 cones, each cone 1 yard (1 m) apart. Step forward quickly and diagonally with your right foot to the right of the first cone, then slide your left foot to the right. Lead with your left foot to the left side of the next cone, and then slide your right foot to the left foot. Zigzag through all the cones quickly and explosively. Repeat.	Week 1	1
		Week 2	2
		Week 3	2-3
		Week 4	3
5. Z-pattern cut	You will need 4 cones. Place 2 cones 5 yd (5 m) diagonally across from each other. Place the next cone 10 yd (9 m) from the second cone. Place the final cone 20 yd (18 m) from the third cone. Start in a two-point stance. Sprint to the first cone, plant on the outside leg, and cut sharply toward the next cone. Walk back to starting point and repeat.	Week 1	1
		Week 2	2
		Week 3	2-3
		Week 4	3

Summary

I'm certain the wide array of agility workouts in this chapter have provided some great training ideas and helped you develop your agility. I hope they also allowed you to see agility for the important athletic component it is and inspired new ideas for training it. Remember, agility is one of the most important physical and movement attributes needed for athletic success, and it requires repetition in order to improve it. Therefore, make sure you always have a little bit of agility training in your athletic development program.

As always, I encourage you to take the workouts and exercises in this chapter and create your own customized agility workouts. For example, take one drill from each workout and create another workout. I bet it will be a killer workout and unique. You will see the greatest gains in performance when you start taking control of the programming aspect of your training. Time and experimentation will lead you to the perfect workout for you. Most importantly, share your newfound love for agility training with the people around you; they will be thankful you did.

PART IV

Athletic Endurance

You can have all the strength, power, speed, and agility in the world and even be the better athlete, but if you run out of gas, you have nothing. It's that simple. How many times has the better athlete lost after being ahead, up to the defining moment when he or she got tired? Part IV is about what I call metabolic training. The name *metabolic* was given to this type of training to distinguish it from cardio. Although there is a cardio component to this training, cardio is not the defining factor. Basically, this has nothing to do with the famous $\dot{V}O_2max$. We called it *metabolic* and the name stuck, but remember, it's just a name. And I cover metabolic workouts for the entire body.

I'm not going to get into the biochemistry of this kind of training because even the biochemistry, all the lactate threshold and fiber research, still can't explain the drastic changes we see in performances at all levels, from recreational to very elite. I'm just going to tell you this training makes you indestructible and changes more than your body and performance. It redefines the human will and changes you from the inside out. We discussed the spiritual changes that hard training can catalyze in the introduction, and I urge you to reread that section before you go on to the training in this section. Just remember, when the sensations associated with accelerated metabolism (i.e., metabolic training) come to your awareness and you want to wince in pain, relax your face because you are not feeling pain. You are feeling accelerated metabolism. Period! The more you practice this form of meditation, if you will, the more you will break through barriers faster than science can explain. Awareness and perception can change in an instant and make the difference.

The lower-body workouts expand on the Vern Gambetta super legs and the subsequent JC leg crank protocols of the 1990s. I've even provided protocols that use specialized equipment, such as the famous Lincoln Navigator push around the IHP parking lot. The upper-body workouts expand on the chisel your chest project and JC meta chest protocols designed in my early days. The specialized equipment in these workouts is readily available and can turn upper-body metabolic training into an exciting aspect of your program. Finally the total-body metabolic chapter introduces the protocols I use to train fighters and members of our special forces. The gauntlet will blow your mind.

Today, a host of workout genres use metabolic training to create training programs, even sports such as CrossFit and obstacle course racing. *Functional Training* has my most popular protocols, such as the JC leg crank, meta chest, meta back, and Gary Gray's dumbbell matrix. I don't want to repeat these protocols, and I urge you to refer to that book for some great metabolic training protocols. To those, I add the ones in this part. Get ready to transform.

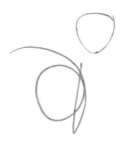

CHAPTER 13

Lower-Body Metabolics

When the legs go, it's over, and it does not matter if you are running, fighting, or playing a sport that requires you to be strong while standing. Therefore, having a lower body that still keeps going when you can't is something just about all athletes will opt for. Having bounce in your legs in the final rounds of a fight, catching up to a tired runner you have been chasing down for a while, or out-hustling the other team in transitions are signs of lower-body metabolic endurance, and that comes from specific training. So this training, like everything, starts early and is nurtured constantly.

Our metabolic training for the lower body was inspired by my kung fu sifus and karate senseis during my early teen years. We did everything from thousand-kick workouts to executing various blocks and punches for an hour from a deep horse stance (wide and deep squat stance), to fast 2-3 mile beach walks in thigh-high water. Vern Gambetta gave us the "super legs" (i.e., 20 squats, 20 lunges, 20 box shuffles, and 10 squat jumps) workout in the mid-1990s, and that inspired a generation of coaches and trainers to develop and expand on his work. Now, let's get to some lower-body metabolic protocols that will take your leg endurance to new heights.

METABOLIC LEGS 1: JC LATERAL LEG CRANK

This 6-week program uses the JC lateral leg crank as a power endurance workout that focuses on lateral movement. All 6 weeks are not necessary for most people, but if you are an ultra-endurance trail runner or obstacle course competitor, for example, all 6 weeks could serve you well in getting across the finish line faster than ever. For most athletes, such as basketball and tennis players, doing 2 sets without rest is about all you will need to accomplish—maybe a third set for good measure. Simply follow the progression indicated in the notes and continue to reduce 15 sec of rest between each exercise each week until you get to no rest between exercises.

Equipment

Medicine ball, plyometric box

Notes

Week 1 (beginner): Rest 45 sec between each exercise.

Week 2 (beginner): Rest 30 sec between each exercise.

Week 3 (intermediate/advanced): Rest 15 sec between each exercise.

Week 4 (intermediate/advanced): No rest between exercises.

Weeks 5-6 (elite): No rest between exercises.

Table 13.1 Metabolic Legs 1: JC Lateral Leg Crank

Exercise	Photo	Instructions	Weeks	Sets × reps
1. MB ABC squat		Stand upright with your feet shoulder-width apart and a medicine ball or weight in both hands. Squat and reach with the medicine ball to your right. Return to standing. Squat and reach with the medicine ball to your left. Repeat.	Week 1	1 × 15 per side
			Week 2	2 × 15 per side
			Week 3	3 × 15 per side
			Week 4	4 × 15 per side
			Week 5	4 × 15 per side
			Week 6	4 × 15 per side
2. Alternating lateral lunge		Stand upright with your feet shoulder-width apart. Laterally step to the left and shift your weight to your left leg as you lower your body as far as you can. As you lower, keep your right leg straight and foot flat on the floor. Push off with your left foot back to the starting position. Repeat with the right leg.	Week 1	1 × 10 per side
			Week 2	2 × 10 per side
			Week 3	3 × 10 per side
			Week 4	4 × 10 per side
			Week 5	5 × 10 per side
			Week 6	6 × 10 per side
3. Alternating lateral box shuffle over box		Begin with your right foot on a box (8-12 in. [20-30 cm] high) and your left foot on the ground. Swing your arms up while laterally jumping to your right. As you land, your left foot should be on the box and your right foot should be on the ground. Replace the foot on the box with the opposite foot every time you jump. Repeat quickly.	Week 1	1 × 10 per side
			Week 2	2 × 10 per side
			Week 3	3 × 10 per side
			Week 4	4 × 10 per side
			Week 5	5 × 10 per side
			Week 6	6 × 10 per side

Exercise	Photo	Instructions	Weeks	Sets × reps
4. Skater		Begin with both feet together and push off laterally with one leg. Upon landing, immediately push off in the opposite direction and continue the drill for either reps or time. To develop quickness, perform as many reps as possible for time (10 sec or less). Repeat.	Week 1	1 × 10 per side
			Week 2	2 × 10 per side
			Week 3	3 × 10 per side
			Week 4	4 × 10 per side
			Week 5	5 × 10 per side
			Week 6	6 × 10 per side

METABOLIC LEGS 2: TRUCK PUSH

This 7-week truck/car push program is one of the workouts we put on the map back in the early 2000s. We eventually used the truck push within many of our circuits, but before that we mastered the truck push around the IHP parking lot (80 yd [73 m] total composed of 25 yd + 15 yd + 25 yd + 15 yd [23 m + 14 m + 23 m + 14 m], down and up hills). I used this progression with my sister 7 weeks after she underwent brain surgery; she eventually mastered one legit truck push. Those with a good fitness base can start at week 2 or 3 if they feel comfortable doing so. Our athletes do it for time and as a prefatigue protocol. Therefore, although pushing a Lincoln Navigator for 80 yd [73 m] is a feat in and of itself, eventually it is done for reps. The IHP elite truck workout is 5 laps around the parking lot with 2-3 min between each lap. That takes about 20 min and involves 800-1,000 reps for the legs (400-500 per leg). If you use a smaller car, like a Toyota Corolla, 2 laps around the IHP parking lot equals one with the Navigator—that's just our crazy estimate. Obviously, you can substitute a sled, such as the Prowler, for the vehicle, but I'm partial to the truck. It reminds me of the 1970s judo training that involved using a judogi to pull an Impala.

A simple application of the truck push as a prefatigue modality is to perform a truck push and then be explosive and do what you normally do for your sport or activity. We use this application for fighters and Special Forces Operators. For example:

1. Truck push in under 1:20
2. Shadow box around the parking lot on the balls of your feet
3. 2 ladder lengths of rotational jumps on the balls of your feet
4. 10 lateral jumps over low hurdle
5. Optional for MMA fighters: 10 hard, low kicks to the bag with each leg

Equipment

Truck or car

Instructions

Simple: Get behind a truck and push (figure 13.1). Make sure the truck is in neutral (so no smoke is blown in your face), put your hands on the bumper (use a towel to protect your hands and vehicle and to keep your hands from slipping), and push from the balls of your feet. Try not to go flat-footed.

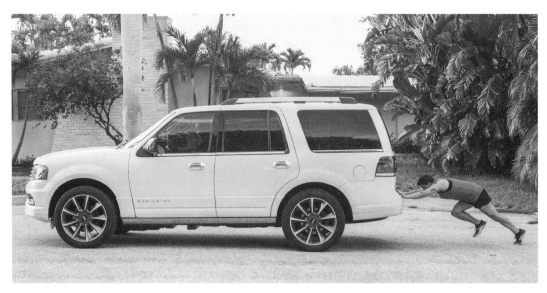

Figure 13.1 Truck push.

Initial Workout

Week 1: 2 × 5 yd (5 m), 3 times per week, 1 min rest between sets

Week 2: 2 × 10 yd (9 m), 3 times per week, 1 min rest between sets

Week 3: 3 × 25 yd (23 m), 3 times per week, 1-2 min rest between sets

Week 4: 2 × 40 yd (37 m), 3 times per week, 1-2 min rest between sets

Week 5: 1 × 65 yd (54 m), 3 times per week

Week 6: 2 × 65 yd (54 m), 3 times per week, 2-3 min rest between sets

Week 7: 1 × 80 yd (73 m), 3 times per week

Elite IHP Truck Workout

Week 8: 2 × 80 yd (73 m), 2 times per week, 3-4 min rest between sets

Week 9: 3 × 80 yd (73 m), 2 times per week, 3-4 min rest between sets

Week 10: 4 × 80 yd (73 m), 1 time per week, 2-3 min rest between sets

Week 11: 5 × 80 yd (73 m), 1 time per week, 2-3 min rest between sets

Week 12 (bonus): 2 × 80 yd (73 m), 1 time per week, no rest between sets

Notes

What makes this workout extra special at IHP is the landscape of the parking lot. Due to drainage design, the push starts slightly downhill and goes through peaks and valleys, but it ends with an uphill and a turn, during which the front tires grab the asphalt and the push slows considerably. The finish is nasty.

METABOLIC LEGS 3: SUPPLEMENTAL LOWER-BODY ENDURANCE

These programs use specialized equipment. Obviously if you don't have any of this equipment, you can drag tires or use stairs or big hills. However, I included this section to give you an idea of what is out there and what to ask for when you are looking for a gym.

VersaClimber (VC): Lower Body Only

The VersaClimber (figure 13.2) may be our single most used piece of equipment in IHP. Using the lower body with the right resistance is as close as you get to stadium runs without going to a stadium. Take a 14- to 18-in (36-46 m) step on a box and feel the resistance in your leg. Set the resistance on the VC as close as possible to what you felt when doing the step-up. Perform an all-out effort for 15 sec using just your lower body. Record how many feet you climbed in 15 sec. Your job is to repeat that effort every time. Allow 1 to 1.5 min of rest between sets. Perform 3-5 sets 2-3 times per week or 2-3 sets after leg day as a flush. In 4 weeks, your legs will be indescribable.

Incline Treadmill Runs

Our goal at IHP is to run on our old incline trainers at 50% set at 6 mph. It's hard to find a new treadmill that provides a 50% incline. If you can't find one, use the highest incline available and adapt the protocol. For example, use an incline of 20%-30% and increase the speed to 8-12 mph. At first, choose a speed and incline that will allow you to barely complete 7-10 sec. Run 10 sec and then use the handles to jump your feet to the side rails and take a complete rest of 50 sec; that's one set. Perform 5-10 sets 2-3 times per week. In 4 weeks, you will be in shape to play any sport.

As an example of what can be accomplished using this protocol, Jeff Monson and other elite UFC fighters have completed up to 20 sets in a conditioning session at 50% incline at 6 mph.

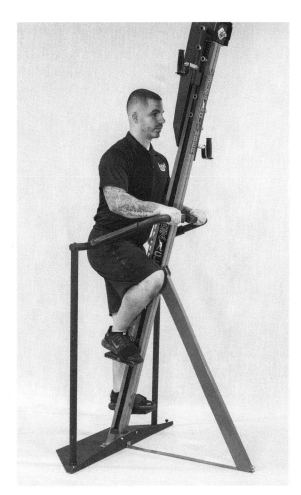

Figure 13.2 VersaClimber.

METABOLIC LEGS 4:
SHUTTLE MVP LOWER-BODY METABOLIC WORKOUT

Many high-level athletes come to IHP when they need to train hard while injured. We also train people who want to train the lower body hard but have conditions that do not allow much compression, especially while standing (e.g., pinched nerves or disc issues). The Shuttle MVP (figure 13.3) is one of our favorite pieces of equipment for many reasons; it can handle the most delicate leg and hip rehab or build fatigue-resistant legs. I have used this protocol with fighters when they could not push the truck or do leg cranks due to disc issues. The protocol is simple: 100 reps in 70-90 sec. We set the back pad so that the athlete is almost in a full squat. We help the athlete extend his or her legs to start the protocol. We start with 50 squats (thighs parallel to foot pad). Then we immediately go to 50 mini jumps while staying on the balls of their feet (knees flex to about 1/4 squat). I experiment with the 50 mini jumps and at times perform any of the patterns one sees when boxers are skipping rope (i.e., split jumps, shuffles). Just 3-5 sets will shred your legs if you use the right intensity. You can perform this workout 2-3 times per week for 4 weeks.

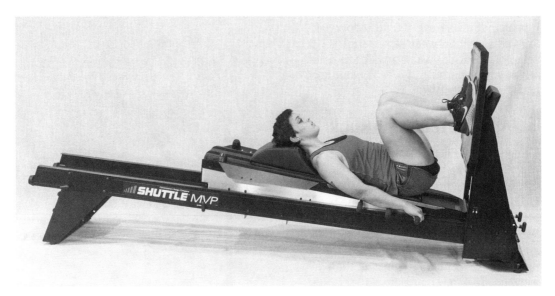

Figure 13.3 Shuttle MVP.

Summary

The protocols in this chapter are greatly responsible for setting the stage for IHP's reputation of making killers. When our athletes set their eyes on a target, their legs always get them there. These workouts are in part what we use to create legs that won't quit. Remember, what initially conditions the legs eventually serves as a prefatigue strategy to technical work. That prefatigue strategy is the magic of our reduced-volume training. Regardless of how you use these workouts, there is no doubt in my mind that you will notice an incredible difference in the way your legs look and function. Remember, when you feel your new killer legs, share the excitement with a friend.

CHAPTER 14

Upper-Body Metabolics

Chapter 13 discussed the importance of lower-body endurance for getting there and firmly standing there in sports. But what happens when you get there? When you do get there, usually it's time to do something with the upper body. Even when the upper body does not need endurance for the activity, it often needs endurance to be able to train at a high level for many minutes or hours. For example, a baseball player does not really need upper-body endurance to hit a ball three to five times during a three-hour game. However, going through a batting cage workout of 50-100 balls three or four times per week requires upper-body endurance. If you don't believe that repetitive training is work, just look at the forearms of professional baseball players who have great batting averages; they're pretty impressive.

Functional Training has several upper-body metabolic protocols, such as the meta chest and meta back. I refer you to that book for a complete explanation of functional training, program design, and over 100 programs that will take your performance to the next level. The workouts in this chapter will provide additional upper-body endurance protocols. I also provide a few supplemental workouts so you can see what other workouts can look like. This is done to provide more content and to ignite the creative process that leads you to design your own metabolic protocols. Remember, if I created all the content in this book through practice, success, and failure, why can't you do the same? Why can't you create personalized workouts that meet your specific needs? You can, and I hope you will.

The equipment used for the protocols in this chapter is simple and easy to get. I love body weight, bands, and medicine balls since these pieces are easy to obtain, cheap, and travel pretty well. Even if you can't get a medicine ball to travel easily, most gyms have them. Therefore, you will be able to pull off these protocols without much difficulty. As always, if you don't have a piece of equipment, either do more reps of something you can do or substitute for a piece of equipment you do have. Making it happen is half the fun, and it's where the learning takes place.

The key thing to the design of our metabolic protocols is to avoid long transitions of even a few seconds that can allow the local muscle environment to recover. There is no rest between exercises or loss of rhythm in movement during the protocols. Constant fast movement is the name of the game in this type of training. Another characteristic is that the sequence we usually follow when working both sides of the body is to include parallel simultaneous movements and alternating limb patterns. We perform the simple, slower movements first and finish with the energy-draining fast movements. An example of this common format is my famous leg crank:

- 24 bodyweight double-leg squats
- 24 bodyweight alternating lunges (12 per leg)
- 24 alternating split jumps (12 per leg)
- 12 squat jumps

When applying this format to the upper body, we start with slow bilateral movements such as a band press or band row, then finish with explosive bilateral movements such as an explosive push-up or explosive swimmer. The upper-body metabolic circuit can last 50 to 70 seconds.

Now, this does not mean we can't break this format, and we do. However, this basic format helps teach the design of metabolic protocols. Once you master this format design, you can start experimenting.

Our most popular metabolic pushing protocols are featured in our chisel your chest project, and I refer you to ihpfit.com for more information on metabolic training for the chest. I provide a couple of additional chest metabolic protocols in this chapter that require nothing but body weight and bands. But I warn you: Metabolic protocols are advanced training, and you need to develop an excellent fitness base before even attempting them. Any protocol involving push-ups requires a person to be able to perform 30-40 push-ups without stopping. For individuals who don't have that kind of strength but still want to experience metabolic training, I recommend you perform the band metabolics so the intensity can be better tailored to individual strength.

UPPER-BODY METABOLIC PUSH 1: JC BAND META CHEST

This 4-week program uses a set of JC bands to provide resistance. I recommend the 4 ft (122cm) orange sports bands for women and the 4 ft green sports bands for men. Set up the band according to manufacturer guidelines. You will need to experiment with the distance you pull the band to get the perfect tension for the entire protocol. This protocol makes for a great flush set after a chest day, to tone your chest during short workouts, or as a prefatigue strategy to technical sports training, such as hitting a speed bag. The tempo is very fast, approximately 2-3 repetitions per second, so the entire protocol is done in about 1 min. Weeks 1 and 2 will be enough for most people, while weeks 3 and 4 should be attempted only by elite athletes or individuals who have years of training behind them.

Equipment

Bands

Notes

Rest 90 sec to 2 min between sets.

Week 1: 1 set, 2 or 3 times per week, using lighter band tension and resting as needed between exercises; exercises 1-3 only.

Week 2: 2 sets, 2 or 3 times per week, using greater band tension and no rest between exercises; exercises 1-3 only.

Week 3: 2 sets, 1 or 2 times per week, using heavy band tension and no rest between exercises; exercises 1-4.

Week 4: 3 sets, 1 or 2 times per week, using heavy band tension and no rest between exercises; exercises 1-4.

Elite: 2 sets back-to-back (all 4 exercises) without rest.

Table 14.1   Upper-Body Metabolic Push 1: JC Band Meta Chest

Exercise	Photo	Instructions	Reps
1. BP staggered stance press		Anchor the band at chest height. Hold one handle in each hand and face away from the anchor point. Create appropriate tension and assume a split stance with your left leg forward. Starting with your hands on the sides of your chest, extend your elbows to perform a double-arm chest press. Flex your elbows to return to the starting position. Repeat for desired reps; switch your foot position and repeat.	20 per foot position (40 total)
2. BP staggered stance alternating press		Anchor the band at chest height. Hold one handle in each hand and face away from the anchor point. Create appropriate tension and assume a split stance, with your left leg forward. Start with your left arm extended and your right hand on the right side of your chest. Simultaneously extend your right elbow to press with your right hand and flex your left elbow to bring your left hand to the left side of your chest. Repeat for desired reps; switch your foot position and repeat.	20 per foot position (40 total)
3. BP staggered stance fly		Anchor the band at chest height. Hold one handle in each hand and face away from anchor point. Create appropriate tension and assume a split stance with your left leg forward. Starting with your arms open, palms facing forward, and elbows slightly flexed, bring your hands together until they almost touch. Open your arms to the starting position. Repeat for desired reps; switch your foot position and repeat.	10 per foot position (40 total)
4. Explosive push-up (optional)		Assume a push-up position, your hands shoulder-width apart. Flex your elbows to lower your body until your elbows are flexed to about 90 degrees, and explode back up as you extend your elbows so that your hands come off the ground. Repeat.	10

UPPER-BODY METABOLIC PUSH 2: CHISEL YOUR CHEST

This 8-week program is made up of two monster workouts; one made it into an issue of *Men's Health*. You can treat each 4-week phase as a separate protocol and even go for the elite version if you like. Just to be able to do either one of these protocols with little to no rest between each exercise is an accomplishment. This strategy of metabolic chest training even has some solid research behind it as well. Dr. Rhadi Ferguson presented his findings on a 3-week version of this protocol for his PhD dissertation (Ferguson, Rhadi. 2009. Use of the medicine ball super arms protocol on the National Football League's 225-lb repetition-to-failure bench press test: Analysis of effects. A dissertation presented in partial fulfillment of the requirements for the degree doctor of philosophy. Capela University), showing a 5.2% increase in the 225 lb (102 kg) bench-press-to-failure in elite football players in 3 weeks, without lifting a weight! The tempo is very fast, approximately 1-2 repetitions per second, so the entire protocol is done in about 50-60 sec. Weeks 1 and 2 will be enough for most people, while weeks 3 and 4 should be attempted only by elite athletes or individuals who have years of training behind them.

Equipment

Small but very firm medicine ball (or 6-8 in. [15-20 cm] step)

Notes

Rest 90 sec to 2 min between each set.

Week 1: 1 set, 2 or 3 times per week, resting as needed between exercises.

Week 2: 2 sets, 2 or 3 times per week, little rest between exercises.

Week 3: 2 sets, 1 or 2 times per week, no rest between exercises.

Week 4: 3 sets, 1 or 2 times per week, no rest between exercises.

Elite: 2 sets back-to-back, no rest between sets.

Table 14.2 Upper-Body Metabolic Push 2: Chisel Your Chest

Exercise	Photo	Instructions	Reps
WEEKS 1-4			
1. Bodyweight push-up		Assume a push-up position, your hands shoulder-width apart. Flex your elbows to lower your body until your chest is 2-3 in. (5-8 cm) off the ground. Straighten your arms and push back up. Repeat.	20
2. Bodyweight lateral shuffle push-up		Assume a push-up position, your hands shoulder-width apart. Place your right hand next to your left hand. Shuffle your left hand to the outside of your left shoulder. Perform a push-up. Repeat.	10 per side (20 total)

Exercise	Photo	Instructions	Reps
3. Diamond push-up		Assume a push-up position, keeping your hands close (i.e., the thumbs of each hand touching). Perform a push-up.	10
4. Explosive push-up		Assume a push-up position, your hands shoulder-width apart. Flex your elbows to lower your body until your elbows are flexed to about 90 degrees, and explode back up as you extend your elbows so that your hands come off the ground. Repeat.	10
WEEKS 5-8			
1. MB (or step) single-arm push-off		Place your left hand on the floor and your right hand on a small medicine ball or small step (4-8 in. [10-20 cm]); put your hands shoulder-width apart. Perform a push-up. Quickly push all the way up until your right arm is straight and your left hand comes off the ground. Perform all repetitions on one side, then switch to the other side.	10 per side (20 total)
2. MB (or step) crossover push-up		Perform a unilateral push-off on the medicine ball or step. While your left arm is locked out, place your right hand next to your left hand on the medicine ball or step. Shuffle your left hand to the left, placing it on the ground at shoulder width. Perform a push-up. Repeat to the right side.	10 per side (20 total)
3. MB (or step) hands-on-ball push-up		Assume a push-up position on the medicine ball or step, keeping your hands close (i.e., the thumbs of each hand touching). Flex your elbows to perform a push-up on the medicine ball or step. Repeat.	10
4. MB (or step) depth jump		Assume a push-up position on the medicine ball or step, keeping your hands close (i.e., the thumbs of each hand touching). Quickly jump your hands off the medicine ball or step and land with your hands to each side of the medicine ball or step. Immediately jump back on to the medicine ball or step. Repeat.	10

UPPER-BODY METABOLIC PULL 1: BAND AND BALL META BACK

This 4-week program uses a set of JC bands to provide resistance and is a mirror of the metabolic push 1 protocol. Again, I recommend the 4-foot orange JC Sports Band for women and the green JC Sports Band for men. Set up the band according to manufacturer guidelines. You will need to experiment with the distance you pull the band to get the perfect tension for the entire protocol. This protocol makes for a great flush set after a back day, to tone your back during short workouts, or as a prefatigue strategy to technical sports training, like swimming. The tempo is very fast, approximately 2-3 repetitions per second, so the entire protocol is done in about 1 min. Weeks 1 and 2 will be enough for most people, while weeks 3 and 4 should be attempted only by elite athletes or individuals who have years of training behind them. Although the parallel stance is used in the protocol, you can certainly perform it with a staggered stance to get more posterior activity (i.e., split sets between foot positions or divide sets in half with each foot position).

Equipment

JC Sports Band (green for men, orange for women), firm medicine ball (2-4 lb [1-2 kg])

Notes

Rest 90 sec to 2 min between sets.

> Week 1: 1 set, 2 or 3 times per week, using lighter band tension and resting as needed between exercises; exercises 1-3 only.
>
> Week 2: 2 sets, 2 or 3 times per week, using greater band tension and no rest between exercises; exercises 1-3 only.
>
> Week 3: 2 sets, 1 or 2 times per week, using heavy band tension and no rest between exercises; exercises 1-4.
>
> Week 4: 3 sets, 1 or 2 times per week, using heavy band tension and no rest between exercises; exercises 1-4.
>
> Elite: 2 sets back-to-back (all 4 exercises) without rest.

Table 14.3 Upper-Body Metabolic Pull 1: Band and Ball Meta Back

Exercise	Photo	Instructions	Reps
1. BP row		Anchor a band at chest height. Hold one handle in each hand and face away from the anchor point. Create appropriate tension. Flex your elbows to row the handles to the sides of your ribs. Extend your elbows to return to the starting position. Repeat.	30
2. BP bent-over alternating row		Anchor a band at chest height. Hold one handle in each hand and face the anchor point. Flex at the hips so that the torso is parallel to the ground, and create appropriate tension in the band. Start with your right arm extended overhead (toward the anchor point) and your left hand on the left side of your chest. Simultaneously pull your right arm to the right side of your chest and allow your left arm to extend overhead. Repeat.	30

Exercise	Photo	Instructions	Reps
3. BP swim		Anchor a band at chest height. Hold one handle in each hand and face away from the anchor point. Create appropriate tension. Stand upright with the arms pointing toward the anchor point. Simultaneously flex your trunk and bring your hands to the sides of your hips so that the band is in contact with the shoulders and your thumbs are near your rear pockets. Return to the starting position. Repeat.	30
4. MB overhead throw (optional)		Stand with your feet shoulder-width apart. Hold a 2-4 lb (1-2 kg) medicine ball in your hands. Bring the ball overhead and throw it to a wall in front of you. (You may slam the ball to the ground away from you if you don't have a wall.) Pick up (catch) ball. Repeat.	10

UPPER-BODY METABOLIC PULL 2: STABILITY BALL AND PULL-UP WORKOUT

This 4-week program uses a stability ball (or wheel) and a pull-up bar as equipment. It requires that you can do 15 pull-ups and 10 stability ball (or wheel) rollouts before you even attempt this baby. I had to pull this one out of our protocol vault since we have not used it in a long time, but I'm not sure why we don't use it more often; it's a beast of a protocol. It was very popular with our combat athletes and probably gave way to newer versions that use our special gripping equipment. The tempo is as fast as you can perform, but due to the higher strength requirements needed for this protocol, the movements are slower that the other protocols. Set up the equipment (or stations) close to each other so you can go from exercise to exercise as fast as possible. Use whatever time between sets and reps you need to complete the protocol; the goal is no rest between exercises or sets. Use 90 sec to 3 min of rest between protocols. Weeks 1 and 2 will be enough for most advanced individuals, while weeks 3 and 4 should be attempted only by individuals who have years of training behind them.

Equipment

Pull-up bar, wheel or stability ball, sports band, medicine ball (2-4 lb [1-2 kg])

Notes

Rest 90 sec to 2 min between sets.

Week 1: 1 set, 2 or 3 times per week, rest as necessary; exercises 1-3 only.

Week 2: 2 sets, 2 or 3 times per week, no rest between exercises, 1-2 min rest between sets; exercises 1-3 only.

Week 3: 2 sets, 1 or 2 times per week, no rest between exercises, 1-2 min rest between sets; exercises 1-4.

Week 4: 3 sets, 1 or 2 times per week, no rest between exercises or between sets; exercises 1-4

Elite: 2 sets back-to-back without rest; exercises 1-4.

Table 14.4 Upper-Body Metabolic Pull 2: Stability Ball and Pull-Up Workout

Exercise	Photo	Instructions	Reps
1. 3D 21 pull-ups		Hang from a pull-up bar, your hands shoulder-width apart. Start with your chin above the bar and perform 7 half pull-ups (from chin above bar to elbows flexed to 90 degrees). Lower your body until your arms are fully extended and perform 7 half pull-ups (from arm fully extended to elbows flexed to 90 degrees). Perform 7 complete pull-ups.	7 + 7 + 7 (21 total)
2. SB (or wheel) roll-out		Assume a plank position with your hands on a wheel or stability ball and your feet on the floor (balance on your knees if your core is not strong enough). Roll the wheel or ball out until your arms are stretched out over your head. Roll back to the starting position. Repeat.	10
3. BP swim		Anchor a band at chest height. Hold one handle in each hand and face away from the anchor point. Create appropriate tension. Stand upright, with your arms pointing toward the anchor point. Simultaneously flex your trunk and bring your hands to the sides of your hips so that the band is in contact with the shoulders and your thumbs are near your rear pockets. Return to the starting position. Repeat.	30
4. MB overhead throw (optional)		Stand with your feet shoulder-width apart. Hold a 2-4 lb (1-2 kg) medicine ball in your hands. Bring the ball overhead and throw it to a wall in front of you. (You may slam to the ground away from you if you don't have a wall.) Pick up (catch) ball. Repeat.	10

SUPPLEMENTAL UPPER-BODY ENDURANCE

The following protocols feature some specialized equipment that we have at IHP. We understand that not every person will have access to this equipment and not every gym has this equipment on the floor. However, as I travel around the world, I'm seeing more gyms step up and offer more interesting equipment to their client bases. I'm also seeing an increasing amount of smaller studios equip themselves with these unique pieces to compete with the bigger gyms that don't have them. Next time you look for a gym or studio, see if it has some of the equipment featured in this section; that will be a sign that the gym is up-to-date.

Hydra-Gym 360

The Hydra-Gym Powermax 360. (go to ihpfit.com to see it in action) is an awesome piece of equipment for the upper body. Like any good piece of equipment, it is a grab-and-go piece that is user-friendly in its application, is super effective, and can train anyone at any level. There are about seven different patterns that can be done with two arms or single arms, for reps or time. Here are two of our favorite applications:

1. Perform 140 altering punches followed by 30 sec of the speed bag, heavy bag, or focused mitt work. This is our standard prefatigue application.

2. Perform as many reps as you can in 30 sec for the patterns in table 14.5. Start with 1-2 sets of 15 sec per exercise and rest about 1-1:30 min between sets. Just about anyone can start with that. You can add one set each week, and add time to the exercise interval, until you are doing 5 sets of 30 hard sec for each exercise. That's right: 35 sets in about 40-50 min was our biggest workout. Perform 2 times each week.

Notes

Week 1: 2 × 15 sec of exercise with 1 min rest.

Week 2: 3 × 20 sec of exercise with 1:30 min rest.

Week3: 4 × 30 sec of exercise with 1 min rest.

Week 4: 5 × 30 sec of exercise with 30 sec to 1 min rest.

Table 14.5 Hydra-Gym 360 Workout

Exercise	Photo	Instructions
1. Simultaneous punch		Stand in a parallel or staggered stance and hold a handle in each hand. Push with both hands simultaneously, then pull with both hands simultaneously.
2. Alternating punch		Stand in a parallel or staggered stance and hold a handle in each hand. Push with your right hand while pulling with your left hand. Repeat.

(continued)

Table 14.5 Hydra-Gym 360 Workout *(continued)*

Exercise	Photo	Instructions
3. Fly		Stand in a parallel or staggered stance and hold a handle in each hand. Keeping your elbows slightly flexed, open your arms wider and close them until the handles almost touch. Repeat.
4. Side to side		Stand in a parallel or staggered stance and hold a handle in each hand. Holding both handles close to each other and keeping your arms almost straight, move both handles as far right as you can, then move them as far left as you can. Repeat.
5. Alternating cross		Stand in a parallel or staggered stance and hold a handle in each hand. With your right hand, push diagonally to your left. As you bring your right arm back, push with your left hand diagonally to the right. Repeat.
6. Inward circle		Stand in a parallel or staggered stance and hold a handle in each hand. Holding both handles close to each other and keeping your arms slightly flexed, simultaneously make a big counterclockwise circle with your right hand and a clockwise circle with your left hand. Repeat.
7. Outward circle		Stand in a parallel or staggered stance and hold a handle in each hand. Holding both handles close to each other and keeping your arms slightly flexed, simultaneously make a big clockwise circle with your right hand and a counterclockwise circle with your left hand. Repeat.

ISOs to Ropes (Isometric Metabolic)

ISOs to ropes is another killer upper-body grind. It involves isometric contractions followed by ropes or a new product called the Inertia Wave, which is an alternative to ropes. Although we call for the alternating up-and-down pattern in the rope drills, you can use other patterns you like. This is just one of the ways we work this protocol, but there are many possible variations. Select a set of dumbbells 15%-20% of your body weight. Set up a 40-50 ft (12-15m) rope looped around a sturdy structure (such as a dumbbell rack) and have a pull-up bar in close proximity. Table 14.6 shows the protocol. Start at any week you think you can do comfortably. You can perform this protocol 2 or 3 times per week.

Equipment

Dumbbells, ropes or Inertia Wave (inertiawave.com), pull-up bar

Notes

Week 1: 2 sets

Week 2: 3 sets

Week 3: 4 sets

Week 4: 5 sets

Week 5: 5 sets

Week 6: 5 sets

Table 14.6 ISOs to Ropes (Isometric Metabolic) Workout

Exercise	Photo	Instructions	Week	Time
1. Isometric DB clinch carry		Hold dumbbells at 90 degrees of elbow flexion. Stand or walk around without allowing your arms to lose the flexed position.	Week 1	5 sec
			Week 2	10 sec
			Week 3	15 sec
			Week 4	20 sec
			Week 5	25 sec
			Week 6 (beast)	30 sec
2. Ropes alternating up and down		With your feet shoulder-width apart and core tight, hold onto the rope ends. Move your arms in opposite directions (right hand up and left hand down) to cause shoulder-height waves in each rope.	Week 1	10 sec
			Week 2	20 sec
			Week 3	30 sec
			Week 4	30 sec
			Week 5	30 sec
			Week 6 (beast)	30 sec
Rest			Week 1	30 sec
			Week 2	30 sec
			Week 3	60 sec
			Week 4	60 sec
			Week 5	60 sec
			Week 6 (beast)	60 sec

(continued)

Table 14.6 ISOs to Ropes (Isometric Metabolic) Workout *(continued)*

Exercise	Photo	Instructions	Week	Time
3. Isometric half pull-up		Hold pull-up at 90 degrees of elbow flexion and hold that position.	Week 1	5 sec
			Week 2	10 sec
			Week 3	15 sec
			Week 4	20 sec
			Week 5	25 sec
			Week 6 (beast)	30 sec
4. Ropes alternating up and down		With your feet shoulder-width apart and core tight, hold onto the rope ends. Move your arms in opposite directions (right hand up and left hand down) to cause shoulder-height waves in each rope.	Week 1	10 sec
			Week 2	20 sec
			Week 3	30 sec
			Week 4	30 sec
			Week 5	30 sec
			Week 6 (beast)	30 sec
Rest			Week 1	30 sec
			Week 2	30 sec
			Week 3	60 sec
			Week 4	60 sec
			Week 5	60 sec
			Week 6 (beast)	60 sec

Summary

I am sure this chapter provided you with some new ideas on how to get your upper body in incredible shape and ready for anything. It does not matter if you just want a finishing pump after your traditional workout or are getting ready for a UFC fight. The protocols in this chapter have delivered in those types of situations, and they will deliver for you. Keep the flame of creativity burning and dare to combine various moves from different workouts to create your own. Challenge your friends to get involved and keep up with you. Make your Saturdays IHP grind day and take these workouts for a spin. It's a great way to kick off the weekend!

Total-Body Metabolics

CHAPTER **15**

This chapter ties it all together—total-body metabolics. When I trained Army Special Forces and many of my fighters, this is what I put them through! Your entire body is a metabolic machine, and training the entire body how to deal with high levels of hydrogen as a result of the dissociation of lactic acid (HLA) into lactate (LA-) and hydrogen (H+) is extremely important. Not only are the metabolic pathways enhanced through this type of intense training, there is the psychological (i.e., spiritual) factor yet to be quantified. As I have previously mentioned, I believe the biggest and fastest adaptation to intense training is resetting the human will, and that is a spiritual transformation, not a physical adaptation. These total-body protocols are not fancy, but they do create what we call IHP cyborgs.

In the old days, we had gut-check Fridays (GCF), a workout that was made up of all our metabolic protocols. This was a brutal workout:

- 6 sets of JC leg cranks (24 bodyweight double-leg squats, 24 [12 per leg] bodyweight alternating lunges, 24 [12 per leg] alternating split jumps, and 12 squat jumps) for 504 total reps for the legs with no rest in about 9 min.
- 5-10 min rest.
- 3 sets of chisel your chest (table 14.2) In weeks 1-4, chisel your chest includes 20 bodyweight push-ups, 20 (10 per side) bodyweight lateral shuffle push-ups, 10 diamond push-ups, and 10 explosive push-ups for 60 total reps. In weeks 5-8, chisel your chest includes 20 (10 per side) MB single-arm push-offs, 20 (10 per side) MB crossover push-ups, 10 MB hands-on-ball push-ups, and 10 MB depth jumps for 60 total reps. Whichever protocol you use, you get 60 total reps for the chest with no rest between exercises and about 2-3 min rest between sets.
- 5 min rest.
- 3 sets of meta back (20 BP rows, 20 [10 per arm and leg] BP staggered stance bent-over alternating rows, 20 BP swims, 10 MB overhead slams) for 70 reps for the back with no rest between exercises and about 2-3 min rest between sets.
- 5 min rest.
- 3 meta abs (10-20 leg raises, 10-20 crunches, 10-20 V-ups) with no rest between exercises, about 2-3 min rest between sets. Start doing the leg raises, lifting legs 8-12 in. (20-30 cm) off the ground. When the leg raises are completed, keep your feet about 12 in. (30 cm) a foot off the ground while doing crunches. When done with the crunches, go straight to V-ups.

Clients took 1-2 months of training just to be able to complete this workout. This workout sent everyone home, ready to call it a day; no happy hour for anyone after this. Since then, we have used versions of these protocols in different combinations. Now, we normally stick with very intense protocols that last 30 sec to 6 mins, depending on what we are trying to accomplish.

Total-body training generally consists of a sequence of intense and continuous upper- and lower-body training. Unless you use specialized equipment, such as an Airdyne or VersaClimber, you are looking at a series of calisthenics strung together in a sequence. *Functional Training* features Gary Gray's dumbbell matrix, which is a 72-rep dumbbell protocol. You can also do Gary's dumbbell matrix with heavy medicine balls or sand bags. However, our premiere protocol, which is actually a test we used with the Navy's SEAL Team 6 and combat-athletes, is the IHP combat-ready rest. This test has been turned into a training workout and consists of a series of metabolic protocols and tests we used individually. Therefore, you don't need much to design a great total-body metabolic protocol. As we always say, your imagination is the only limitation to program design. Now, let's rock total-body metabolic training.

TOTAL-BODY METABOLIC 1: IHP COMBAT READY (OR RING READY) TEST

This is the test of all tests. It's a two-in-one tool for IHP combat athletes and Army Special Forces. This test is not only a great way to assess the readiness of an individual but also a great workout that requires no equipment—all you need is a watch, a 25-yard runway, and a willing body. This test serves as a general physical assessment to evaluate ring readiness for combat athletes. The exercises were chosen so that everyone could perform them with no equipment and in any environment. In very simple terms, practicing an activity is the best way to get good at doing that activity. Therefore, practicing the components of the IHP test is the best way to prepare for the ring. This creates a great advantage: The test is the workout, and the workout is the test! The times listed are the times that most of the athletes in our initial database completed the test. It provides a rough idea of how your performance stacks up to all the IHP clients that participated in the initial data collection.

Table 15.1 IHP Combat Ready Test

Event time	Event
70 sec	300 yd (274 m) shuttle (25 yd [23 m] 12×)
5 sec	2-5 sec transition
20 sec	Ab blast: 10 leg raises, 10 crunches, 10 V-ups
5 sec	2-5 sec transition
60 sec	Squat thrust inferno (10 frog squats, 10 burpees, 10 squat thrust jumps)
5 sec	2-5 sec transition
20 sec	Push-ups (20 reps)
5 sec	2-5 sec transition
90 sec	JC leg crank (24 squats, 24 lunges, 24 split jumps, 12 squat jumps)
5 sec	2-5 sec transition
80 sec	300 yd (274 m) shuttle (25 yd [23 m] 12×)
Total: 365 sec (6:08)	

Recommended Completion Times for Elite Athletes

Lightweights (< 170 lb [77 kg]): < 4:30

Level I (170-190 lb [77-86 kg]): < 5:00

Level II (191-210 lb [86-95 kg]): < 5:30

Level III (211-230 lb [95-104 kg]): < 6:00

Level IV (> 230 lb [104 kg]): < 6:30

Need help getting there? Here is how to do it! Follow this 8-week schedule:

Weeks 1-2: Perform 1 set of each exercise with ample rest between exercises. Do this 3 times per week.

Weeks 3-4: Perform 2 sets of each exercise with ample rest between exercises. Do this 3 times per week.

Weeks 5-6: Perform 2 sets of each exercise with 90 sec of rest between exercises. Do this 3 times per week.

Week 7: Perform 1 set of the circuit 2 times per week.

Week 8: Set personal records on each circuit.

300-Yard (276 m) Shuttle (25 yd [23 m] 12×)

Mark two Xs on the ground 25 yd (23 m) apart from each other. Start with your right hand on the starting X. Run to the other X (25 yd [23 m] away) and touch it with your left hand. Repeat 12 times (6 round trips) until you cover all 300 yd (274 m).

Ab Blast

Lie with your legs 8 in. (20 cm) off the ground and your hands by the sides of your head (as if you were protecting your head from punches). Perform 10 **leg raises,** bringing your feet from the 8 in. (20 cm) height to about 24 in. (61 cm) high. Holding your feet at the 8 in. (20 cm) mark, perform 10 **crunches** by reaching your hands toward the ceiling. Without putting your feet down, finish with 10 **V-ups,** reaching as close to your feet as your flexibility allows.

Squat Thrust Inferno

Stand with your feet shoulder-width apart (or slightly wider). For **frog squats,** squat 10 times, touching the ground between your feet with both of your hands on each squat (i.e., the frog position—all fingers must touch the ground). After completing the squats, immediately perform 10 **burpees** by putting your hands between your feet, thrusting back into a push-up position, tucking back into the frog position, and standing up straight. Immediately follow with 10 **burpees (squat thrust) to jumps** (i.e., add a jump to the end of the burpee or squat thrust).

Push-Ups

Start in a plank position. Lower your chest until it touches the ground. Press back to a straight-arm position.

JC Leg Crank

Perform 24 bodyweight double-leg squats. Do 24 bodyweight alternating lunges (12 per leg) with the rear knee 6-8 in. (15-20 cm) from the ground. Do 24 (12 per leg) alternating split jumps with the rear knee 12-18 in. (30-46 cm) from the ground. Finish with 12 squat jumps, with 90 degrees of knee flexion.

TOTAL-BODY METABOLIC 2: FIGHTING CIRCUIT

This 5-week program is a sample of one of the many MMA protocols we have used with UFC fighters such as Cezar "the Mutant" Ferreira. As you can see, it's a series of multiple metabolic protocols with various pieces of equipment to create multiple rounds just under 6 min each. This training is harder than any sparring and much safer. If you don't have specific equipment, see the suggested equivalent exercises you can use. Set the stations as close to each other as possible, and always set them up the same way so you can accurately compare the circuit times between training days. Jog from station to station with your hands up to guard your face. Perform 3-5 circuits per workout. Perform 1 or 2 workouts per week, depending on your weekly schedule and training volume. Total circuit time should be under 6 min.

Equipment

VersaClimber, low hurdles (6-8 in. [15-20 cm]), barbell, dumbbells, medicine balls, Hydra-Gym Powermax 360, pull-up bar, bands

Notes

If performing the workout twice a week, time one workout and use that as your test. Use the other workout for training (don't time it).

Week 1: Rest 3 minutes between rounds.

Week 2: Rest 2 minutes between rounds.

Week 3: Rest 1 minute between rounds.

Week 4: Rest 1 minute between rounds; wear a tight weight vest that is 3%-5% of your body weight.

Week 5: Rest 1 minute between rounds; no weight vest.

Table 15.2 Total-Body Metabolic 2: Fighting Circuit

Exercise	Photo	Instructions	Reps and time
1. VersaClimber or burpees		Step onto the VC steps, strap in your feet, and set the handles to the appropriate level. Pump your legs and arms simultaneously at a rate of 210-250 ft (64-76 m) per min (or 105-125 ft [32-38 m] in 30 sec).	30 sec at over 220 ft (67 m) per min
2. JC leg crank		24 bodyweight double-leg squats, 24 (12 per leg) bodyweight alternating lunges, 24 (12 per leg) alternating split jumps, 12 squat jumps.	84 total

Exercise	Photo	Instructions	Reps and time
3. Low-hurdle lateral jump		Jump laterally over a 6-8 in. (15-20 cm) hurdle, land with both feet, and immediately jump back over the hurdle. Repeat.	10 total (5 per side)
4. Barbell deadlift (or pick up a partner)		Load the barbell with 110%-120% of your body weight. Place the bar in front of you, touching your shins. Grab the bar with your palms facing you, and keeping your back straight, lift to a fully extended body position.	10
5. DB clinch walk (or pick up and hold a partner)		Choose dumbbells that are 15%-20% of your body weight. Hold the dumbbells with your elbows bent at 90 degrees without losing the flexed arm position.	30 sec
6. Sprawl		A fighter's version of a burpee. Stand in an athletic position, jump your legs back so you land in a push-up position and immediately jump back up to the standing position.	10
7. MB get-up		Lie face up and hold a medicine ball that weighs 3%-5% of your body weight in your left hand. Using your right hand for assistance, get up to a full standing position. Lie down and repeat. Switch to the other hand.	5 per side (10 total)
8. Upper-body metabolic push 2		20 bodyweight push-ups, 20 lateral shuffle push-ups (10 per side), 10 diamond push-ups, 10 explosive push-ups.	60 total

(continued)

Table 15.2 Total-Body Metabolic 2: Fighting Circuit *(continued)*

Exercise	Photo	Instructions	Reps and time
9. 360 alternate punching (or punch with bands)		Stand on a 360 platform in a parallel or staggered fighting stance. Holding a handle in each hand, punch in an alternating fashion.	140 punches
10. BP alternating downward punch		Secure a band such as the JC Predator Jr. (triple 2 in. [5 cm]) from a pull-up bar. Holding a handle in each hand, perform alternating downward punches. You may use a punching bag as a target.	50 punches

SUPPLEMENTAL TOTAL-BODY ENDURANCE

Some total-body protocols use specialized equipment. Some are used in the MMA circuit and are worth mentioning separately with full workout suggestions. Once upon a time, specialized equipment was not found anywhere, but now that has changed. Look for a gym that has some of this equipment; it shows it is on the cutting edge. If your gym does not have it, talk to the owner and show him or her what it can do; the owner may buy it for the gym.

VersaClimber (Total-Body Climber)

Here it is again, the VersaClimber (go to the equipment link at ihpfit.com to see it in action). I first saw this equipment in the early 1990s when visiting a gym during personal training certification. I started to use it in 1994 and fell in love with it. I made up my mind that I would have several if I ever had a gym. Now, it is a go-to piece at IHP for total-body strength and cardio. Here are two of our favorite applications.

As a HIIT workout, work up to 10 sets of 30 sec, over 110 ft (33 m) climbs (over 220 ft/min [67 m/min] pace), with 60-90 sec rest between sets. This is a 2 day per week, 4-week progression.

- Week 1: 4 sets of 30 sec, try to get 90 to 100 ft (27-30 m), rest 2 min between sets
- Week 2: 6 sets of 30 sec, try to get 95 to 105 ft (29-32 m), rest 2 min between sets
- Week 3: 8 sets of 30 sec, try to get 100 to 110 ft (30-33 m), rest 90 sec to 2 min between sets
- Week 4: 10 sets of 30 sec, try to get 110 ft (33 m), rest 60-90 sec between sets

The Gauntlet (Body Weight)

I invented this protocol to keep wrestlers with shin splints busy while the rest of the team ran 400-meter laps around the track. It cured shin splints in one session. Now, a version of this is part of the combat ready circuit. However, this is a more expanded version that deserves special mention. Obviously, smaller individuals do better with the times than bigger individuals. Small men weighing 135-145 lb (61-66 kg) can eventually get close to 1:35. Big men weighing 230-250 lb (104-113 kg) may take as much as 2:45-3:00 minutes. But seeing a man that size move nonstop for 3 min is a sight to see.

- 20 frog squats (squat and touch ground between feet) (20-30 sec)
- 20 bodyweight push-ups (20 sec)
- 10 burpees (20 sec)
- 10 jump squats (10-15 sec)
- 10 burpees with push-up to jump (25-35 sec)

The complete protocol should take 1:45 to 2:15, including short transitions. Because of its constant nature, the difficulty feels similar to a hard period of high school wrestling. Perform 3 protocols, with 30-60 sec rest between each, and you are ready to start wrestling season.

- Week 1: 2 gauntlets (no time requirement) with 3 min rest, 3 times per week
- Week 2: 3 gauntlets (no time requirement) with 2 min rest, 3 times per week
- Week 3: 3 gauntlets (under 2:30) with 60 sec rest, 2 times per week
- Week 4: 3 gauntlets (under 1:45-2:15) with 30-60 sec rest, 2 times per week

Rope Gauntlet

This killer workout combines the gauntlet and rope work. Since the gauntlet has a lot of lower-body work and level changes, the ropes give it a nice upper-body twist. If you don't have a rope, use a DB clinch carry or a partner carry as your upper-body endurance work. This is a great workout for obstacle course athletes, people getting ready for the fire or police academy, or as part of a boot camp using 30 sec station intervals. You can use multiple sets as shown here or you can use one round as a flush conditioning protocol as a portion of a total workout. Feel free to experiment combining this protocol with the ISO ropes of the upper-body metabolics; they are a perfect match and work well together.

Table 15.3 shows a 6–week progression. Start at any week you think you can perform comfortably. Use this protocol 1 or 2 times per week.

Equipment

Ropes

Notes

Week 1: 2 sets, 15 sec rest between exercises, 2 min rest between sets.

Week 2: 2 sets, 15 sec rest between exercises, 1 min rest between sets.

Week 3: 3 sets, no rest between exercises, 1 min rest between sets.

Week 4: 3 sets, 15 sec rest between exercises, 30 sec rest between sets.

Week 5: 4 sets, 15 sec rest between exercises, 15 sec rest between sets.

Week 6: 5 sets, 15 sec rest between exercises, 15 sec rest between sets.

Table 15.3   Rope Gauntlet

Exercise	Photo	Instructions	Week	Time
1. Frog squat		Stand with your feet shoulder-width apart (or slightly wider). Flex your knees to squat, touching the ground between your feet with both of your hands on each squat (i.e., the frog position—all fingers must touch the ground).	Week 1	10 sec
			Week 2	15 sec
			Week 3	15 sec
			Week 4	20 sec
			Week 5	20 sec
			Week 6 (beast)	30 sec
2. Ropes alternating up and down		Hold on to the rope ends with your feet shoulder-width apart and core tight. Move your arms in opposite directions (right hand up and left hand down) to cause shoulder-height waves in each rope.	Week 1	15 sec
			Week 2	20 sec
			Week 3	20 sec
			Week 4	30 sec
			Week 5	30 sec
			Week 6 (beast)	30 sec
3. Burpee		Put your hands between your feet, thrusting back into a push-up position, tucking back into the frog position, and standing up straight.	Week 1	10 sec
			Week 2	15 sec
			Week 3	15 sec
			Week 4	20 sec
			Week 5	20 sec
			Week 6 (beast)	30 sec

Exercise	Photo	Instructions	Week	Time
4. Ropes alternating up and down		Hold on to the rope ends with your feet shoulder-width apart and core tight. Move your arms in opposite directions (right hand up and left hand down) to cause shoulder-height waves in each rope.	Week 1	15 sec
			Week 2	20 sec
			Week 3	20 sec
			Week 4	30 sec
			Week 5	30 sec
			Week 6 (beast)	30 sec
5. Jump squat		Stand with your feet parallel. Flex your knees to perform a squat to parallel position, then immediately jump as high as you can. When you land, immediately lower into the squat and jump back up.	Week 1	10 sec
			Week 2	20 sec
			Week 3	20 sec
			Week 4	20 sec
			Week 5	20 sec
			Week 6 (beast)	30 sec
6. Ropes alternating up and down		Hold on to the rope ends with your feet shoulder-width apart and core tight. Move your arms in opposite directions (right hand up and left hand down) to cause shoulder-height waves as in each rope.	Week 1	15 sec
			Week 2	20 sec
			Week 3	20 sec
			Week 4	30 sec
			Week 5	30 sec
			Week 6 (beast)	30 sec
7. Burpee to jump		Put your hands between your feet, thrusting back into a push-up position, tucking back into the frog position, and jump up. Repeat burpee to jump sequence.	Week 1	5 sec
			Week 2	10 sec
			Week 3	10 sec
			Week 4	15 sec
			Week 5	15 sec
			Week 6 (beast)	30 sec
8. Ropes alternating up and down		Hold on to the rope ends, keeping your feet shoulder-width apart and core tight. Move your arms in opposite directions (right hand up and left hand down) to cause shoulder-height waves in each rope.	Week 1	15 sec
			Week 2	20 sec
			Week 3	20 sec
			Week 4	30 sec
			Week 5	30 sec
			Week 6 (beast)	30 sec

Jeff Monson Tire and Truck Workout

This monster workout was designed for Jeff Monson in 2005 to get him ready for his heavyweight five-round title fight in UFC 65. We later used this workout to train SEAL Team 6 members for some of their most important missions. At the time, nobody had even come close to this, and when UFC found out about what we were doing, they featured our training in a UFC 65 Countdown segment. Until then, we did not know it if was humanly possible, but it was. Jeff was in the best shape of his life for that fight. Unfortunately, he did not end up with the title, but if he would not have been in the kind of shape he was in, he would have gotten seriously hurt that night. I truly believe this conditioning saved his life. Table 15.4 shows one of the 3 weekly workouts Jeff performed during his 5-week power endurance phase. Once the circuit begins, you walk or jog from one exercise to the other with no additional rest. Perform exercises 1-3 twice for 1 set. If possible, try to jog between exercises so you get minimum rest between exercises.

Table 15.4   Jeff Monson Tire and Truck Workout

Exercise	Week 1	Week 2	Week 3	Week 4	Week 5
1. Drag a 140 lb (64 kg) tire 10 yd (30 m) + 10 bob and weaves	3	3	3	3	3
2. Flip a 600 lb (272 kg) tire	2	2	2	2	2
3. Navigator push (80 yd [24 m])	1	1	1	1	1
2 rounds without rest = 1 set	repeat	repeat	repeat	repeat	repeat
Total sets (2 rounds of 1-3)	3	4	4	5	5
Rest progression (rest between exercises/rest between sets)	3-5 / 2 min	3-5 / 1 min	3-5 / 1 min	3-5 / 1 min	3-5 / 1 min

Summary

I hope this chapter gave you some insight into what is possible when it is time for total-body metabolic conditioning. The mind can be a limiting factor to exercise programming; it can take years to find out what people are capable of in a new area and to evolve training to those levels. I still remember not knowing if Jeff Monson was going to survive the training we pioneered in 2005 for his run at the UFC 65 heavyweight title. It has taken us the better part of two decades of pushing the envelope in metabolics to get a glimpse at how the human will can evolve with training. Now, with the workouts presented in this book, especially the intense ones in these last few chapters, your training will be accelerated by knowing what has been done before, sparing you decades of experimentation. Take these protocols for a ride and witness the evolution of the human will beyond that of which any physiological parameters measured can explain.

PART V

Putting It Together

This is a very special part because it ties together everything in this book. Part V kicks off with nutrition and recovery, two of the most important elements of body transformation. Nutrition is certainly the most important factor in fat loss, even more important than exercise. Recovery is the most important factor in performance. The nutrition and recovery chapter covers why I have these strong opinions. In this chapter, I elicit the help of professionals I consider gurus in the areas of nutrition, recovery, and anti-aging to ensure I bring you the latest and most accurate information available. They help me cover some conventional nutrition information, but also provide unique perspectives on nutrition and its spiritual component. By the end of the nutrition and recovery chapter, you will know how to eat better, but you will also understand why the window to the soul could very well be the mouth.

The programming chapter will teach you all you need to know to use the workouts in this book. Many people can perform a workout, but most don't know how to create or combine workouts to create programs. Even fewer know how to put together a program to peak for a specific event. This chapter covers exactly those topics in a very practical and effective manner.

You will learn the basic principles of periodization and program design and how those principles work within today's gym environment. The chapter expands the weekly workout and shows how it can concentrate on a weak body. It describes how to combine workouts to create a more balanced, total-body program. The workouts covered in this chapter range from bodybuilding programs to agility and speed programs, and some incorporate a little of both.

This chapter will teach you how to take a weekly workout and expand it to a monthly program that covers an entire cycle. It will also teach you how to set up a series of cycles to create a long-term program that can fit any time frame or type of activity. The chapter ends with workouts from some of the industry greats to further illustrate how to use the exercises and workouts in this book to take your performance to its highest level, while developing a body that looks as good as it functions.

CHAPTER 16

Nutrition and Recovery

With contributions from Jose Antonio, PhD; Cliff Edberg, RD; Douglas Kalman, PhD, RD; and Dave Woynarowski, MD

Iknow it may be strange hearing this from an exercise guy, but the most important component of health and body composition is nutrition. What goes into your body has a profound effect on how you look and feel. I'm not saying that exercise is not important, because it is. Exercise is the foundation of fitness, and it can have a protective effect against diseases such as obesity and diabetes. However, a huge component of the cause for these diseases is what you ingest into your body. Therefore, if you like the "ounce of prevention is worth a pound of cure" proverb, then nutrition is your ounce of prevention, and it can be worth a ton of cure, not a pound.

Name any major chronic disease plaguing modern society, and you'll see a trail that leads to what that person has consumed. Of course, some things are harder to trace back to nutrition, but in this book, we are talking about the majority. Even conditions not considered a disease state, like inflammation, can end up being problematic down the road, both from a health standpoint and certainly from an aesthetic standpoint.

Any figure or bodybuilding competitor will tell you that nutrition makes or breaks the performance on stage. It not only supplies the nutrients to help build muscle and provides energy for workouts but also can dictate the storage of fat. Since much of this book focuses on transformation workouts, there is no way we can get away from talking about nutrition. Unless you have incredible genes and can eat anything you want and still have a six-pack, you will have to manage the nutritional component of your appearance. I will give it to you straight: If you are like most people, you will have to be very conscious of the way you eat, or you will wear it where you don't want to!

Traditional Nutrition Education

To set the stage for the more involved nutrition topics in this chapter, we'll start with general nutrition facts that are important to understand. There are three major categories of nutrients, known as macronutrients. Each macronutrient has a specific calorie density and a specific thermic effect on the body. In other words, each macronutrient provides calories and requires a specific percentage of its energy for digestion, absorption, and disposal of ingested nutrients. This is called the thermic effect of food (TEF). Table 16.1 shows the three main macronutrients, their calorie densities, and their thermic effects. We have also included whey protein since we will refer to it later and use it as a nutritional supplement.

Food also contains micronutrients, which are vitamins and minerals. They are essential for good health and support a host of important processes in the body.

Table 16.1 Macronutrients and Thermic Effect

Macronutrient	Calories/gram	Thermic effect
Whey protein	4	30%-40%*
Protein	4	20%-35%
Carbohydrate	4	5%-20%
Fat	9	1%-5%

* Personal communication with Jose Antonio, PhD.

You can eat a higher volume of food if you focus on protein and veggies because they not only have fewer calories per volume of food but also require more calories to digest. You can also increase your thermic effect of food if you add whey protein to your diet. Remember that just because fat is calorie dense does not mean it's bad. We all need good fats for many functions in the body, including transporting fat-soluble vitamins and proper immune and hormonal function.

Of particular importance is how the body spends energy. Learning about this can help you take small steps that lead to big changes over time. These are the best changes. The body spends calories in four basic ways. Basal metabolic rate (BMR) is the energy the body uses to stay alive at rest (such as when you are sleeping). Then you have TEF, which is the energy your body uses to break down and digest food. Obviously, exercise is a well-known energy expenditure, although it may not use as much energy as you think it does. However, the one way that the body spends energy that many people don't know about (even though it is the make it or break it energy expenditure) is your nonexercise activity thermogenesis (NEAT). NEAT is all the other life-related activity you do that is not exercise, like walking at work, working around the house, etc. This component of energy expenditure is where most people can really affect their weight; getting your steps in each day is where it's at with NEAT. Figure 16.1 shows you these four components and their approximate percentages of calories expended each day. (This approximation is for illustrative purposes only. All people are different in how, where, and when they move.)

Later in this chapter, we will show you how to alter each of the components of your daily energy expenditure so that you can reach your ideal weight and achieve your transformation goals.

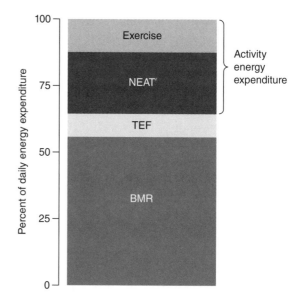

Figure 16.1 Energy expenditure.

Role of Hormones

I don't want to turn this into a biochemistry lesson, so I want to speak generally yet clearly in a way you can understand. The body is a survival machine, and it does not care about the things you care about. It does not care about a six-pack, putting on five pounds (2 kg) of muscle, or running a 4.4 forty. The body loves fat because it is its energy bank account, and it hates muscle because it's not needed as much as we like to think and also costs a lot of energy to maintain. The body has very efficient ways to regulate energy balance and even limit muscle growth. Hormones like leptin, ghrelin, insulin, glucagon, and many others regulate when you are hungry, what you are hungry for, and how what you eat gets used or stored. The myostatin gene limits muscle growth, making sure that a gym rat does not end up with 30-inch arms. So, the way you look and what you eat are hugely affected by your hormonal environment and your genetics, and you must keep that in mind. Your genetics in turn are affected by your epigenetics (the stuff that controls gene expression), and nothing (including exercise) will affect your epigenetics or your genes as much as what you eat! At the end of the day, you may fool your body and its hormones for little while, but they will win in the long run. Yo-yo dieters are a perfect example of temporarily winning the weight-loss battle but losing the hormone war. The take-home message is that you can't starve yourself into looking good for the long haul; your body will detect what you are doing and use its hormones to survive. The end result is usually a lower metabolic rate (mediated by the thyroid and various metabolic mechanisms) that leads you into something like a hibernation state. This explains how a bear can go into a cave for several months, not die, and come out and regain all the weight lost by only consuming a few more calories than normal. You are fighting hormones with your nutrition, and you can't railroad your body into losing weight or fat. Unless you are willing to live a calorie-restricted diet the rest of your life, you will not win in the long term and may end up getting fatter on the rebound.

Inflammation

We hear a lot about inflammation these days—it's a new buzzword. The body experiences good and bad inflammation. Good inflammation is usually acute, and it's one of the first healing responses. However, the inflammation we refer to as bad inflammation is the chronic inflammation that results when your immune system is dealing with a constant invader such as an allergen. Inflammation is now thought to be a precursor and foundational dysfunction associated with many chronic diseases such as diabetes, high blood pressure, and even arthritis.

Inflammation may be caused by something you are ingesting that you have some kind of sensitivity to. However, finding the culprit of the inflammation is another story. At this time, the research is lacking in pinpointing which foods cause inflammation. Therefore, this book will not deal with diagnosing allergies (inflammation), sensitivities, or complicated nutritional issues. We are going to deal with the basics in sound and healthy nutritional practices for most people.

Just about anything a person is sensitive to can trigger an inflammatory response: a food, any chemical added to something we ingest, or any agent we come in contact with. This includes toothpaste, deodorant, detergent, makeup, food, drinks, and even the air we breathe. Here are some of the most common foods and substances thought to cause inflammation in the body:

- **Sugar**—It's probably one of the biggest addictions in our modern-day society and the biggest cause of inflammation via excess insulin (the hormone used to store fat).
- **Artificial sweeteners**—If you think that a product is safe because it is labeled as zero carbs, it may not be! These artificial additives are sensed by the bacteria in your gut (called the microbiome), and some artificial sweeteners can be poison for the bacteria and thus, for you!

- **Artificial additives**—If you can't pronounce an ingredient on a nutrition label, it's probably bad for you.
- **Refined flour**—Refined means that most of the nutrients of the grain have been removed, and your body has to deal with what's left.
- **Gluten from common store bread**—Altered processing procedures leave higher gluten levels in bread that can cause irritation in your GI tract and cause inflammation.
- **Processed meats**—These products often contain additives to preserve color, texture, and taste along with whatever the animal was injected with, not to mention a good dose of saturated fat. Thus, this is also the mystery-meat classification.
- **Conventional grain-fed meats**—Sweet grains are not what grazing animals are supposed to eat. They eat grass! Grains make them fat quickly, compromise their immune systems, and create a need for high amounts of antibiotics. You consume all these pleasantries.
- **Saturated fats**—Saturated fats get a bad rap when it comes to heart disease, and there is evidence that it causes inflammation in fat tissue itself (i.e., white fat tissue).
- **Fried foods**—Vegetable-oil fried foods, as well as foods that are cooked at high temperatures, pasteurized, dried, smoked, or grilled, contain high levels of inflammatory end products. Vegetable oils are high in omega 6 (inflammatory) and low in omega-3 (anti-inflammatory). The American diet is high in omega-6, and the ratio of omega-6 to omega-3 is as high as 15-20:1 when it should be closer to 1:1.
- **Trans fats**—These fats (partially hydrogenated oils, PHO) are not made by the body, so the body finds the oils difficult to break down, causing inflammation.
- **Fast foods and containers**—It's not only the food, but the container the food is in! Plastic containers used at fast-food chains have phthalatēs (thal-ates) that leech out, especially when heated. Phthalates can disrupt your endocrine system and thus cause inflammation.
- **Dairy**—We are not talking about good yogurt with its good gut bacteria. Dairy has a good amount of saturated fat, which can be inflammatory. Also, some people are sensitive to lactose or casein proteins.
- **Excessive alcohol**—While a little bit may be helpful in controlling inflammation, too much takes you in the other direction and possibly damages the liver and weakens the immune system. Everything in moderation.

I'm not saying these foods are evil, but I can make a strong argument that avoiding them will result in better health. In essence, try to avoid these foods and aim to eat whole foods as much as possible. But we understand you don't want to live in a cave and graze off the land; most of us just don't live in that environment. So, do the best you can and try to stay away from or greatly reduce the foods listed above. If you eat these foods now but cut them out of your diet, you could lose two to five pounds (1-3 kg) of toxic water you don't need. People say, "It's just water, it's not fat." To them, I say it's weight you don't have to carry, and it's an indication of compromised health. Losing it will benefit you. So, lose the water and keep it off; you will look better and, more importantly, improve your health!

Fat Loss

Let start off by understanding how the body responds to hunger, stress, and even boredom. We have to understand that we are not the first people to reach for sugary and fatty foods when we are stressed, bored, or starving from not eating for four to eight hours. Sugar has an enormous impact on the pleasure centers of our brains and is addictive. We are wired to want sugary and fatty foods when starved, since our brains run on glucose and our bodies use sugar for immediate energy, and the body wants fat to store for future famines. That's why pizza, cookies, burgers, fries, and ice cream are the all-time favorites to reach for when you are anxious, bored, celebrating, or starved. As you can see, stress, boredom, and starvation can have a huge impact on what and when we eat. So, let's try to keep ourselves from getting so hungry, bored, or anxious, and always have healthy nutritional alternatives available everywhere for when those moods hit. That way, we don't sabotage our health and fitness goals.

This is the tricky part and where we detour from standard nutritional dogma. Fat loss occurs when your body has to use stored fat because it is not getting enough calories to sustain life; to the body, this is called starvation. What you see as a positive in reducing the number of calories you take in so you can lose weight, the body (the ultimate survival machine) sees as a negative. Your body does not know you are on a diet, that you will feed it regularly, or that you have goals. Your body only knows it's not getting enough fuel. It's like a bear caught in a trap. When you try to free it, the bear attacks because it doesn't understand your motives. In the same way, the hormonal machine that is in charge of keeping the body alive reacts to what it perceives as starvation. When your body sees the caloric deficit needed to lose fat, the hormone machine lowers your metabolic rate, causing you to plateau. Now, you need to burn more calories or eat fewer calories to drop more weight. A continued calorie deficit doesn't fix the problem and actually digs you deeper into a hole.

So, how do we lose fat without alarming the body or making it think it is starving? Here is where our approach and philosophy to weight (fat) loss takes a different course than your standard nutrition dogma. First, we feel that a slow and steady approach to weight loss and not the blistering 2 pounds (1 kg) a week (500-calorie deficit per day) approved by some organizations is a better approach for ridding your body of fat without significant hormonal and organ disruption. We also believe that the natural "cheat" foods or meals (e.g., homemade pizza, pasta, non-dairy ice cream) everyone lives with can keep the body from freaking out hormonally and actually reset some hormones, like leptin.

We believe—although this is not yet scientifically proven—that the body knows the difference between abundance and scarcity. We believe the body hormonally acts differently when it knows that there is an abundance of frequent and nutritious food versus when it feels there is not enough food (i.e., a diet or starving). The thought of food, the sight of food, the smell of food, and chewing food all signal that food is coming. We strongly believe and have witnessed that the body sees frequent nutrient-rich feedings as a state of abundant nutrition and is more willing to give up fat when that is the world it lives in. We have also witnessed the opposite, where people drop weight in aggressive calorie-restricted diets and look "thin-fat." In our opinion, when people practice severe calorie-restricted diets (e.g., below 1,200 for women and below 1,500 for big men), they get thin but still store fat in places they don't want it, such as their faces, necks, torso, and lower body. Some experts have referred to this type of unpleasant fat storage as the "cortisol fat deposition (storage) pattern." The stress of starving, not to mention the stress of life, can spike cortisol, the stress hormone, and it can do a number on how you look and feel. So, the key to permanent fat loss is to frequently feed your body nutritious, highly thermic (meaning it increases your metabolism) food, and make it feel like it's in a state of abundance. Good foods that are highly thermic nourish the body and require calories to digest. We will talk about this later in this chapter.

Muscle Gain

The body does not like to put on muscle; it sees muscle as a luxury, not a necessity. That's not to say that added muscle is bad for you or that you should not aspire to gain muscle; it's just not a top priority for the body. If you want to add muscle, you want to ensure that your body gets enough calories and enough protein in addition to an aggressive muscle-building weight-training program. In our supersize-me world and with the advent of nutritional supplements, neither of these should be a problem unless you are a hard gainer.

Muscle gain, although not favored by the body, can be easier to accomplish than fat loss. The body has a much easier time of putting on weight than taking it off, partly because the body sees "abundance" as a better option than starvation. One nutrient you will need in order to add muscle is protein. Protein is broken down into amino acids, which are the building blocks of muscle and are needed to repair the muscle you are disrupting when you train. Good fats are also a favorite food group when building muscle due to their concentrated calories. In general, sufficient calories and protein are your key nutritional components to developing muscle through a transformation program.

Health and Recovery

We have talked about proper nutrition for fat loss, muscle gain, and inflammatory control. This dovetails nicely into recovery, which is essential to meeting your health and fitness goals. When you eat foods that are good for you, you nourish your body. Food, often foods that are not as nutritious, can also be used as a way of entertaining yourself when you are bored or calming yourself when you are anxious—and those uses of food will not help you improve your fitness. We will talk more about this distinction later on in this chapter. Nutrition is about repair and recovery. When you are feeding yourself natural or healthy foods, you are giving your body the best possible chance to recover and adapt to the stresses the workouts in this book impose on the body. It's that simple. If you put crap products into your car, it runs like crap—and the same goes for your body. It's so ironic to see people insist on high-grade, premium gasoline and oil for their cars as they eat doughnuts to fuel their bodies. To those people I say, "Treat your body more like you treat your car, and you are off to a good start." Crazy, but true.

Conscious Awareness

You are forewarned: This is where it gets a little crazy, so bear with us. We often hear that the obesity epidemic is a matter of education, or lack thereof. Well, I say it depends on what you consider education. When people talk about nutrition education, they usually mean the mechanics and science of nutrition. In all my years of education, every nutrition class or course has dealt with the same things you read in books: the biochemistry of nutrition. This covers everything from how many calories are in the three macronutrients to their molecular composition. The basic digestive process is covered in most courses as well. The more practical courses deal with actual food prep, meal planning, grocery shopping strategies, and portion control. Still, in spite of a historical amount of nutrition education at everyone's fingertips, the obesity problem has reached staggering heights. If obesity was due to a lack of traditional education, it would have been solved by now. But the weight-loss industry is an utter failure, in spite of its multibillion-dollar yearly market value.

According to a study by Marketdata Enterprises Inc. (*The U.S. Weight Loss & Diet Control Market, 14th edition.* https://www.webwire.com/ViewPressRel.asp?aId=209054), the U.S. weight-loss industry is a $66 billion machine and climbing at about 3 percent per year. This industry serves a population of people, 40 percent of whom are overweight. Although the figure can be debated, some experts claim 95 percent of individuals who lose weight from dieting gain the weight back within three years! Why is this? Well, my opinion is that we have not dealt with why people eat and are obese, and let's face it, we have a ruthless, profit-driven marketplace that does not care whom they prey on to make a profit. We also have a society that talks a good talk but does not walk the walk; we market sugar-filled products to children, and politicians slash physical education budgets in schools. We are starting the race 10 yards behind the starting line.

There is a common saying, "The eyes are the window to the soul." Maybe we should rephrase this to, "The mouth is the window to the soul" in our "I'm stressed out, so supersize me so I will forget about my stress" world. Many people may not even realize that much of their food consumption is chemical, habitual, emotional, and even psychological (or spiritual, if you will), having nothing to do with a lack of traditional nutritional education or nourishing the body. I believe that is very hard for addicts to take control of an addiction, especially if they are not even aware there is an addiction. Therefore, once people are aware of how they are using food, they can make conscious decisions to control not only their nutrition but also their health and their lives.

How do people become aware of their nutritional habits in a way that can really help them understand how to take control of their health and appearance? I think the first step is to create an awareness of what drives us to eat, and beyond that, to eat certain foods. Then we create a nutritional conscience or inner voice of reason. Believe it or not, our conscience can be exercised, and like all things that are worked, it can get stronger. There are seven logical steps to creating this nutritional awareness and conscience.

SEVEN STEPS TO AWARENESS AND A NUTRITIONAL CONSCIENCE

1. The body does not take in foods; it takes in and uses the chemicals (the compounds) in food. You have to see food as a compound you put in your body for the right reason: to nourish it.

2. One of society's biggest issues is the addiction to certain compounds, such as opioids and illegal drugs. People medicate themselves to blunt emotions or escape life's challenges.

3. Sugar is a powerful compound that acts on the same reward centers of the brain as other addictive drugs such as nicotine, cocaine, and opioids. In my opinion, and some experts agree with me, sugar may well be addictive. It is legal, available everywhere, and found in many foods. Sugar is also what the brain runs on, so when you have not eaten in many hours, sugar is what you reach for first.

4. Stress or boredom often manifest as an oral fixation (sensation), such as how a baby stops crying when you put a pacifier in his or her mouth. Humans also often drink, eat, smoke, or chew gum to help them calm down when they are anxious.

5. Society associates large food quantities of high-calorie foods with a good experience (a good time or a good deal), as in the food quality and quantity at an event or restaurant. So, you are culturally driven to consume large quantity of rich foods to celebrate. We don't blow out birthday candles on a salad!

6. Every time you feel the urge to eat, ask yourself, "Am I hungry, bored, or anxious?" If you ate a few minutes or even an hour ago, you probably aren't physically hungry. More likely, you are feeling an emotion such as boredom or anxiety.

7. Every time you eat, ask yourself, "Am I medicating, entertaining, or celebrating with food? Or am I nourishing my body?"

Being aware of the first five steps above allows you to exercise your nutritional conscience in the last two. When you feel the need to eat, think about how long ago you ate and what you ate. If you ate a good meal (over 300 well-proportioned calories) 30 minutes ago, you are probably anxious, not hungry. But if you ate a salad (about 150 calories) within the last 90 minutes, then you could be hungry.

If you determine that you are legitimately hungry, then eat. If you are not sure, drink 8-10 ounces of water and wait five minutes. The water fills you up a little, plus it helps with the oral sensation that boredom or stress can create. The pause makes you aware of how you feel, instead of being compulsive; this is a practice. If after five minutes you still don't know, drink a protein shake (200-300 calories with 20-40 grams of protein). That should do it. But if you still want what you want, then eat it and be done with it.

The more you practice these conscious decisions, the better you get and the quieter the inner dialogue becomes. Eating well becomes easier when it becomes a lifestyle, and you work your own program. The following section will cover the strategies you can implement to create your unique program.

Strategies for Optimal Health and Fat Loss

As we mentioned, four factors involved in energy expenditure regulate your weight and health: BMR, TEF, exercise, and NEAT. Burning more calories will help you lose weight and, more importantly, fat, although BMR slows down with age and when dieting. However, BMR can be boosted by putting on muscle and eating frequent and nutritious meals with sufficient calories. This is where our muscle-building workouts and nutritional strategies come into play. TEF can be boosted by consuming more protein and veggies and less refined and processed foods while reducing caloric intake. The exercise component can be boosted by performing workouts from this book 3 or 4 times per week, and if you can't get to your workout, walk. Walking is one of the most effective activities to drop weight and keep it off. Walking uses a good amount of calories without stressing the body. Finally, buy a smartwatch or any other device that monitors steps and get your steps in. Nothing under 6,000 steps six days a week is acceptable!

If you follow these guidelines, your total daily energy expenditure increases. Let's consider the example of a person who weighs 200 pounds (91 kg), is sedentary, has 20 percent body fat, and eats highly processed foods. Since he does not move much, his total caloric expenditure is 2,300 calories per day, consisting of 1,650 calories in BMR, 0 from exercise, 500 calories from NEAT, and a TEF of about 150 calories (figure 16.2).

Two months later, he has put on some muscle, eats highly thermic foods, and gets in more walking with the dog, parking further way, taking stairs, shopping in the mall, and other activities. His pattern (figure 16.3) looks totally different. The added

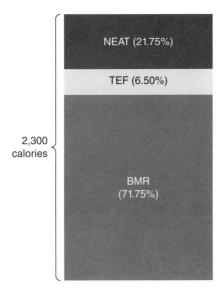

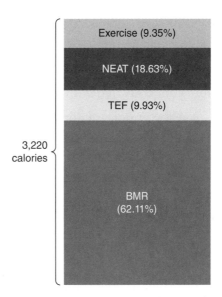

Figure 16.2 Energy expenditure of a 200-pound (91 kg), sedentary man who eats processed foods.

Figure 16.3 Energy expenditure of a 200-pound (91 kg), active, moderately muscled man who eats highly thermic foods.

muscle from the workouts and better eating habits elevates his BMR to a whopping 2,000, exercise adds a modest 300, his NEAT is now at 600, and he has more than doubled his TEF to 320. His total caloric expenditure is up to 3,220. He is not counting calories and can barely keep up with eating the great foods he is consuming. He craves nothing because he can have anything he wants in moderation and with good planning.

If you want to get lean and healthy, you have to plan and execute. It's just like going to work because you need to pay the bills; you go to work and make that money then budget your money so your bills are paid on time. Losing weight takes no less planning.

Programming Nutrition

Just like we program training, we can program nutrition. There are three variables in the programming of nutrition: frequency, quality, and quantity. We work them in this order because success in one leads to an automatic success in the other.

Frequency is important because it regulates hunger, hormones and, to a certain degree, energy expenditure. The rule is that you can't skip a meal, no matter what. When constantly fed, you are calmer. You are in a nutritional-abundance state of mind, so you binge less, and you make better choices. This leads to a change in the quality of food. When you are calm, not starving, and thinking about nourishing your body, you automatically choose healthier foods. These healthier foods add more volume and nutrients to your food intake while reducing the caloric density of the food. Your quantity is taken care of; more food of better quality, with fewer calories. Now, let's talk some simple techniques that can help you practice using your conscience!

Nutritional Techniques

Everyone should practice these techniques since they are centered around conscious nutrition, not impulsive nutrition. Whether you are gaining muscle or reducing fat, what you put into your body matters, so create an environment that helps you make good choices.

- Ask the important question: Am I hungry, anxious, bored, or celebrating? Then, practice the water and protein shake strategies on page 228 as needed.

- Keep a bottle of water at your desk, in your car, and in your backpack/gym bag. Drinking water throughout the day is the single most effective strategy to reduce the oral sensation associated with anxiety and reduces hunger while keeping you hydrated. It's a win-win all around.

- Have healthy food options with you at all times: in your purse, console of your car, gym bag, office, home, etc. Protein powders, ready-to-drink meal replacements, protein bars, fruits, almonds, and prepared foods will help you maintain frequency of eating.

- Reduce the availability of unhealthy foods. This is simple: If it does not belong in your stomach, don't have it in the house or office! If you want it badly enough, drive (or better yet, walk) to get it.

- Never shop for groceries while hungry. If you had a rough day and could not eat something before grocery shopping, go into the store for a protein shake or other healthy snack, and then shop the perimeter of the store for veggies and protein before shopping the middle aisles. This keeps your hunger from doing the shopping and allows your conscience to take over.

JC's Prep for a Big Meal or Party

To reduce the negative impact of sugar, consume foods rich in fiber and oils (for example, cruciferous vegetables and fish oils). Both lower the glycemic index of sugary meals. Not too hard to follow, right? To preserve your health during holidays or vacations, here are three tips that combine eating strategies with exercise.

Tip 1: The day before the big meal, get in an extra 30 to 40 minutes of walking and drink 80 to 100 ounces of water. Have a healthy dinner the night before, and consume fiber-rich foods and 3 to 6 grams of fish oils throughout the day.

Tip 2: The day of the eating event, wake up 20 minutes earlier and use that time to walk. Keep consuming water (up to 120 ounces) throughout the day. The liquid in shakes counts, so drink up. Don't skimp on eating before the big dinner. I recommend having the JC Smoothie for breakfast; a protein shake for a snack; and salad and chicken with 3 grams of fish oil for lunch. Walk for 30 minutes before the dinner. When you get home, drink a protein shake or water, with food that has 2 to 3 grams of fiber and 3 to 4 grams of fish oil. Go to dinner and enjoy.

Tip 3: The day after the event, repeat the healthy eating, water drinking, and walking you performed the day of the event. If you overate at the event, repeat tip 3 for 2 or 3 days.

- Before going to a party or restaurant, drink a protein shake or eat a serving of almonds. The protein drink may keep you from quenching your thirst with alcohol or sodas, and having something in your stomach can help you to minimize the calorie-rich party or restaurant foods you may want to eat. You can enjoy the party or restaurant and taste your food, not scarf it down.

- Buy a blender and make nutritious smoothies. These can be part of your daily routine, and certainly before you go to a party or to a restaurant. Here is my favorite smoothie recipe, called the JC Smoothie. Start with 20-50 grams of protein (I like Labrada Lean Body), 1 cup kale or spinach, 1/2 cup carrots, 1/2 cup celery, 1/2 cup tomato, 1/2 cup blueberries, 1/2 cup raspberries, 1/2 cup banana, 1/4 cup beets, and a small cube of ginger. I freeze all my veggies and fruits so they make the drink cold and thick.

- Finally, I'm the only person I know who does this so it may not work for everyone, but I believe in my fish oil sandwich. Nothing can make a bad meal healthy, but if anything can make it less bad, it's fish oil. I call these better bad choices. If I know I'm going to tear up the town on food consumption such as Christmas Eve at our Cuban get-together, I take 3 grams of fish oil before the party and 3 grams when I get back. The oil will blunt the glycemic spike of carbs, and will help with the ratio of bad fats to good fats.

These are the big strategies that will help you stay on track while being able to enjoy life. Nutrition and life are about steady progress and balance. Nothing good in life comes fast or easy: All beautiful things, like a loving relationship and job fulfillment, take time to develop. Work your program, and it will pay off.

Menus

This section is not meant to provide detailed menus, food prep, or even a grocery shopping list. We just want to provide a general example of two of the most popular menus we use at IHP. These meal plans are based on meal frequency and nutrient timing. We emphasize small meals eaten at moderate to high frequency throughout the day with no gap between meals/snacks lasting more than 3 hours in order to control your metabolism and ultimately hunger and cravings. Most women will lose weight with the 1,500-calorie menu and gain muscle with the 2,000-calorie intake. Most men will drop weight with 2,000 to 2,300 calories daily and gain weight with a daily intake of 3,000 calories. To turn the 2,000-calorie menu into a 2,300-calorie menu, simply add a Labrada Lean Body 40 ready-to-drink shake at the end of your workout or before going to sleep. To turn the 2,000-calorie menu into a 3,000-calorie menu, increase each portion by 50 percent. This means a 4-ounce fillet becomes a 6-ounce fillet, and 3 cups of veggies become 4.5 cups of veggies! Anything beyond this general recommendations can be figured out using an app or website such as MyFitnessPal or CalorieKing.

The 40 percent protein, 30 percent carb, and 30 percent fat plans included in this section are a good start to behavioral modification toward a healthier and fitter lifestyle because of the fundamental balance in macronutrients. These plans are relatively easy to initiate and maintain, making them a perfect starting point for most people. Both plans consist of moderate carbohydrate plus a good amount of protein and fat. As with any dietary recommendation, it is important to express the importance of macronutrient quality: lean protein sources, complex carbohydrates, fibrous and colorful fruits and vegetables, and healthy unsaturated fats.

1,500 Calories (40%C/30%P/30%F) Moderate CHO

Basic meal plan and calorie breakdown for a possible weight-loss program for a woman.

Shake

> 1 scoop whey protein isolate
>
> 1 cup frozen blueberries
>
> 8 ounces almond milk

Breakfast

> 1 piece of Ezekiel toast
>
> 1 egg, scrambled or fried
>
> 1/8 of an avocado
>
> 1 teaspoon raspberry preserves (no sugar added)

Lunch

> 3 ounces grilled chicken
>
> 2 cups mixed greens and baby spinach
>
> 2/3 cup of kidney beans
>
> 1 ounce reduced-fat cheese
>
> 1 teaspoon of balsamic vinegar and 1/2 teaspoon of olive oil

Snack

> 1/2 cup plain nonfat yogurt
>
> 1 tablespoon chopped walnuts
>
> Cinnamon to taste

Dinner

> 3 ounces grilled salmon
>
> 1 cup cooked string beans
>
> 1/2 cup cooked brown rice
>
> CHO: 140 g
>
> Pro: 111 g
>
> Fat: 52 g

Hydration is extremely important when changing your eating behavior. Being and staying hydrated will help control cravings, curb appetite, improve digestion, and help to generally detoxify the body. Hydrate via herbal teas and mineral and seltzer water. Be mindful that calories from liquids add up fast. It's better to eat 4 apples than to have 8 ounces of apple juice.

2,000 Calories (40%C/30%P/30%F) Moderate CHO

Basic meal plan and calorie breakdown for a possible weight-loss program for a man.

Shake

　　1 scoop of whey protein isolate

　　1 cup frozen blueberries

　　8 ounces of almond milk

Breakfast

　　2 pieces of Ezekiel toast

　　2 eggs, scrambled or fried

　　1/2 of an avocado

　　1 teaspoon of raspberry preserves (no sugar added)

　　1/2 of a grapefruit

Lunch

　　3 ounces grilled chicken

　　2 cups mixed greens and baby spinach

　　2/3 cup of kidney beans

　　1 ounce reduced-fat cheese

　　1 teaspoon of balsamic vinegar and 1/2 teaspoon of olive oil

Snack

　　1 cup plain nonfat yogurt

　　1 tablespoon chopped walnuts

　　Cinnamon to taste

Dinner

　　4 ounces grilled salmon

　　1 cup cooked string beans

　　1 cup cooked brown rice

　　CHO: 209 g

　　Pro: 143 g

　　Fat: 69 g

Supplementation

Like the menu section, this supplement section deals with the essentials—what we recommend for most people. Before taking any supplements, it is important to talk with your doctor or dietitian to ensure that adding these substances to your diet is healthy for you. We do not provide an all-inclusive list of effective supplements here. Rather, we refer to the International Society of Sports Nutrition (ISSN) for the latest in nutrition and supplement education and research. Their certification is a must for all personal trainers. Here are the basic supplements and their scientifically proven therapeutic dosage ranges according to the ISSN, not the U.S. RDA recommendations.

Protein

Whey and casein proteins are two of the protein supplements used most often. Whey (isolate) is the fastest acting and works well as a workout drink (before, during, or after your workout) and fast snack. Whey protein includes high levels of all the essential amino acids and branched-chain amino acids. Casein protein is rich in glutamine and is slow acting. It's an excellent choice as a late-evening snack. Supplementing protein can ensure you get the protein you need to put on muscle each day. My recommendation for protein intake for active people who are strength training is based on their body weight in grams. A person with 150 pounds (68 kg) of lean body weight should consume up to 150 grams of protein per day.

Fish Oils

Fish oils are rich in omega-3 fatty acids, which are a combination of EPA and DHA (best ratio is 2:1). The best sources of omega-3 are from fish oils, not plants or nuts. The best food sources are fatty fish (e.g., salmon, tuna, herring, mackerel, sardines). Therapeutic dosages can run from 2 to 6 grams EPA + DHA for high levels of support. This level may pose some potential health problems if you are on blood-thinning medicine like aspirin, so always consult your doctor, but make sure he or she knows a little bit about supplements!

Vitamin D, Vitamin D3 (cholecalciferol)

This is the most recommended version because this is the type our body naturally makes from sunlight. Sunlight represents 80 to 90 percent of our intake of vitamin D. The recommended dosage of vitamin D is 800 to 1,000 IU for adult men. For women, the dosage is 2,000 IU combined with calcium.

Multivitamin/Mineral

If you have a healthy and balanced diet, you should not need a multivitamin. However, most people do not eat well all the time, so it is important to cover nutritional gaps with a multivitamin and mineral supplement. A basic Twinlab Daily or Klean multivitamin are our standard recommendations. I myself have been on the Twinlab daily (no iron for men and with iron for women) for 10 years.

Supplements for Sport Performance and Muscle Gain

Many supplements can be used to improve performance, add muscle, and help you recover. However, there are also things one can do to help the body recover and create an environment for optimal performance. The following are my favorite go-to supplements and strategies for optimal muscle building and recovery. We give it to you simple, practical, and effective.

Creatine

Creatine is one of the most extensively studied nutritional supplements, and most findings indicate it works. Creatine improves muscle performance during high-intensity exercise and supports hypertrophy. Vegetarians may have a greater response to supplementation because of their limited intakes of dietary creatine. It's not necessary to load creatine, and 3 to 5 grams daily will improve strength and speed while increasing muscle size.

Beta-Alanine/Carnosine

Beta-alanine is an amino acid combined with histidine, another amino acid, to form carnosine. Carnosine helps to buffer hydrogen that results from the disassociation of lactic acid, therefore allowing muscles to work longer at high intensity before high hydrogen concentration shuts them down. There is also evidence showing a combination of beta-alanine and creatine will help you gain more muscle mass and lose more body fat than if you took creatine alone, so both make a good "stack." Take 1 to 2 grams of beta-alanine immediately before and after every workout in addition to your shakes and creatine. On nonworkout days, take 2 grams with breakfast, along with 3 to 5 grams of creatine.

Recovery and Stress Management

Few people have died or even gotten sick from not working out, but the same can't be said about not recovering and being all stressed out. I think science would back me up in this: out-of-shape, calm people outlive in-shape, stressed-out people. Stress in any form, even from lack of sleep, is a killer. Often more sleep and better stress management are a better option than joining a gym and staying all stressed out.

Life in the modern world is hectic. Long work hours, chronic stress, late-night shifts, and a multitude of other factors are robbing us of the ability to unwind and shut off our minds. People are stressing out over work, not having enough money, not looking and feeling their best, and not having enough time to really enjoy life. With today's extended workweek and 24-hour access to phones, texts, and social media, what else do you think is on the rise? You got it: Stress! Our growing dependence on our constantly present electronic devices is possibly one of the biggest obstacles to controlling stress and recovering. Smartphones, TVs, video games, and laptops dominate every feature of our daily living, and the constant images and data that electronics throw at us keep us stimulated and stressed out for prolonged periods of time.

There are some indicators that our society is stressed out and not recovering. One indicator is the increased use of mind-numbing drugs, from heroin to opioids! What's on the decline? You got it: Sleep and relaxation (stress management). Many people head to gyms to exercise and "get rid of stress." For some, that works. Although exercise will help you deal with stress, exercise itself is a stressor, and using up what little sleep and rest time you may be getting to hit the gym just may push your immune system overboard! Trying to fix your stressed-out and out-of-control life with exercise is like trying to take supplements to undo a crappy diet! It's not going to work.

Stress Hormones and Health

There are two types of stress: acute (short term) and chronic (prolonged). The acute stuff happens to everyone. It's short-lived, and the body will naturally return to normal. However, when stress takes over your life, and you are stuck in the fight mode of the fight-or-flight response to stress, you could be in trouble. Chronic stress does a number on your body, cranking out hormones like glucagon, epinephrine (adrenaline), norepinephrine, cortisol, and growth hormone, just to name a few. Constant, high levels of these hormones can lead to long-term health problems such as chronic fatigue and inflammation, suppressed immune function, poor sleep, weight gain, various endocrine dysfunctions, increased anxiety, and poor performance in all aspects of life. Therefore, no matter how hard you work out, if you don't recover from workouts and your active life, your workouts and active life can end up doing you more harm than good. Getting your stress under control will ensure that practicing the training and nutritional strategies contained in this book will pay off big dividends.

Stress Management: 3-2-5 Breathing

There are many aspects to stress, its hormonal response, and the various ways you can manage it. In general terms, some of the basic things you can do to manage your stress include:

- Eating a healthy diet and getting regular exercise and plenty of sleep.
- Practicing relaxation techniques such as deep breathing.
- Taking time for relaxing hobbies, such as reading a book or listening to music.
- Fostering healthy friendships and laughing with friends.

Of all these, the one I love to teach my athletes and friends is the 3-2-5 breathing technique. This is a simple technique that can be done anywhere and can help you lower your heart rate by as much as 30 to 40 percent if you get really good at it. It's simple:

- Push your tongue to the roof of your mouth.
- Breathe in deeply for a slow three count.
- Hold for two seconds.
- Breathe out through pursed lips for a slow five count.
- Perform five rounds five times per day. The slower the count, the better.

This is your stress management workout! You can do this in your car when stressed out if you are late or irritated due to heavy traffic, during a lunch or work break, before sleep, and during any moment of anxiety.

Note: Put five daily alarms on your phone that say 3-2-5 and do it; it will change your life.

If you are really stressed out, put the 3-2-5 on steroids and practice present moment awareness (PMA), or the now, as Eckhart Tolle would call it. I learned this technique from Sharon Byrne of Life Mastery, one of my many spiritual coaches. Although some spiritual gurus can spend hours in meditation, I have meditation ADD and need something shorter. Therefore, my basic form of PMA lasts as little as 90 seconds, but I usually do 2-3 minutes.

- For 30 to 60 seconds, look at everything around you. Don't assign it a name, meaning, or identity. Just look at colors, shapes, and movement. You just see and acknowledge everything there is to see.

- For the next 30 to 60 seconds, start listening to everything around you. Don't assign it a name, meaning, or identity. Just listen to sounds, volume, and location. By now you should be seeing, hearing, and acknowledging everything there is to see and hear.

- For the next 30 to 60 seconds, add feeling all the sensations you are feeling (the touch of your clothing on your body, the breeze or temperature on your skin, the ground under your bare feet, and even whatever tension you may be feeling and its location in your body). Don't assign the feeling or sensation a name, meaning, or identity, just acknowledge it. By now you should be seeing, hearing, feeling, and acknowledging everything there is to see, hear, feel.

The 3-2-5 breathing and PMA are the two single most powerful stress management strategies I have ever come across, and they have helped my clients calm their stressful lives. Practicing stress management in this fashion has helped me get off the sleep medications I used for 10 years. If it worked for my severe stress, it probably can do you some good, too. Try it for 2 weeks. I bet you will feel better.

Sleep

The last thing this chapter covers is sleep, something most people don't get enough of. As I tell my athletes, the stimulus happens in the gym, but the adaptations occur while you sleep. That's right; you don't get bigger and stronger in the gym. You get bigger and stronger while you sleep. Although everyone inherently knows the importance of good sleep and rest, few people in our technologically driven society get enough sleep and rest. Insomnia (not being able to sleep) is becoming increasingly common these days, and it negatively affects our society, from work productivity, to personal safety, to health care costs.

Some of the basic causes of insomnia are:

• **Technology**—Our addiction to electronic devices may be one of the biggest obstacles to restful sleep. Smartphones, TVs, video games, and laptops pretty much rule our everyday lives.

• **Persistent stress at work or at home**—Everyday problems (e.g., pressures of work or relationships) that are not addressed plague our subconscious and can keep us anxious without us even knowing why.

• **Poor sleep hygiene**—Those who don't have a sleep routine keep their rooms full of light, noise, or physical distractions that can cause trouble falling asleep or staying asleep.

• **Other health issues**—Some health problems such as sleep apnea, depression, chronic pain, digestive issues, or urinary problems can wreak havoc on getting a good night's sleep.

• **The graveyard shift**—For an animal who is programmed to be up with the sun and down with the sun, working the night shift can create a host of problems in getting adequate sleep.

• **Genetic causes**—We did not know this previously, but new evidence indicates that there is a genetic link that predisposes people to insomnia.

So what can you do? Your best allies against insomnia are quiet, comfort, relaxation, and good sleep habits (i.e., a routine).

• **Make your bedroom a recovery sanctuary.** Your bedroom should be quiet, dark, cool, comfortable, and relaxed. I like the idea of using the bedroom for sleeping, relaxing, and sex. I prefer no TV, computers, or any other electronic distractors in the room. Teach your body that the bedroom is for recovery, and it will respond with better sleep.

• **Create a relaxing sleep routine.** A good sleep routine creates a habit and sleeping is exactly that—a good habit. Whatever works for you is fine, such as reading or meditation 30 minutes before lights out. Try to go to bed and wake up close to the same time every day.

• **Turn off all screens at least an hour before bed.** Electronic screens emit a blue light that disrupts your body's production of melatonin and combats sleepiness. So instead of watching TV or spending time on your phone, tablet, or computer, choose another relaxing activity, such as reading a book or listening to soft music.

• **Avoid anything that cranks you up or makes your mind busy.** This includes avoiding all electronic communication devices and social media activities, big discussions or arguments with your spouse or family, or work-related activities—all can wait until the morning. Also, although naps can help you catch up on sleep, they can interfere with your night sleeping so be careful with naps if you have problems with night sleeping.

Summary

Nutrition is the most important aspect of developing a great looking, highly functioning body. We must address the enormous emotional component of nutrition if we are going to really understand weight management and good health. Techniques and strategies that support nutritional consciousness help us make better decisions. Supplements can help us achieve health and fitness goal, but can never undo bad nutritional choices. You cannot make up for a bad diet with exercise or supplements.

Stress is also a major factor that impacts looks and performance. I believe the conditions that result from stress are some of the biggest, if not the biggest, health problems our society faces today. Although a good fitness workout can help with stress, we can't expect to manage our stress with just exercise, especially if extra time is limited or nonexistent. Of course, life will have its challenges and stressful moments, but scheduling your life so that you can deal with stresses when they come, yet be able to sustain a fit, healthy, and peaceful existence, is doable and should be at the top of everyone's list. Good nutrition and proper stress management make up a huge part of any performance enhancement program.

CHAPTER 17

Programming for Success

Since you might have skipped to this section before reading other important sections of this book, I will take this opportunity to remind you of some of my most common strong recommendations. Let's start with this one: Take it easy and progress slowly. Follow the recommendations I gave you. Each chapter features a beginner workout that acts as a prerequisite. Please make sure you are easily beyond that point in training before you attempt the workouts. If you are a beginner, or if you have never done serious, supervised training, make sure you follow all my recommendations and always take a conservative approach. It's wise to hire a professional certified trainer, even if just for 30 minutes, and show him or her what you want to do. Your trainer can teach you the correct movements and help you progress through the workout.

This chapter ties the entire book together. I want to bring in a few of my industry friends and fitness superstars to add some variety and spice. Generally, the workouts in this book are intense and focused on a body part or performance outcome. This is especially true when it comes to weeks 3 and 4 for most of the workouts. Therefore, a beginner can use this book, and the workouts quickly take you to the professional level of IHP's elite athletes if you follow all the recommendations.

Programming still challenges most trainers and fitness aficionados. Putting together a workout seems to be the biggest request I get from fans and clients. Creating a solid monthly or yearly plan is something that virtually everyone struggles with. Therefore, I'm going to try to help you develop a weekly, monthly, and yearly training plan.

Daily, Monthly, and Yearly Programming

Most of the people I know cycle their training, sometimes by default, not design. Some plan their training around vacations or get sick or busy and can't train. Whether it's planned or by circumstances, life assures us that there are high and lows in our training. However, when the highs and lows and the stuff in between is planned, gains come bigger and faster and with fewer injuries. *Functional Training* includes an extensive review of programming and periodization and has all the information you need to vary programming deliberately. That book focuses on sports, but the periodization and programming guidelines can be used for fitness programming as well.

The concept of managing training over time is called *periodization.* Periodization is the art and science of manipulating the training variables intensity (load), volume (sets × reps × load), and frequency (number of workouts) over time. Many people do the same thing every workout until they get sick, hurt, tired, or bored or take a vacation.

Then they start up and do it all over again; that's their idea of periodization. However, there is a way to plan training so you don't get sick, hurt, tired, or bored, and vacation is a planned off-season. This is how to do it.

Traditional periodization has four basic periods of training:

1. Hypertrophy or conditioning to create a base of training. Repetitions of traditional exercises are in the 8 to 15 range with moderate weight for 12 to 20 weekly sets.

2. Strength to get as strong as possible. Sets and reps are cut in half. Repetitions of traditional exercises are in the 4 to 6 range with the heaviest weight possible for 10 to 12 weekly sets.

3. Power to gain power and speed through explosive training. Five repetitions of traditional exercises with moderate weight are used, followed by a 1-minute rest and a light, explosive exercise similar to the traditional exercise. Weekly sets are 8 to 12.

4. Power endurance to create resistance against fatigue and hit the nitrous oxide button with metabolic training. This is the best period to burn fat and get ready for a photo shoot or a hard event. But you can't stay in this phase forever; you will crash after a month or so. Five repetitions of traditional exercises with moderate weight is used, followed by an explosive exercise similar to the traditional exercise. Weekly sets are 8 to 12.

I like to do three- or four-week cycles of each phase, but you can do two if you are tight for time or are just not interested in that phase.

Chronic Programming

Planning a few months or a year is easy once you understand that a month of training is as easy as a week of training performed four times. Once you have the four phases, and assuming you want to perform all cycles, a training block can look like this:

1. Hypertrophy: 2-4 weeks
2. Strength: 2-4 weeks
3. Power: 2-4 weeks
4. Power endurance: 2-4 weeks

The training block (multiple cycles in sequence) can be repeated as desired. You may take a week off every couple of cycles or at the end of a block. Prioritize training according to your needs. If you need more size, extend the hypertrophy phase. If you are big and strong but need more power and power endurance, shorten the first two phases and lengthen the power and power endurance phases.

If you want to cycle only hypertrophy and strength, it can look like this:

1. Hypertrophy: 2-4 weeks
2. Strength: 2-4 weeks
3. Hypertrophy: 2-4 weeks
4. Strength: 2-4 weeks
5. Repeat

This example is typical for bodybuilders, but most other athletes use all four cycles. If you come off a competition and need to peak again quickly, execute the power and power endurance phases if you have more than five weeks:

1. Competition
2. Power: 1-2 weeks
3. Power endurance: 3-4 weeks
4. Competition

If you have less time, repeat a few weeks of the power endurance phase to keep your peak:

1. Competition
2. Power endurance: 2-3 weeks
3. Competition

Let's look at a sample year from someone who runs 10k and Obstacle Course Racing (OCR) races. This is how he or she can get ready for races and even take a vacation:

1. Hypertrophy: 3 weeks
2. Strength: 4 weeks
3. Power: 4 weeks
4. Power endurance: 4 weeks
5. Competition
6. Power: 2 weeks
7. Power endurance: 3 weeks
8. Competition
9. Vacation
10. Hypertrophy: 1-2 week
11. Strength: 2 weeks
12. Power: 2-3 weeks
13. Power endurance: 4 weeks
14. Competition

As you can see, once you know when to peak and when to wind down, scheduling training becomes easy. You can prioritize and dedicate ample time to the type of training you need. Continue to cycle your training, and you reduce the chances of overtraining so you can peak at the right time.

Managing a Workout

Many people don't have the time or physicality to perform the final weeks of the workouts in this book (e.g., weeks 3 and 4 of the four-week progressions could take 90 to 120 minutes). For people with limited time or recovery capacity, the volume of the first two weeks is perfect; just substitute and change exercises. Even using portions of the workouts or combining exercises from different workouts can create the perfect workout for a special situation. This is especially true if you want to tackle multiple body parts in one day. Let's look at how to create short, grab-and-go workouts from the workouts in this book.

Let's create a half-hour chest routine and a one-hour chest and back routine so you can see how this works. For example, we can create a short, 30-minute chest routine by taking his chest workout 3 (page 115) and chopping it down to the basics: selecting exercises 1a, 2a, and 3a and performing the volume in week 2. That's 9 sets of 12 reps for the chest. Taking 3 minutes per set gives you 27 minutes; that's an easy day.

If you want to work your chest and your back in about an hour, you can combine the *his* chest workout 3 (page 115) and *his* back workout 4 (page 135). Taking major, compound exercises from each workout, we can create a shorter workout by taking exercises 1a, 2a, and 3a from the *his* chest workout 3 and exercises 1, 2, and 3 from the *his* back workout 4. Again, most people will do very well staying within the volumes outlined in weeks 1 and 2. If you choose the volume of week 2 of each workout, you get this nice routine for the chest and back.

1a. DB incline bench press 3 × 10-12

1b. DB bench press 3 × 10-12

1c. DB decline bench press (or weighted dips) 3 × 10-12

2a. Wide-grip pull-down 3 × 10-12

2b. Cable V-handle row 3 × 10-12

2c. Barbell bent-over row 3 × 10-12

If you are in a hurry, you can superset 1a and 2a, 1b and 2b, and 1c and 2c. At four minutes per superset, three supersets per number, and three sets each superset, you get 36 minutes. If you have more time, you can perform each exercise in the order presented with plenty of rest between each set. At two to three minutes per set, six exercises, and three sets each exercise, you get 36-54 minutes.

Another great example of combining the workouts in this book is to combine synergistic body parts, such as combining chest, shoulders, and triceps, and combining back, rear shoulders, and biceps. The advantage of combining synergistic body parts is its efficiency; exercises for the preceding body part prefatigue the subsequent body part, requiring less work from each of the subsequent body parts. For example, doing chest presses also works the shoulders, so the front shoulders are already pumped by the time you get to shoulder presses. Likewise, both the chest and shoulder presses work the triceps, so after doing a few sets of chest and shoulder presses, your triceps are cooked, and only a few sets are needed to finish them off. The same thing goes for the back pulling muscles and the biceps. Basically, take two of the major traditional strength exercises for each body part, and put them in a series. Start with the bigger muscle group and work toward the smallest. Table 17.1 shows two very common combinations and synergistic workouts for the pushing and pulling musculature.

Table 17.1   Synergistic Workouts for Pushing and Pulling

COMBINED PUSHING WORKOUT (CHEST, SHOULDERS, TRICEPS)		COMBINED PULLING WORKOUT (BACK, BICEPS)	
Exercise	Sets and reps	Exercise	Sets and reps
Barbell bench press	3 × 10	Lat pull-down	3 × 10
DB incline fly	3 × 10	Seated machine row	3 × 10
Machine shoulder press	3 × 10	Low rope face pull	3 × 10
DB lateral fly	3 × 10	Cable reverse fly	3 × 15
Triceps push-down	3 × 10	EZ-bar curl	3 × 10
Flush: diamond push-up on bench	1 × failure	Flush: neutral grip cable rope curl	1 × failure

This is how easy it is to create new workouts from the workouts offered in this book! So, what does a week look like? That is as easy as drag and drop.

Managing a Week and a Month

People often walk into IHP and either want to work out by themselves or want things they can do on days they are not training with one of our personal trainers. The training plans in this section will be a big help if this describes you. It should be noted that once we create a week, that becomes the monthly workout; the only things varied are load and possibly reps. Normally we increase weight a little (about 2.5 to 5 percent) each week and keep the same sets and reps or increase weight significantly (5 to 10 percent) and drop a couple of reps each week if we want to build more strength.

First, I want to show you a hybrid week since this is 90 percent of what goes on at IHP. The IHP hybrid training methodology was covered extensively in *Functional Training*, and I refer you to that text for a complete discussion on the topic and dozens of hybrid workouts. Tables 17.2 and 17.3 show the basic workout scheme.

During the power phase, rest one minute between exercises 1 and 2. During the power endurance phase, transition from exercise 1 to 2 without rest.

Table 17.2   IHP Hybrid Workout: Hypertrophy and Strength

Monday	Wednesday	Friday
Legs with functional chest, back, and core	Chest with functional legs, back, and core	Back with functional legs, chest, and core)
Circuit 1 × 3-4 rounds Barbell squat: 8-15 BP alternating press: 10 per arm SB roll-out: 20 Circuit 2 × 3-4 rounds DB lunge: 8-15 per leg BP single-arm row: 10 Cable short rotation: 20 Circuit 3 × 3-4 rounds Barbell deadlift: 8-15 Suspension recline row: 10 Hanging knee-up: 10-15	Circuit 1 × 3-4 rounds Barbell incline bench press: 8-15 Single-leg anterior reach: 10 Roller IT massage: 10 sec per leg Circuit 2 × 3-4 rounds Machine chest press: 8-15 BP alternating row: 10 per arm BP low-to-high chop: 20 Circuit 3 × 3-4 rounds Dip: 8-15 DB single-leg alternating curl: 10 per leg 45-degree bench extension: 15	Circuit 1 × 3-4 rounds Machine pull-down: 8-15 MB lateral reaching lunge: 10 per leg Kneeling hip flexor stretch: 10 sec per leg Circuit 2 × 3-4 rounds BP seated row: 8-15 BP single-arm fly: 10 per arm BP high-to-low chop: 20 Circuit 3 × 3-4 rounds DB upright row: 8-15 Runner's reach: 10 per leg SB reverse hyperextension: 10-15

Table 17.3   IHP Hybrid Workout: Power and Power Endurance

Monday	Wednesday	Friday
Legs with functional chest, back, and core	Chest with functional legs, back, and core	Back with functional legs, chest, and core
Circuit 1 × 3-4 rounds Barbell squat: 5 Vertical jump: 5 SB roll-out: 20 Circuit 2 × 3-4 rounds DB lunge: 5 per leg Split jump: 5 per leg Cable short rotation: 20 Circuit three × 3-4 rounds Barbell deadlift: 5 Burpee: 5 Hanging knee-up: 10-15	Circuit 1 × 3-4 rounds Barbell incline bench press: 5 MB chest throw: 5 Roller IT massage: 10 sec per leg Circuit 2 × 3-4 rounds Machine chest press: 5 Explosive push-up: 5 BP low-to-high chop: 20 Circuit 3 × 3-4 rounds Dip: 8-15 MB explosive crossover push-up: 3-5 per side 45-degree bench extension: 15	Circuit 1 × 3-4 rounds Machine pull-down: 5 MB overhead throw: 5 Kneeling hip flexor stretch: 10 sec per leg Circuit 2 × 3-4 rounds BP seated row: 5 BP swim: 5 BP high-to-low chop: 20 Circuit 3 × 3-4 rounds DB upright row: 5 per arm BP explosive single-arm upright row: 5 per arm SB reverse hyperextensions: 10-15

This is the most popular scheme our trainers use at IHP. It has rehabilitated bad backs, taken off pounds of fat (with the right diet), and helped fighters win championships. The workouts are performed for two to four weeks for hypertrophy or conditioning. For a two- to four-week strength phase, drop the number of reps on exercises 1 to 4 to 6. The power and power endurance phases can last two to four weeks each. You can perform cardio and enjoy active hobbies on days you do not work out. You can add workouts from the agility, quickness, and metabolic chapters of this book if you want to add more days to your training. Most of the plans include a blend of conditioning and bodybuilding.

The workout shown in table 17.4 helps you to stay active and healthy. It works well if you don't have specific aesthetic or performance goals.

Table 17.4   Two Days of Functional Training

Monday	Tuesday	Wednesday	Thursday	Friday	Saturday	Sunday
Total-body functional*	Agility	Metabolic	Speed	Total-body functional*	Fun day	Recover
Choose 1 or 2 functional exercises from each of the 7 transformation workouts (see chapters 4-9), and perform 2-3 sets of 10-20 reps	Choose one of the agility workouts in chapter 12, and perform 1-2 sets	Choose one metabolic protocol for the legs, push, pull, and total-body sections from chapter 12, and perform 1-2 sets of each	Choose one speed protocol from chapter 11, and perform 1-2 sets of each	Choose 1 or 2 functional exercises from each of the 7 transformation workouts (see chapters 4-9), and perform 2-3 sets of 10-20 reps	Partake in an active hobby or slow, long cardio (bike ride, brisk walk, etc.)	

* If you choose 8 different functional exercises from the transformational workouts in chapters 4-9, set up 2 circuits, each with 4 exercises (each with a lower body, push, pull, core, or arms exercise). Perform each exercise for 10-20 repetitions and complete 2-3 sets of each circuit.

Here are some suggestions for creating a full schedule of functional training to do on your own:

- If time is tight, do the workouts listed for Monday and Friday.
- For a three-day workout, add Wednesday or Saturday. The order of these two days can be switched.
- For a four-day week, perform Monday, Wednesday, Friday, and Saturday.
- The agility and quickness workouts can be added last, depending on how much training is desired.

The workout shown in table 17.5 can be cycled month to month by switching the emphasis between body parts (i.e., weak body parts), by dropping the reps to 4-6 during a two- to four-week strength phase, or by adding metabolic training during a power endurance or fat-cutting phase.

Table 17.5   Workout to Grow Muscle and Lose Fat

Monday	Tuesday	Wednesday	Thursday	Friday	Saturday	Sunday
Weak body part (e.g., legs)*	Other body parts (e.g., chest, shoulders, and triceps)	Fat burn and core	Weak body part (e.g., legs)*	Other body parts (e.g., back and biceps)	Fun day and core	Recover
Choose *his* or *her* workout 4 from the leg chapter (see chapter 4) for your weakest body part that you want to concentrate on and follow the progression provided in workout	Combination pushing workout (see chapters 7 and 8)	Slow, long cardio (bike ride, brisk walk, etc.) Choose any core workout (see chapter 5) and follow progression	Choose *his* or *her* workout 5 from the leg chapter (see chapter 4) for your weakest body part that you want to concentrate on and follow progression provided in workout	Combination pulling workout (see chapter 9)	Partake in an active hobby or slow, long cardio (bike ride, brisk walk, etc.) Choose any core workout (see chapter 5) and follow the progression	

* This may be a weak body part you want to give more attention to; we used legs as an example.

This workout is for someone who wants to add size to a body part (e.g., legs) while dropping body fat. Other body parts are worked on other days, and cardio is added to help with fat loss. This is how you can approach this workout.

- Perform the big, high-volume workout for your body part of emphasis on Mondays and Thursdays. Usually workouts 4 and 5 are big-volume, bodybuilding workouts.
- On Tuesdays and Fridays, combine body parts into pushing and pulling.
- If you have five days to train, add Saturday.
- If time permits, add 20 minutes of light cardio three or four times per week after each workout. This will go a long way to accelerating the fat loss.
- Wear some kind of step-counter to motivate you to increase your nonexercise activity thermogenesis (NEAT).
- For fat loss, women can have 1,500 calories per day, and men can have 2,000 to 2,500 calories per day. I also recommend beta-alanine for sustained performance and fat loss. This eating recommendation should work for most people. Athletes or people with metabolic disorders will differ in energy requirements.

The workout in table 17.6 can also be cycled month to month by switching the emphasis between body parts (i.e., weak body parts) or by dropping the reps to 4-6 during a two- to four- week strength phase.

This workout is for someone who wants to add size to a body part (e.g., chest) while adding body weight, such as a high school athlete trying out for the football team. I combine body parts on four days to add as much muscle-building stimulus as possible.

Table 17.6 Workout to Build Muscle and Add Weight

Monday	Tuesday	Wednesday	Thursday	Friday	Saturday	Sunday
Weak body part (e.g., chest)*	Other body parts (e.g., legs and hips)	Other body parts (e.g., arm and core)	Weak body part (e.g., chest)*	Other body parts (e.g., back)	Other body parts (e.g., shoulders)	Recover
Choose *his* or *her* workout 4 from the chest chapter (see chapter 8). Perform the volume for the week you feel suits your level of training.	Choose *his* or *her* workout 4 from the legs chapter (see chapter 4). Perform the volume for the week you feel suits your level of training.	Choose *his* or *her* workout 4 from the arms chapter (see chapter 6). Perform the volume for the week you feel suits your level of training.	Choose *his* or *her* workout 4 from the chest chapter (see chapter 8). Perform the volume for the week you feel suits your level of training.	Choose *his* or *her* workout 4 from the back chapter (see chapter 9). Perform the volume for the week you feel suits your level of training.	Choose *his* or *her* workout 4 from the shoulder chapter (see chapter 7). Perform the volume for the week you feel suits your level of training.	

* This is a weak body part you want to give more attention. I used the chest as an example.

This is how to approach this workout:

- If you have four days to train, perform the Monday, Tuesday, Thursday, and Friday workouts.
- If you have five days to train, add Wednesday or Saturday.
- If you have six days to train, obviously add the remaining day.
- If time permits, add two, three, or four 10-second, all-out sprints (one-minute rest between each run) on inclined treadmill after each workout to help maintain conditioning level. Use the maximum incline and maximum speed you can handle at that incline for 10 seconds.

For weight gain, try to consume approximately 15 to 20 times your body weight for calories per day (usually 2,000 to 2,500 for women, 3,500 to 4,000 for men). I also recommend the creatine and beta-alanine combination for weight gain and sustained performance. This eating recommendation should work for most people; special populations and specific situations will have different requirements.

Table 17.7 shows a week for someone training hard and devoted to bodybuilding. Many people who concentrate on bodybuilding cycle only between hypertrophy and strength. For example, they do four weeks of bodybuilding (8 to 15 reps) and four weeks of strength by dropping the reps to 4-6 during a two- to four-week strength phase. Even for people not interested in performance, I still recommend regular metabolic training a couple of times per week; just throw in some sprints at the end of a workout. Sprints provide the cardio you need to push your body during muscle-building workouts.

This is how you use the workouts:

- This is a hard schedule that requires time and total dedication, plus at least five days of training.
- If you only have five days to train, you can sprinkle the abs and core work throughout the week at the end of each workout.
- If time permits, add 20 minutes of light cardio three or four times per week or after every workout, if possible.

For weight gain, try to consume 2,000 to 2,500 calories per day for a woman or 3,000

Table 17.7 Bodybuilding Cycle

Monday	Tuesday	Wednesday	Thursday	Friday	Saturday	Sunday
Legs/hips	Chest	Back	Shoulders	Arms	Abs and core and supplemental	Recover
Perform *his* or *her* legs/hips workouts in chapter 4. Perform the volume for the week you feel suits your level of training.	Perform *his* or *her* chest workouts in chapter 8. Perform the volume for the week you feel suits your level of training.	Perform *his* or *her* back workouts in chapter 9. Perform the volume for the week you feel suits your level of training.	Perform *his* or *her* shoulders workouts in chapter 7. Perform the volume for the week you feel suits your level of training.	Perform *his* or *her* arms workouts in chapter 6. Perform the volume for the week you feel suits your level of training.	Perform *his* or *her* abs and core workouts in chapter 5. Perform the volume for the week you feel suits your level of training. Supplemental can be anything, like calf work.	

to 3,500 calories per day for a man. I also recommend creatine and beta-alanine supplementation for weight gain and sustained performance. This eating recommendation should work for most people; special populations and situations will have different requirements.

More Programming Ideas From JC's Friends

What better way to provide you with more programming ideas than to share training plans from some of the big guns in the industry who serve as advisors and colleagues to me. I respect these individuals and always look forward to our talks and collaborations.

SANCHEZ SHAPE

Let's look at one of the split workouts Carla Sanchez uses for some of her bikini competitors and personal training clients who want to look and feel their best. This is a 4- to 6-week cycle, focusing on different body parts.

Alternate pull/push training split, 3 days per week

Day 1: Legs, back, and abs

Hex bar deadlift 3 × 10-12

SB hamstring curl 3 × 10

V-bar pull-down 3 × 10-12

Suspension recline row 3 × 10-15

EZ-bar biceps curl 3 × 10-12

SB crunch to SB knee tuck superset 3 × 15 + 15

Day 2: Push and abs

Goblet squat and vertical jump 3 × 10-12 + 10

Banded barbell hip thrust and banded hip abduction 3 × 15 + 30

DB incline press 3 × 10-12

BP triceps extension 3 × 10-12

Hanging knee tuck 3 × 10-15

Day 3: Booty, back, and abs

Barbell hip thrust 3 × 25

Romanian deadlift and KB swing 3 × 10 + 10

Pull-up with band assistance 3 × 10-12 reps

T-bar or landmine row 3 × 10-12

DB single-arm row 3 × 10-12

JC's meta abs (leg raise, crunch, and V-up superset) 3 × 10 + 10 + 10

Bicycle crunch 1 × 50-100

EDBERG BUILT:
MEN'S PROFESSIONAL BODYBUILDING WORKOUT

This workout (table 17.8) is from my good friend and fitness/nutrition genius, Cliff Edberg. This weekly workout is part of his elite training for on-stage bodybuilding and physique competition performance. Four weeks of this, and you are ready for the final stages of dieting to get on stage and win. Cliff is one of the many trainers who uses the time-under-tension approach. He feels he can get people to maximize focus on the targeted muscle if they slow down and concentrate on what they are doing. Cliff feels that heavier weight can force some people to compensate and lose form and tension on targeted muscles. I agree with him and referred to this several times throughout this book. His preference is to make sets last 30 to 40 sec. Not too many people have the patience for this, but if you give it a try, you will get a great pump with minimal abuse to your joints. Try a two- or three-count eccentric movement (lowering the weight), zero- or one-count at the bottom, and a one- or two-count concentric movement (lifting the weight) so your sets last about 30 to 40 sec. Play with the tempos shown in the workout so that it fits well with your preference.

This workout uses a superset format for many of the movements, supersetting agonist and antagonist muscles or upper and lower body. This approach to training keeps the body moving and is very demanding, providing a huge hormonal response, stimulating muscle growth, and accelerating fat burning.

Table 17.8 Edberg Built: Men's Professional Bodybuilding Workout

MONDAY				
Lift: total upper	Sets	Reps	Tempo	Rest
A1. Barbell bench press	4	6	3,0,1,0	1 min
A2. Barbell bent-over row	4	6	3,0,1,0	
B1. Barbell incline bench press	3	6	3,0,1,0	1 min
B2. Weighted chin-up	3	6	3,0,1,0	
C1. Weighted dip (bent over)	3	8-10	2,0,1,0	1 min
C2. BP row	3	8-10	2,0,1,0	
D1. Barbell shoulder press	3	10	2,0,1,0	30 sec
D2. Barbell curl	3	10	2,0,1,0	
D3. Barbell lying triceps extension	3	10	2,0,1,0	
E1. DB lateral raise	3	10	2,0,1,0	30 sec
E2. DB incline curl	3	10	2,0,1,0	
E3. EZ-bar skull crusher	3	10	2,0,1,0	

TUESDAY				
Lift: total lower	**Sets**	**Reps**	**Tempo**	**Rest**
Deadlift	4	6	3,0,1,0	2 min
Leg press	4	6	3,0,1,0	1 min
A1. Barbell front squat (elevated heels)	3	8 to 10	2,0,1,0	1 min
A2. Romanian deadlift	3	8 to 10	2,0,1,0	
B1. Lying leg curl	3	10	2,0,1,0	30 sec
B2. Walking lunge	3	10	2,0,1,0	
C1. Leg extension	3	10	2,0,1,0	30 sec
C2. Glute bridge	3	10	2,0,1,0	
D1. Weighted hyperextension	3	10	2,0,1,0	30 sec
D2. Seated calf raise	3	10	2,0,1,0	
WEDNESDAY: OFF				
THURSDAY				
Chest and biceps	**Sets**	**Reps**	**Tempo**	**Rest**
A1. DB incline bench press	3	6	3,0,1,0	30 sec
A2. DB incline biceps curl	3	6	3,0,1,0	
B1. DB bench press	3	6	3,0,1,0	30 sec
B2. EZ-bar narrow grip curl	3	10	2,0,1,0	
C1. Weighted bench dip	3	10	2,0,1,0	30 sec
C2. DB preacher curl	3	10	2,0,1,0	
D1. Pec deck fly	3	10	2,0,1,0	30 sec
D2. BP single-arm curl	3	10	2,0,1,0	
FRIDAY				
Legs and shoulders	**Sets**	**Reps**	**Tempo**	**Rest**
A1. Hack squat (glute focus)	4	12	2,0,1,0	30 sec
A2. Cable rear delt	4	12	2,0,1,0	
B1. Barbell walking lunge	3	12	2,0,1,0	30 sec
B2. Machine lateral raise	3	12	2,0,1,0	
C1. 45-degree bench extension	3	10	2,0,1,0	30 sec
C2. Cable shoulder front raise	3	10	2,0,1,0	
D1. Machine leg curl	3	12	2,0,1,0	30 sec
D2. Upright row	3	10	2,0,1,0	
E1. Standing calf raise	3	15	2,0,1,0	30 sec
E2. Arnold press	3	10	2,0,1,0	
SATURDAY				
Back and triceps	**Sets**	**On**	**Tempo**	**Rest**
A1. Lat pull-down	3	6	3,0,1,0	30 sec
A2. Machine dip	3	10	2,0,1,0	
B1. DB incline bench row	3	6	3,0,1,0	30 sec
B2. DB or barbell skull crusher	3	10	2,0,1,0	
C1. Neutral grip pull-down	3	8	3,0,1,0	30 sec
C2. Wide pronated triceps extension	3	10	2,0,1,0	
D1. T-bar row	3	10	2,0,1,0	30 sec
D2. Rope triceps extension	3	10	2,0,1,0	
SUNDAY: OFF				

HURRICANE ROONEY

This workout is from my friend and one of the most inspirational coaches I know, Martin Rooney. This workout is known as *hurricane training*. In hurricane training, rest for 30 sec between each set and 1 min between each round. If it is too difficult, you can add more rest. Complete this workout once or twice a week for 4 weeks in addition to your other training. For more information on hurricane training, visit Martin at www.trainingforwarriors.com.

Sample Hurricane

Round 1: Perform the round 3 times

Sled or sprint or treadmill run for 30 sec

Bench press × 8

Chin-up × 8

Round 2: Perform the round 3 times

Sled or sprint or treadmill run for 30 sec

Dip × 8

Overhead press × 8

Round 3: Perform the round 3 times

Sled or sprint or treadmill run for 30 sec

MB slam × 10

DB curl × 10

Hurricane rules

Get a good 15-20 min warm-up.

Keep intensity as high as possible while still maintaining good form.

Select rest periods according to ability.

Attempt to use light to moderate weights in order to move as fast as possible.

Perform the hurricane a maximum of 2 times per week to avoid overtraining.

LANDOW SPEED

The next workout is a simple speed workout from one of the best performance coaches in our industry, Loren Landow. This 4-week speed progression can be performed 2 or 3 times per week. In the first week, perform 3 sets of all 4 drills, then add a set each week. By the time week 4 rolls around, you will be much faster and in great shape. This is one of those simple workouts that shows you don't have to make things complicated to make things great. Execute this workout with intense and perfect execution, and you will be faster.

Sample speed workout: Use the warm-up from the agility chapter (page 176)

1. A skip 10 yd (9 m) × 3-6 (rest 60 sec between reps)
2. Wall run single exchange 3-6 × 5 per leg (rest 60 sec between sets)
3. 20-yard sprint from two-point start at 85%+ × 3-6 (rest 90-120 sec between reps)
4. Power skip 20 yd (18 m, distance emphasis) × 3-6 (rest 90-120 sec between reps)

DARRYN'S FOUR-DAY SPLIT

This workout (table 17.9) is from my colleague and, in my opinion, one of the greatest minds in muscle physiology, Dr. Darryn Willoughby. Darryn also practices what he researches, having competed in many bodybuilding shows. He competed in the super heavyweight division for standard bodybuilding and recently won his pro card in the Global Bodybuilding Organization.

Table 17.9 Darryn's Four-Day Split

MONDAY				
Legs, shoulders, abs	**Sets**	**Reps**	**Tempo**	**Rest**
Deadlift	3	8-10	3,0,1,0	2-3 min
Barbell squat	3	8-10	3,0,1,0	2-3 min
Lunge	3	8/leg	3,0,1,0	1-2 min
Barbell seated military press	3	8-10	3,0,1,0	2-3 min
DB front raise	3	8-10	2,0,1,0	1-2 min
BP upright row	3	8-10	2,0,1,0	1-2 min
Hanging knee raise	4	10-15	2,0,1,0	1-2 min
TUESDAY				
Chest, triceps, calves	**Sets**	**Reps**	**Tempo**	**Rest**
Barbell or DB bench press	3	8-10	3,0,1,0	2 min
Barbell or DB incline bench press	3	8-10	3,0,1,0	2 min
Cable fly	3	8-10	2,0,1,0	1-2 min
Cable triceps push-down	3	8-10	2,0,1,0	1-2 min
Close grip triceps press	3	8-10	1,0,1,0	1-2 min
Standing calf raise	4	15	3,0,1,0	1-2 min
WEDNESDAY: OFF				
THURSDAY				
Legs, shoulders, abs	**Sets**	**Reps**	**Tempo**	**Rest**
Leg press	4	12-15	3,0,1,0	2-3 min
Bulgarian squat	4	10/leg	3,0,1,0	2-3 min
Leg extension	4	12-15	3,0,1,0	1-2 min
Leg curl	4	12-15	3,0,1,0	1-2 min
DB seated press	4	12-15	3,0,1,0	2-3 min
DB lateral raise	4	12-15	2,0,1,0	1-2 min
Smith machine shrug	4	12-15	1,0,1,0	1-2 min
Crunch	4	10-15	2,0,1,0	1-2 min
FRIDAY				
Back, biceps, lower back, calves	**Sets**	**Reps**	**Tempo**	**Rest**
Wide-grip pull-down	3	8-10	3,0,1,0	2 min
BP row	3	8-10	3,0,1,0	2 min
Single-am bent-over row	3	8-10	2,0,1,0	2 min.
Barbell curl	3	8-10	2,0,1,0	1-2 min
Incline (preacher) curl	3	8-10	2,0,1,0	1-2 min
45-degree back extension	4	10-15	2,0,1,0	1-2 min
Standing calf raise	4	15	3,0,1,0	1-2 min
SATURDAY AND SUNDAY: OFF				

Darryn likes this workout because it incorporates moderate-intensity (higher-volume) days and higher-intensity (lower-volume) days. He feels that the variation this type of workout provides during the week is helpful in fully activating muscle fibers and is also appropriate recovery between training sessions. He also feels the time-under-tension strategy for the moderate-intensity (higher-volume) training day is a great tool to concentrate on a muscle group while sparing extreme wear on the joints.

Summary

Programming can be a daunting task for just about anyone, even personal trainers. I hope the ideas provided in this chapter simplify the process of programming so that creating a workout is doable, not impossible. As you can see from some of the best in the industry, and as I have stated throughout this book, the workouts and exercises we have presented can provide an infinite number of workouts, from very simple to more complex.

Remember that none of us who are really good at programming did it overnight. I have been programming for 45 years! I have practiced it, prescribed it, studied, and traveled all over the world learning from many professional trainers, from the Chinese Olympic coaches, to Russia's elite coaches, to Brazil's and South America's top guns, and of course the incredible professionals here in the United States. Even with the benefit of such experience, I'm still learning and learning a lot! So, don't get frustrated or feel like you don't know anything or will never get it; you will get it. Just stay with it, read, share, and practice. Maybe one day, I'll be reading your book and learning from you!

Contributors

The following colleagues provided programs, advice, support, and their expertise to enhance the material in *JC's Total Body Transformation*. I am grateful for their contributions and encouragement.

Former Mr. USA **John DeFendis** (www.defendis.com; facebook.com/john.defendis; defendis@aol.com) generously let me include the concept he developed called the DeFendis rep in chapter 3.

These gifted trainers provided programs:

Bret Contreras, His Legs and Hips 5: Bret's Weights Workout, and Her Legs and Hips 2: Bret's At-Home Workout, chapter 4; www.bretcontreras.com; bretcontreras@hotmail.com

Cliff Edberg, MS, RD, Her Abs and Core 5: Heavy Abs, chapter 5, and Edberg Built: Men's Professional Bodybuilding Workout, chapter 17; CEdberg@lifetimefitness.com

Cem Eren, Her Legs and Hips 6: Cem's Fitness Competition Workout, chapter 4; www.Diamondglutes.com; Cemcondition83@gmail.com

Loren Landow, Landow Speed, chapter 17; www.landowperformance.com; Lmlandow@gmail.com

Martin Rooney, Hurricane Rooney, chapter 17; www.trainingforwarriors.com; mrooney@trainingforwarriors.com

Carla Sanchez, Sanchez Shape, chapter 17; www.Performanceready.com; glamourjock@gmail.com

Dave Woynarowski, MD, Darryn's Four-Day Split, chapter 17; www.darryn_willoughby@baylor.edu; www.baylor.edu/chhs/index.php?id=940465

These professionals lent their expertise to make chapter 16, Nutrition and Recovery, as comprehensive and accurate as possible:

Jose Antonio, PhD; www.theissn.org; exphys@aol.com

Cliff Edberg, MS, RD; CEdberg@lifetimefitness.com

Douglas Kalman, PhD, RD; www.theissn.org; dkalman@nova.edu

Dave Woynarowski, MD; www.thelongevityedge.com; doc@drdaveshealthsecrets.com

About the Author

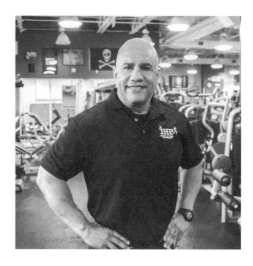

Juan Carlos "JC" Santana, MEd, CSCS,*D, has authored 17 books and manuals and produced over 70 DVDs. He has published more than 300 articles, many in peer-reviewed journals such as the NSCA's *Strength and Conditioning Journal*. His texts have been used internationally in over 20 universities.

Santana is the founder and director of the Institute of Human Performance (IHP) in Boca Raton, Florida. For the last 17 years, IHP has been consistently recognized as one of the top training facilities in the world and the best core-training facility in the United States. His IHP certification system has certified over 10,000 trainers worldwide in over 15 countries, including more than 200 Olympic coaches in China and South America. His IHP mentorship program has welcomed over 400 fitness professionals from over 20 different countries.

Santana has been part of the strength and conditioning programs for several Florida Atlantic University sports teams for over two decades. He was responsible for the strength and conditioning programs for men's basketball, men's and women's cross country and track and field, women's volleyball, and men's and women's swimming.

Santana is a Certified Strength and Conditioning Specialist with distinction (CSCS,*D) and a fellow (FNSCA) of the National Strength and Conditioning Association (NSCA). He is also certified as a health fitness instructor by the American College of Sports Medicine. In addition, he is a certified senior coach and club coach course instructor with the U.S. weightlifting team and a USA Track and Field level 1 coach.

Santana has served two terms on the NSCA board of directors. For eight years, he was the sport-specific conditioning editor for the *NSCA Journal*. His professional responsibilities have included serving as NSCA's vice president, chairman of the NSCA Coaches Conference, a member of the NSCA Conference Committee, and NSCA state director for Florida. As a college adjunct professor, he has taught strength and conditioning at Florida Atlantic University (FAU). An FAU graduate with bachelor's and master's degrees in exercise science, Santana is involved in several ongoing research studies with numerous universities and is working on his PhD in exercise physiology.

Founded in 2001, IHP provides an unparalleled training environment for elite athletes, including Olympic athletes in a variety of sports; world-class tennis champions; NFL, NHL, and MLB players; world champion Brazilian jujitsu and mixed martial arts fighters; numerous NCAA Division I teams; and hundreds of nationally ranked teen hopefuls from a cross-section of sports. IHP also handles delicate spinal rehab cases as well as serving the local community gym.